# SECRETS
## FROM THE
### EATING LAB

# SECRETS FROM THE EATING LAB

**The Science of Weight Loss, the Myth of Willpower,
and Why You Should Never Diet Again**

......................................................

# TRACI MANN, PH.D.

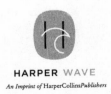

HARPER WAVE

*An Imprint of* HarperCollins*Publishers*

This book is written as a source of information only. The information contained in this book should by no means be considered a substitute for the advice of a qualified medical professional, who should always be consulted before beginning any new diet, exercise, or other health program. All efforts have been made to ensure the accuracy of the information contained in this book as of the date published. The author and the publisher expressly disclaim responsibility for any adverse effects arising from the use or application of the information contained herein.

SECRETS FROM THE EATING LAB. Copyright © 2015 by Traci Mann. All rights reserved. Printed in the United States of America. No part of this book may be used or reproduced in any manner whatsoever without written permission except in the case of brief quotations embodied in critical articles and reviews. For information, address HarperCollins Publishers, 195 Broadway, New York, NY 10007.

HarperCollins books may be purchased for educational, business, or sales promotional use. For information, please e-mail the Special Markets Department at SPsales@harpercollins.com.

FIRST EDITION

*Designed by William Ruoto*

Library of Congress Cataloging-in-Publication Data

Mann, Traci.

  Secrets from the eating lab : the science of weight loss, the myth of willpower, and why you should never diet again / Traci Mann, PhD.

     pages cm

  ISBN 978-0-06-232923-3 (hardback)

  1. Reducing diets—Social aspects. 2. Reducing diets—Psychological aspects. 3. Weight loss—Social aspects. 4. Weight loss—Psychological aspects. I. Title.

  RM222.2.M3257 2015

  613.2'5—dc23

                    2014049872

15 16 17 18 19   OV/RRD   10 9 8 7 6 5 4 3 2 1

*In memory of my mother, Jacklyn Rosen Mann, who always wanted me to write a book.*

*Not this book. But some book.*

*And for my husband, Stephen Engel, for making it possible.*

# CONTENTS

## PART FOUR: YOUR WEIGHT IS REALLY NOT THE POINT

# PREFACE

*"You study self-control? You should study me.*
*I have great self-control."*
—NOBODY, EVER

There is no sign on the door of the Health and Eating Lab at the University of Minnesota. That's my lab, and if I want to learn about people's eating habits, I can't let on that I am studying—or even noticing—what people are eating. It would make them self-conscious and stop them from eating the way they normally do. Instead, my students and I tell our research participants that we are studying other things entirely, such as their memory, or their moods, or how they communicate with their friends. But being the hospitable people we are, we just happen to offer them some snacks while we study them. They have no idea that it's what they do with those snacks that we're really studying.

For more than twenty years, I have been doing research on eating, both with sneaky studies in my eating lab on campus, and in that other eating lab known as "the real world," where I have studied dieters going about their normal daily routines, kids eating in school cafeterias, visitors to the annual feeding frenzy that is the Minnesota State Fair, and even astronauts on the International Space Station. Much to my surprise, I've learned that nearly everything I thought was true about eating was false, including the three pillars of the commercial diet industry: that diets work, that dieting is good for you, and that obesity is deadly. The truth is that diets do not work and may be bad for you, and obesity is not going to kill you. I also learned that despite what most people assume, a lack of self-control is not why people become fat and "harnessing" willpower is not the way to become thin.

Along the way I've also learned that many people have a vested interest in all of us believing those things are true. The obesity research community, in particular, is not delighted that my students and I dare to question their three sacred cows. I've had a well-known diet researcher publicly accuse my young graduate student of doing a disservice to the field by suggesting that diets don't lead to long-term weight loss. I've gotten such vitriolic reviews of manuscripts that journal editors have called me before sending the reviews to prepare me for what I was about to read. I've had journal editors unable to find scholars willing to provide reviews of my work (even negative reviews) out of fear of getting involved in a controversy. And I've received lots of hostile and decidedly nonscholarly feedback when I've spoken up about these things in the media. Some people discount my research by suggesting I must be a bitter fat person (as if fat people cannot be scientists). One online commenter said I was just looking for an excuse to continue stuffing myself "like a Thanksgiving turkey."

I'm not obese, but I am a science nerd, obsessed with research methods and data, and the results of my studies don't lie (or have anything to do with what I weigh). I can't ignore them and I do not want to, because my research points the way to living a healthy life without suggesting that dieting is the answer. And that way to living a healthier life is what I'll share with you in this book.

In Part I, I'll share the research that proves diets don't lead to long-term weight loss and explain why this is so. If you lost a lot of weight and then gained it back, it is not because you lack self-control. In fact, I suspect you used more self-control than the people who accuse you of not having any. But it doesn't matter either way. Self-control is not the problem, and harnessing it is not the solution.

In Part II, I will make the case that diets are neither harmless nor necessary for optimal health, and that most people simply should not go on restrictive diets. My argument is based on the scientific criteria doctors use when they decide whether to recommend treatments (such as drugs) to patients for other conditions: Does the treatment work? Is it safe? Does it have side effects? For some reason, people rarely ask these questions before urging everyone to diet, but my students and I asked them, and the answers are clear: no, not necessarily, yes.

I understand that we all have an image in our mind about what we want to weigh. The problem is that for many of us, that image is outside of our biologically set weight range. It is possible to maintain a weight outside that range—a small minority of dieters does—but to do so, you would have to make weight maintenance the central focus of your life, above all others, including your relationships with your family and friends, your work, and your emotional well-being. It would be a life of agonizing self-denial, and for what purpose?

Instead, I suggest we aim to live at the low end of our set weight range, which is our leanest livable weight. At that weight you can be happy and healthy, and you can maintain it without making it your life's work. In Part III we will look at twelve scientifically supported strategies for painlessly getting to that weight and staying there. These strategies don't involve calorie restriction or require willpower, because relying on willpower is foolhardy, and this is not a diet. Remember, I run an eating lab, not a dieting lab.

You won't find this set of strategies elsewhere, because most of them are based on the research conducted in my lab over the last two decades. Not only will the results of this research surprise you, but I suspect the methods we use in these studies will as well. A rule of thumb in my lab is that if there is a fun way to do a study and a boring way to do a study, we go with the fun way. And as we've learned, there's always a fun way. But rest assured, the methodology we use is rigorous. In fact, the goofier the methods, the more rigorous the study needs to be to get published in leading academic journals, as these studies are.

Finally, once you are effortlessly maintaining your leanest livable weight, in Part IV I'll urge you to forget about the numbers on the scale and get on with your life. That means you need to forget about other people's weight, too. Rebel against our weight-obsessed culture by fighting weight stigma, and shift the focus to your health and well-being instead of your weight. I'll introduce you to the reasonable—yet oddly unnoticed—notion that doing healthy things is healthy, whether or not they make you model-thin. Let's get started.

# PART ONE

# WHY DIETS FAIL YOU

# CHAPTER 1

# DIETS DON'T WORK

Diets don't work. There. I said it. Maybe that's not what you wanted me to say, but I'm here to tell you the truth, according to science, without sugarcoating it. Like most simple-sounding scientific points, of course, it is more complicated than it seems. The reason for the complexity comes from the word "work." What you mean when you think of a diet "working" is not the same as what, say, the CEO of a diet company or an obesity researcher means.

I suspect that for you, a diet works if you lose a lot of weight and keep it off. If that's the case, I can tell you definitively: diets don't work. The diet company CEO might define "works" a little differently: for him or her, a diet may work if people lose any weight at all for any length of time. And for obesity researchers, a diet might work if test subjects lose slightly more weight than people who are not dieting. CEOs and obesity researchers say diets work because people do lose weight—and more weight than non-dieters—during the early months of most diets. Since the 1940s, hundreds of studies have shown that dieters lose an average of five to fifteen pounds over the first four to six months on a diet.[1]

This seems to be the case no matter what type of diet you try, whether you go low calorie, low fat, or low carb, or whether you attempt whatever fad diet is currently popular. There are diets that require you to fast for hours or days at a time,[2] diets that require you to consume only liquids, diets that suggest you eat like a caveman, or even diets that restrict your food intake solely to grapefruit, cabbage soup, or Snickers bars.[3] There are also diets that promise to publicly humiliate you if you fail,[4] or jolt you with electric shocks whenever you attempt to eat certain foods. As recently as 2014, a doctor in the United States was sewing patches onto people's tongues to cause them stabbing pain whenever they ate.[5]

The CEOs and obesity researchers who support these different types of diets are not technically lying when they say their diets are effective, because diets do lead to weight loss in the short term. But there are two problems with saying these diets work: people don't lose enough weight, and they don't keep it off.


## WHAT DOES IT MEAN FOR A DIET TO "WORK"?

Although it seems like a no-brainer to most dieters, it has been surprisingly difficult for the medical community to decide what constitutes a successful diet. Even deciding what counts as a "normal" weight is not as simple as you might think. The World Health Organization (WHO) currently classifies people's weights based on their body mass index, or BMI,[6] which is a measure of weight that takes height into account. The use of BMI is controversial because the formula for calculating it is not based on any understanding of how height and weight relate to each other, and because people who have high muscle mass tend to get categorized as overweight, despite having very little fat.[7] Nevertheless, according to the WHO,[8] the cutoff between what it calls normal weight[9] and overweight is a BMI of 25, and between overweight and obese is 30. Anything under 18.5 is considered underweight.

Originally, the goal of a diet was to achieve what was known as your "ideal weight." Starting in the 1940s, this weight was determined by the height and weight tables in your doctor's office. They offered a heavier ideal weight for large-framed women than for medium-framed women (which is larger than the ideal for small-framed women). For most of us, it was difficult to look at these tables without concluding one must be large-framed.

According to these ideal height and weight tables (which have been criticized for being methodologically flawed and have been abandoned by researchers),[10] an average-height woman (five feet, five inches tall) should weigh between 117 and 130 pounds if she is small-framed and from 137 to 155 pounds if she is large-framed.[11] The problem was, obese people tended to start diets weighing well above these somewhat unrealistic ideal ranges, and they rarely lost enough weight to reach them. Eventually researchers and physicians realized this, and they did the only thing they could do to increase the number of successful dieters: they changed the definition of success to one that was easier to achieve, which was losing 40 pounds. It's like a pole-vaulter lowering the bar when he realizes he cannot leap over it where it is.

According to an influential review from the 1950s, however, 95 percent of dieters failed to achieve this standard as well.[12] The response from the medical community was simply to lower the bar again. So for the next several decades, a diet that resulted in weight loss of 20 pounds was considered a success.[13] Of course, a 20-pound weight loss means something very different to a 300-pound man than it does to a 100-pound girl, and in the 1970s, researchers quite sensibly started describing weight-loss goals in relation to a person's starting weight (and later included a person's height in the calculation as well). Stated in these terms, losing 10 percent of one's starting weight was considered a successful diet. Only about 20 percent of dieters manage to achieve that goal, though,[14] and in 1995, the Institute of Medicine lowered the bar again. They decided that the goal of weight loss programs would be to lose 5 percent of one's starting weight,[15] which is just 10 pounds for a 200-pound person. At this point, our pole-vaulter probably no longer needs the pole to clear the bar.

Although researchers have continually lowered their standards, dieters have not lowered theirs. Not one dieter in a survey of 130 dieters said he would be satisfied with a 5 percent weight loss, and only one said he would be satisfied with a 10 percent weight loss.[16] Heartbreaking evidence of dieters' high (and unfulfilled) standards comes from a study that surveyed sixty obese women about their weight loss goals when they started a new diet, and then checked in with them a year later to see how much weight they lost.[17] When they were surveyed before the diet, the women selected their goal weight for the diet, and then listed their dream weight, their acceptable weight (defined as a weight they could accept, even though they would not be happy with it), and a weight that would be considered their disappointed weight—one that they "could not view as successful in any way," although less than their current weight.

The women started the diet weighing an average of 218 pounds, and their goal was to lose more than 70 pounds. They defined their acceptable weight loss as losing 55 pounds, and said they would be disappointed if they lost less than 38 pounds. In fact, the women on this diet lost an average of 36 pounds, making this an incredibly successful diet compared to the ones I summarized earlier (which averaged a 15-pound weight loss). But despite the comparative success of these women, very few were satisfied with the outcome. As shown in Figure 1, none of the women achieved the weight those height and weight tables would have defined as ideal back in the 1940s (that's why there's no bar there), none achieved her dream weight, and only 9 percent achieved their goal

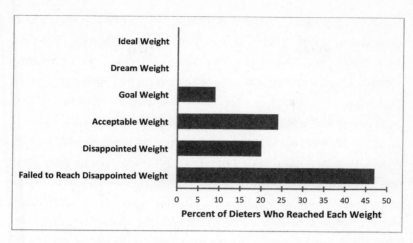

FIGURE 1. Percent of dieters reaching their ideal weight, dream weight, goal weight, acceptable weight, disappointed weight, and none of those weights.

weight. Twenty-four percent of the women achieved their acceptable weight, and 20 percent achieved their disappointed weight. That means that 47 percent of the women—nearly half—did not even lose enough weight to reach their disappointed weight.

That's the first reason why we can't say that diets work. Although people nearly always lose enough weight for researchers to consider the diet successful, they rarely lose enough weight to satisfy themselves. The second reason why we can't say diets work is that dieters do not keep off the weight that they lose.

## DO DIETS WORK IN THE LONG TERM?

For most dieters, the goal is not to lose weight temporarily, nor is it to remain on a strict diet their entire life. Yet for much of the last century, researchers focused primarily on the results from the first three to six months of diets—the part of the diet where a small amount of weight is lost relatively quickly—but did not track participants for much longer. Do dieters continue to lose weight? Does some of the lost weight return? Do some dieters gain back more weight than they lost? These important questions about diets have not been examined in most diet studies. Perhaps not surprisingly, commercial diet companies like Weight Watchers, Jenny Craig, or Nutrisystem, which could provide a wealth of information on their clients' weight changes over many years, claim they are unable to collect long-term data on the effectiveness of their diets.[18] Which raises the question: unable or unwilling?

In the 1990s, when the Federal Trade Commission (FTC) began to increase its scrutiny of the weight loss industry's marketing practices, it asked a panel of experts to create guidelines for advertising weight loss products. This expert panel included representatives from several commercial diet programs, and those representatives insisted that advertisements should not have to include information about the effectiveness of a program. They said they would not offer data on the efficacy of their diets in the short term or the long term, or even the number of people who completed their programs after starting them,[19] which are pretty much the exact facts potential customers would want to know.

The representatives of the diet programs gave amazingly unconvincing reasons for why they should not have to provide this information. First, they argued that it was too costly and difficult to collect such information, even though many of them already had the information on hand. Second, they said, dieters don't need this information because they have had lots of experience with diets and are already very knowledgeable about them. Their third argument, however, was the most illuminating. They said, as recorded in the FTC report, "Dieters will be discouraged if they are provided with realistic outcome data."[20] This was nothing less than an admission that their programs were not effective. The diet companies won the battle—they still do not have to disclose any of this information in their ads. But their unwillingness to report on whether their diets are effective makes it clear that they do not have much confidence in their diets, and they don't want you to know it.

If their products were effective in leading to long-term weight loss, of course, they would soon put themselves out of business. These companies count on repeat customers for their very existence. Richard Samber, the longtime financial chairman of Weight Watchers, likened dieting to playing the lottery. "If you don't win, you play it again. Maybe you'll win the second time."[21] When asked how the business could be successful when only 16 percent of customers[22] maintained their weight loss, he said, "It's successful because the other 84 percent have to come back and do it again. That's where your business comes from."[23] And come back they do. As stated in Weight Watchers' business plan, "Our members have historically demonstrated a consistent pattern of repeat enrollment over a number of years. On average . . . our members have enrolled in four separate program cycles."[24] Clearly, if long-term weight loss were achieved, their members would not need to reenroll.

## The Evidence

Although diet studies have been published regularly in the scientific literature since the 1920s, very few long-term follow-up studies of diets were conducted before the 1990s, and not many have been published since then.[25] Tracking dieters in the years after a diet ends is crucial, because what happens after a diet ends, as most dieters know, is that the lost weight returns. The more time that passes, the more weight is regained. In one study, for example, a group of obese people volunteered to be starved (in a hospital) for about thirty-eight days.[26] After the starvation period, they were tracked for varying lengths of time. Among those who were followed for less than two years, 23 percent gained back more weight than they had lost. Among those who were followed for two or more years, 83 percent gained back more weight than they lost.

Even in the studies that track people for the longest periods of time (four or five years), the amount of weight regained doesn't appear to level off.[27] This is important, because it suggests that if people were followed for even longer, they may be found to have kept gaining weight. Researchers imply that their participants' weight at the end of a study is the most they'll weigh, but the end of a diet study simply means that researchers will no longer see how much more weight participants gain—it doesn't mean that participants will stop gaining weight.

To find out how effective diets are in the long term, the graduate students in my Psychology of Eating seminar and I decided to track down every study that followed dieters for at least two years after a diet began. During class discussion one day, we had concluded that what really mattered about diets was *keeping* the weight off, not just *taking* the weight off, and we were curious to find out what the research showed. We assumed there would be many articles that reviewed the research on this topic, because no matter how esoteric or narrow the research question, a paper reviewing it always seems to already exist. In this case, with such a straightforward, obvious (to us), and important question, in a field with huge amounts of research, we were shocked to find that there was no such review. So we did it ourselves. Had we known what a massive undertaking this seemingly simple project would be, we probably would have convinced ourselves not to bother. Being naive about the research on dieting, we went for it.

Most diet studies are conducted by researchers who have a vested interest in a particular outcome. I'm not saying that diet researchers would purposely tilt their findings toward showing diets work, but despite one's best intentions, bias does creep into research.[28] It's true for all of us researchers all of the time, so not having a preference for any particular outcome in this project helped us in our effort to look at the research as objectively as possible.

We hunted through the research for studies that tracked participants for at least two years after they started a diet, and that used the gold standard research design, called a randomized controlled trial. This kind of study assigns participants to either be put on a diet right away, or be wait-listed to go on the diet sometime in the distant future. The researchers can then compare the results of these two groups over time.

The crucial factor that separates randomized controlled trials from other kinds of studies is that neither the participants nor researchers have any control over whether participants are assigned to the diet or to the wait list. It is done randomly. Although it may seem counterintuitive, this makes the groups as *similar* to each other as possible. If participants picked their groups, those who were most motivated and eager to diet would select the diet condition, and those less interested would put themselves on the waiting list. It wouldn't really be fair to compare these two groups to each other, because they would each start out with different kinds of people.

There are many hundreds of diet studies, but even with six of us hunting through them thoroughly, we were able to find only twenty-one studies that satisfied our criteria.[29] The diets in these studies varied from 800-calorie-a-day "very low calorie diets" to low calorie, low fat, low carbohydrate, or combinations of these, and several also included other dietary changes such as reduced sodium, reduced cholesterol, or reduced alcohol. Some diets featured support services as well, such as group counseling or weekly phone calls.

The studies we looked at ranged from two to ten years (lasting an average of 3.6 years), and we found that at the end of that time, dieters had managed to keep off, on average, a measly two pounds.[30] Nearly half of the participants, or about 40 percent, actually weighed *more* at the follow-up than before they went on the diet. Obesity researchers know that dieters keep off only a small amount of weight, but they justify these small weight losses by suggesting that these individuals would surely have gained lots of weight if they had not participated in the diet. That's a perfectly reasonable possibility to consider. The type of study we required in our review, the randomized controlled trial, is set up to test that very question, and we found that this was clearly not the case. Participants in the no-diet conditions of these studies gained an average of just one pound. Dieters went through all that effort and self-denial, and in the end they weighed only the tiniest bit (three pounds) less than the non-dieters.[31]

Now for the really bad news. The truth is, most diets are probably even less successful than these gloomy findings suggest. The results I just described almost certainly inflate the success of these diets. Despite using the gold standard of research design, these studies have three serious flaws—flaws that are mostly unavoidable—that tilt them toward showing that diets work.[32] Each of these flaws adds to the false impression that people can keep off the weight they lose.

The first of these flaws is that the people who start and finish these studies are not necessarily typical dieters. Many people who volunteer to participate in weight loss studies are rejected from participating before the study begins. In some studies, for example, researchers only allow people to join if they are able to diet successfully in a "tryout" period for a month or more before the study starts.[33] In those cases, the people who struggle the most with dieting don't even make it into the studies. It's like giving a class a test but not letting the D and F students participate. Your class average will look impressive, but only because you have excluded those who would have scored the lowest.

That's not the only reason participants are different from typical dieters. Many of the people who do make it into studies do not stick around for the full duration of the study. They often stay on the diet for the first six to twelve months, but then do not return for the follow-up measures a year or two after that. In essence, they drop out. In these studies, an average of about 20 percent of participants dropped out.[34]

Dropping out of diet studies is so common that researchers have carefully studied the question of how dropouts might change the results. For example, researchers have compared participants who returned to be weighed two years after a diet started to those who did not, and found that the people who returned had lost more weight[35] and kept it off longer[36] than people who did not return. It seems logical, doesn't it? Imagine if you had been a part of a diet study a few years ago and had regained a lot of the weight you lost. Wouldn't it be tempting to ignore the researchers' request to come back and be weighed? You might feel embarrassed about regaining the weight and probably wouldn't be eager to face them. This is understandable, but we do need to acknowledge that studying only the people who get selected for a diet study and finish the diet gives a false impression of what happens to most people on diets. It makes diets seem more effective than they are.

The second serious flaw with these studies is that most of the participants are not weighed *in person* by the researchers at the end of the study. Instead, they weigh themselves and communicate their weight to researchers over the phone or by email. Over half of the dieters in the studies we analyzed reported their weight instead of being weighed by researchers in a lab.

This is problematic partly because people may take a guess at their weight rather than weighing themselves, or weigh themselves with an inaccurate scale. Even if they use a highly accurate scale, they still may not admit their true weight to the researchers. People tend to say they weigh less than they do. This has been documented in several studies in which researchers ask people their weight over the phone, and then—surprise!—show up on their doorstep with a scale soon after. When they compare what people said they weighed to the number on the scale, they found that, on average, non-obese people report that they weigh about five pounds less than they do, and that obese people say they weigh about eight pounds less than they do.[37] Remember that the participants in the diet studies (most of whom were obese) only maintained a weight loss of about two pounds. If they actually weighed eight pounds more than they reported to researchers, it is possible the average weight change was a six-pound weight *gain*, rather than the two-pound loss.

The third flaw in these studies is that 20 percent to 65 percent of participants went on at least one other diet while the original diet was being studied. This makes it appear as if the original diet had led to sustained weight loss, when, in fact, any weight loss is almost certainly attributable to the beginning stages of another diet. The weight hasn't stayed off; it's been regained and then lost all over again. In one of the studies, participants reported that they didn't go on another diet until they had gained back *all* the weight they lost on the diet that was being studied.[38] And in another, the researchers stated that if they had not taken into account what participants weighed when they started an additional diet, they would have falsely concluded that the diet they were studying had worked.[39] Because nearly all studies fail to take this behavior into account, diets end up looking more effective than they are.[40]

Without taking these flaws into account, the most rigorous diet studies find that about half of dieters will weigh more four to five years after the diet ends than they did at the start of the diet. This conclusion must, unfortunately, be considered a low estimate of how many people's diets will fail, since it comes from studies so strongly biased toward showing that diets work. The true number of people who fail on diets is probably much higher.

The fact that diets don't lead to long-term weight loss isn't news to diet researchers. In 1991 researchers stated that "it is only the rate of weight regain, not the fact of weight regain that appears open to debate."[41] Ten years before that, another researcher pointed out that "If 'cure' from obesity is defined as reduction to ideal weight and maintenance of that weight for 5 years, a person is more likely to recover from most forms of cancer than from obesity."[42] Researchers have known for a long time that diets don't work. Now you know it, too.

.............................................................

# CHAPTER 2

# WHY DIETS DON'T WORK: BIOLOGY, STRESS, AND FORBIDDEN FRUIT

I've given you the bad news: diets fail in the long run. Now, let's try to understand why.

In social psychology we often say that if you find that most people behave in the same way, then the explanation for their behavior has very little to do with the kind of people they are. It has to do with the circumstances in which they find themselves. For example, most students in class raise their hands and wait quietly to be called on before speaking. It's not that they are all timid or overly polite types of people. It's that the classroom setting is sufficiently powerful that without really thinking about it, nearly everyone ends up following the same unwritten rules. When we think about people who regain weight after dieting, it's a similar principle. It's not that they have a weak will or lack discipline, or that they didn't want it enough, or didn't care. It's about the circumstances in which they find themselves, and the automatic behavior that is provoked by those settings. In other words: if you have trouble keeping weight off, it is not a character flaw.

When it comes to keeping weight off, a combination of circumstances conspires against you. Each one on its own makes it difficult, but put them together and you are no longer in a fair fight. One circumstance that makes things hard is our environment of near-constant temptation (we'll talk more about this in Chapter 3). Two others are biology and psychology. I realize it may seem odd to you that I am calling these things "circumstances," but, like a classroom setting and the behavior it produces, we need to acknowledge the context in which you regain weight.

To an important extent, weight regain after a diet is your body's evolved response to starvation. When you are dieting, it may feel as though you are about to starve to death, but you know that you can open the fridge at any time and find more to eat, if you really wanted to. Your body doesn't know this, however, and you have no way to tell it that you just want slimmer hips or a flatter stomach. All your body knows is that not enough calories are coming in, so it kicks into survival mode. From an evolutionary perspective, the bodies that were best able to survive in times of scarcity (and then pass their genes on to future generations) were those that could use energy efficiently in order to get by on tiny amounts of food. Another quality that would have helped you survive was psychological: a single-minded pursuit of more fuel—and once you located it, the overwhelming urge to eat lots of every type of food you found.

Together, these biological and psychological forces make regaining lost weight all too easy. Let's take a closer look at the biological ones first, because they set the stage for everything else.

## YOU CAN (PARTLY) BLAME BIOLOGY

Your genes play an important role in determining how much you weigh throughout your life. In fact, your genetic code contains the blueprint for your body type and, more or less, the weight range that you can healthily maintain. Your body tends to stay in that range—which I will refer to as your set weight range—most of your adult life. If your weight strays outside it, multiple systems of your body make changes that push you back toward it. While this may seem controversial—aren't we all in control of our own weight?—the role of your genes in regulating weight is backed up by solid evidence. And we don't even need to rely on high-tech gene mapping to understand this; we just need to study people who share the same genetics.[1]

One classic study compared the weight of more than 500 adopted children with that of their biological parents and that of their adoptive parents.[2] Obviously, if genes matter more to weight than does environment, the children's weight should be similar to the weight of their biological parents. If learned eating habits have more of an impact on weight, their weight should be more like their adoptive parents. In fact, researchers found that the children's weight correlated strongly with the weight of their biological parents and not at all with the weight of their adoptive parents.

That evidence always blows me away, but if that's not persuasive enough for you, there's also evidence from studies of twins. Twin studies are commonly used to see how much genes matter in all sorts of human features, from personality traits to psychological disorders to physical diseases. The problem for eating studies is, while identical twins share all of the same genes, they also typically share the same eating environment. So if features are common in both twins, it is possible that they are the result of a shared environment.

To tease apart the effects of genes from the effects of the shared environment, researchers located identical twins that were raised in separate homes without knowing each other. It may seem surprising that there are enough sets of twins that meet this criteria, but there are. This type of twin research was partly pioneered in the very psychology department in which I work, at the University of Minnesota (coincidentally located in the twin cities of Minneapolis and St. Paul). If you go up to the fifth floor, the walls are covered with photographs of identical twins that were separated at the age of five months (on average) and had been apart for about thirty years before being reunited as adults. The visible similarities are remarkable, as are the many documented behavioral similarities.[3]

The crucial twin study of body weight (which comes from the Swedish Adoption/Twin Study of Aging) included 93 pairs of identical twins raised apart (and 154 pairs of identical twins raised together). Sure enough, the weights of identical twins, whether they were raised together or apart, were highly correlated. That study, along with several others, led scientists to conclude that genes account for 70 percent of the variation in people's weight.[4] Seventy percent! What is truly remarkable is that this is only slightly lower than the role genes play in height (about 80 percent of the variation).[5] Don't get me wrong. I'm not saying you can't influence your weight at all, just that the amount of influence you have is fairly limited,[6] and you'll generally end up within your genetically determined set weight range.

Okay, so maybe you can't easily influence your weight to achieve long-lasting losses, you might say, but it seems all too easy to influence it in the direction of weight gain, right? Actually, it's not as easy as you might think. Researchers have studied that side of the equation, too—instead of having people *lose* weight and then try to maintain the *thin* weight, they had people *gain* weight and then try to maintain the *fat* weight. Staying fat shouldn't be that difficult, should it? In one set of studies, researchers tried to make people fat by overfeeding them. They didn't want exercise to get in the way of weight gain, so they did these studies with people they could prevent from doing any exercise at all: prisoners.[7] I'm not wild about using prisoners in research because it is often hard for them to refuse to participate, but the researchers explained their plans fully and got permission from each prisoner.

Several fascinating things happened next. First of all, it was remarkably difficult to make the prisoners fat. The prisoners had to eat enormous quantities of food—some of them over 10,000 calories per day, for four to six months—to gain 20 percent of their starting weight. That's a lot of extra calories, considering men in the United States tend to average about 2,500 daily calories. Some of the prisoners could not gain that much weight, despite eating huge amounts of food, and the prisoners gained much less weight than the researchers predicted based on the amount of calories they consumed. And most surprising, once the prisoners had gained weight, it was very difficult for them to keep it on. They had to continue eating a large number of calories per day (at least 2,700) just to maintain it; otherwise they would lose the weight. When researchers tried the same study with dedicated student volunteers who were free to walk around and exercise some, they were actually *unable to turn them obese*.[8] In another study, researchers fed twins an additional 1,000 calories per day over what they would need to eat to maintain their weight. They did this for 100 days. Like the prisoners, these twins were unable to maintain the higher weights.[9]

In addition to showing why it is so difficult to maintain a weight higher or lower than is dictated by our genes, these kinds of studies also offer evidence that our genes control *how much* weight we gain. Even when study participants were fed the same amount of calories, they gained varying amounts of weight. The pairs of twins that were overfed 1,000 calories per day gained anywhere from 9 to 29 pounds. In other words: the same number of calories led some people to gain three times as much weight as other people. Moreover, each twin gained nearly the same amount as their own twin, even though each pair of twins gained different amounts of weight than the other pairs of twins.[10] All of these studies are evidence that your body is trying to keep you within that genetically determined set weight range.[11] When our weight is within this range, we don't have to fight to maintain it. It's easy. We can eat a little more or a little less, exercise a little more or a little less—and it won't have much of a lasting impact. The hard part is trying to get out of that range, because to do so, you have to battle biology. Your body uses many biological tricks to defend your set range, particularly if you get below it, because this is when your body thinks you are starving to death. To save you, it makes you eat more food, and stores some of the energy you consume in case of emergency.

When you are dieting and hungry, your brain responds differently to tasty-looking food than it does when you are not dieting. The areas of the brain that become unusually active make you more likely to notice food, prompt you to pay more attention to it when you find it, and make it look even more delicious and tempting than usual.[12] These are potent signals to eat. At the same time, activity is reduced in the prefrontal cortex, the "executive function" part of the brain that helps you make decisions and resist impulses.[13] Either one of those responses would make you more likely to indulge, but when you put them together, you don't stand a chance. Your ability to resist is taking a snooze exactly when you most want its support. To make matters worse, this response has been found to be particularly strong in obese people—and it also gets stronger the longer you diet.[14]

Another way your body defends your set range is through hormonal changes. As you diet and lose weight, you lose body fat.[15] Many of us think of body fat as blubbery stuff that just sits there under our skin and makes us look fat, keeps us warm, and helps us float in the ocean, but body fat (also called adipose tissue) is an active part of the endocrine system.[16] It produces hormones that are involved in the sensations of hunger and fullness, and as you lose body fat, the amount of these hormones circulating in your body changes. The levels of hormones that help you feel full (including leptin, peptide YY, and cholecystokinin) decrease. The levels of hormones that make you feel hungry (including ghrelin, gastric inhibitory polypeptide, and pancreatic polypeptide) increase.[17] Just like with the changes in brain patterns, these hormone changes give you an urge to eat, and to eat a lot. One study found that these changes in hormone levels were still detectable in people a year after they stopped dieting.[18]

While these changes in brain reactivity and hormone production are pushing you to eat more, your metabolism also betrays you. It changes partly because you are thinner, and partly due to the effects of (what it perceives to be) starvation. Whether or not you are dieting, your metabolism is affected by your weight. It takes energy to run all of the metabolic processes in your body every day; the more you weigh, the more energy (calories) your body burns just to keep you alive. When you lose weight, even if starvation has no effect on your metabolism, your body will still burn fewer calories, simply because it is now a smaller body to run. This means that the number of calories you ate to lose weight eventually becomes too many calories to eat if you want to *keep* losing weight.[19]

On top of that, starvation also has an effect on your metabolism. Because there is not enough food coming in, your metabolism slows down to conserve energy. Unfortunately, this doesn't make you feel full longer or help you lose weight. Quite the opposite. It uses each calorie in the most efficient manner possible, which allows your body to run on even fewer calories than it would need just based on the size of the body. More calories are left unused and can be stored as fat.

The consequences of these changes are problematic, to say the least. When you aren't taking in enough calories, your body makes storing those calories as fat the top priority, regardless of the dietary fat content of whatever you ate.[20] That's right, in certain cases, even non-fat foods can get stored as fat. And more alarmingly, this means that a person who loses weight to reach 150 pounds, for example, is not the same, physiologically, as a person who normally weighs 150 pounds.[21] To maintain 150 pounds after dieting down to that weight, dieters must eat fewer calories per day than people who were 150 pounds all along (not to mention fewer calories per day than they ate to get to that weight) or else they will gain weight.[22]

You know what I find the most infuriating about this situation? People will blame the weight regain on your self-control, even though you are probably eating less food than they are! To maintain your new weight, you have to fight evolution. You have to fight biology. You have to fight your brain. You have to fight your metabolism. These are the ways your body tries to protect you from starvation, and it is not a fair fight. You have to respect this miracle of being human, but you don't have to like it.

## SAVE SOME OF THE BLAME FOR PSYCHOLOGY

The other foe in the long-term weight loss battle is psychology. When people are dieting and hungry, psychological changes take place. We learned about a lot of these changes from a groundbreaking semi-starvation study that was conducted in the 1940s by Ancel Keys, a professor in the School of Public Health at the University of Minnesota.[23] In it, thirty-six men volunteered to be starved for six months as a humanitarian act so that researchers could test the best ways to help starving people throughout the world. Although this study is always referred to as a starvation or semi-starvation study, I think of it as a diet study, because the men were allowed nearly 1,600 calories per day.

All sorts of things happened to the men during the study, which I will talk more about later, but the most common *psychological* response was an obsession with food. Before the study started, the men had many interests. They actively followed current events; they were curious about the new city they were living in; and they wanted to become acquainted with each other. Some of them even signed up to take classes on campus. But when the men were starving, the only thing they wanted to think about, or could think about, was food. They lost interest in their humanitarian mission, stopped attending classes, and even lost interest in sex. Their conversations with each other centered on food, their dreams were about food, and their spare time was occupied with thoughts of wonderful meals they had in the past, or plans for what they would eat someday in the distant future. Several of the volunteers vowed to take up careers in the food industry when the study ended—to open a grocery store or restaurant, become a chef, or work on a farm. Even those who had never cooked before started clipping recipes and reading cookbooks (including one volunteer who collected more than twenty-five cookbooks).[24]

This type of behavior would have been useful for our ancestors during times of starvation. Individuals who focused exclusively on food and how to access it would have been more successful at finding some and, therefore, would be more likely to survive than their peers who were able to distract themselves from thoughts of food. But today, it just means that the less we try to eat, the more obsessed we become with food.

To take a closer look at this phenomenon, a collaborator[25] and I examined what happens when people are denied a particular kind of food. We asked the students in my research methods class to participate, and they roped their friends into helping us, too. We had them record how many times they thought about a particular food, every day for three weeks. One of those weeks they were told they were forbidden from eating that food. Sure enough, they thought about the food more often that week than either of the other weeks.[26] This shouldn't come as a big shock. One of the first stories in the Bible is of Eve struggling not to eat the forbidden fruit. What is surprising, though, is that unlike Eve's fixation on that delicious, tantalizing apple, the students thought about an off-limits food more frequently even if it was a food they didn't like very much.

The problem for diets is that almost by definition, you have to forbid yourself from eating all sorts of foods, and for a period longer than a week. On a diet, you will think more about food in general, because you are hungry, and you will especially think about the very foods you have forbidden yourself from having. This just makes the job of avoiding and resisting those foods even harder.

## ONE MORE THING TO BE STRESSED ABOUT

There are biological reasons why you regain lost weight, and there are psychological reasons why you regain lost weight. And then there is stress, which combines both of these forces in a uniquely powerful way. You probably don't need me to define stress. It's one of those "I can't define it but I know it when I see it" sorts of things. But when psychologists talk about stress, we are referring to a negative emotional response that leads to a specific set of physical, cognitive, and behavioral changes.[27] These changes are thought to have evolved to help us handle one particular form of stress—stress that comes on suddenly and needs a quick, powerful mobilization of energy, such as fleeing from a woolly mammoth or other fast-moving predator.[28] But that is not the kind of stress we routinely encounter in our day-to-day life. The kinds of stressors we experience don't start and end quickly or suddenly. They tend to be ongoing, such as chronic worry over our finances, our jobs, or our families.

Among the physical changes that stress initiates is the release of a hormone that you've probably heard about if you've ever tried to lose weight: cortisol. This particular hormone has made headlines for its link to belly fat. That's because one of the many things cortisol does to help you flee the mammoth is to make energy—in the form of glucose—available for use in your bloodstream. But if the cause of your stress isn't chasing you across the tundra, this newly available glucose isn't needed to combat the stress right away. Instead it ends up getting stored in your belly, as fat.[29] So on a chemical level, stress causes weight gain.

Stress also leads people to act in ways that cause weight gain. Studies have shown that stress causes us to overeat,[30] exercise less, and sleep less. It is no surprise that eating more and exercising less leads to some weight gain, but many people underestimate the role of sleep when it comes to weight maintenance. Your brain responds to sleep deprivation in a similar way as it responds to hunger, even if you aren't hungry. If you are sleep deprived, even for one night, the sight of enticing food elicits a stronger-than-normal response in a part of your brain that motivates eating, and a weaker-than-normal response in the prefrontal cortex, that area of your brain that controls impulsive behavior.[31] In one sleep study, when participants were allowed to sleep only for five hours a night, they gained about two pounds in five days. But when they were allowed to sleep for nine hours a night, they had no trouble maintaining their weight over five days.[32]

So, let's think about this: Stress leads to weight gain. Most of us consider ourselves to be under stress at various points in our lives, but what about dieters? While many people on a diet will tell you that dieting is stressful, is it accurate to say that the act of dieting alone promotes a stress response?

For her dissertation, my brilliant student Janet Tomiyama set out to see if dieting actually causes that physiological chain reaction that is part of the stress response.[33] If it did, she also wanted to know what exactly about dieting was causing the problem. There are two main rules you have to follow on any diet: you have to restrict what you eat, and you have to monitor your food intake. Restricting what you eat means that you can't always have the things you want, that you have to politely say "no" when someone offers you a slice of cake at a birthday party, and that you often feel hungry. Monitoring your food intake means that you have to keep careful track of what you eat, count calories, and plan meals. These tasks could be considered stressful, or at least a giant hassle.

Janet sought out women who wanted to start a diet, and then she had her study participants restrict their calories, monitor their eating, both, or neither. Specifically, some of the women had to restrict their eating to 1,200 calories a day and also monitor their eating by keeping a daily food diary. One group had to restrict their eating to 1,200 calories a day but *not* monitor their eating. (That part was tricky—how do you get people to eat exactly 1,200 calories without tracking their calories? For those women, Janet provided 1,200 calories a day of prepackaged food, so they didn't need to keep track of anything.) Another group had to monitor their eating by keeping a daily food diary, but they were not asked to restrict their eating to 1,200 calories. And some of the women weren't required to do any of these things.

Because Janet was interested in whether dieting caused a physiological stress response, she needed to measure the cortisol in the dieters' saliva. To do that, the women would need to provide saliva samples six times a day for a few days before and after the diet. Whenever it was time for them to give a saliva sample, they had to chew on a cotton pad called a Salivette until it was totally saturated with saliva, and then spit the whole soggy thing into a little plastic tube. It's a bit icky, but the women in the study were troupers and did this without complaint.

Until Janet could test the samples, they needed to be kept frozen. Janet ran half of the study in my old lab at the University of California, Los Angeles, and Jeff Hunger, my lab manager at the time, ran the other half in my new lab in Minnesota. Our regular freezer was full of ice cream for another study, so we acquired a special freezer solely for storing saliva samples. Rules of scientific conduct require that things researchers intend to serve people to eat may not occupy the same freezer as samples of human bodily fluids (which is not a bad rule of thumb for home freezers, either). Once the freezer was full of saliva, Jeff packed all those tubes of Salivettes in dry ice and shipped them to Janet in Los Angeles; she then did whatever one does with saliva samples to test them for cortisol (I try to avoid that sort of thing).

What Janet found is that whether or not her subjects monitored their calorie intake, the act of restricting calories led to a physiological stress response.[34] This was the first human study to prove that diets are stressful (though around the same time it was shown in mice).[35] I think its findings add an important wrinkle to how we think about dieting. It's not just that people should try to avoid stress while dieting. It's that stress *cannot be avoided when you are dieting*, because dieting itself causes stress. Dieting causes the stress response that has already been shown to lead to weight gain.

Remember, this stress response is just one of the many biological and psychological changes that happen when we restrict our eating. Each one on its own creates an obstacle to keeping off weight. Perhaps you can surmount one of these obstacles, or even two, for a while. But all of them, all of the time? It is unrealistic to expect people to succeed when they are up against evolution, biology, and psychology. It's time to try something different.

## MEET YOUR NEW BEST FRIEND: YOUR SET WEIGHT RANGE

Any time I talk to people about the idea of a genetic set weight range, they focus on the bad news—that if they lose so much weight that they fall below their set range, they will gain it back. But don't forget about the good news. As we learned from the study of the prisoners who were purposely overfed, it is harder to gain a lot of weight than people realize. (It can happen, though, so I wouldn't recommend trying this one at home.) If you gain a lot of weight so that you are above your set range, you have to consume more calories to maintain it than someone who was that weight all along, or you will lose weight. Many people monitor their eating carefully and believe that if they didn't, they would gain a lot of weight. They are probably wrong. They would likely gain weight, but not enough to drastically change them.

So how do you determine your set range? It's more of an art than a science, at least given the current state of knowledge, but we do know that it will encompass the weights you tend to be at when you are not dieting and not engaging in extreme overeating. If there is a particular weight that you seem to keep coming back to after changes in either direction, it might be in the middle of your set range. One expert says that you can comfortably lose about fifteen pounds[36] below your set point before your body starts trying to defend a higher weight. (Of course that assumes you weigh enough to begin with—if you weigh 100 pounds, losing 15 pounds is almost certainly outside your set range.) If it works the same on the high end as on the low end, that would mean that your set range reasonably covers about thirty pounds.

Unless you want to battle evolution, biology, and psychology and be hungry every single day of your life, I wouldn't suggest trying to live below your set range. I understand that for many people, the goal is simply to be thin, but you also want to enjoy your life. Losing some weight but staying within your set range is a healthy goal; getting so thin that you are below this range is a very difficult and self-defeating one. For all of us, the aim should be to live at the low end of our set range. We'll call that weight our leanest livable weight, and it's perfectly reasonable to aim for it, and to make some lifestyle changes to get there.

But first, I want to talk a little bit more about what's *not* the cause of your weight regain: your inability to control yourself. Lack of willpower is not why people can't lose weight or maintain weight loss on a diet, and strong willpower is not why thin people stay thin. The idea that willpower is the key to weight control is misguided. It's time we set the record straight.

# CHAPTER 3

# THE MYTH OF WILLPOWER

Life would be a lot easier if I liked sorbet. I am constantly finding myself in ice cream shops with my two sons, and if I actually liked sorbet, I would eat it. Fruity, lower-calorie, low-fat sorbet.[1] Instead, I have to try to resist ice cream, and I inevitably fail. Because I don't have enough willpower. Neither do you. Even without meeting you, I know this is true, because very few people do (and those people are probably not reading this book). The unfortunate fact is that hardly anybody has enough willpower to resist tempting foods if they are routinely confronted with them. And we *are* routinely confronted with them, because we live in an environment[2] in which the most tempting, most difficult-to-resist[3] foods (those with lots of fat and sugar) are inexpensive and readily accessible.

Dieting requires you to resist temptation every time. No exceptions. Esteemed obesity researcher John Foreyt said in *Living Without Dieting*[4] that dieting is like holding your breath. At some point, you have to breathe. When a food is present, you don't have to resist it just one time to be successful. You have to resist it an hour from now and ten minutes from now and one minute from now and one second from now. As long as the food is there, you have to resist it as often as you take a breath. And therein lies the problem.

Imagine you are a master of self-control. Nobody's perfect at anything, but suppose you are so good at self-control that you can successfully resist temptation 99 percent of the time. If a cookie is next to your desk while you are working, you have to resist that cookie every time you notice it—every time you look up from your computer. I don't know about you, but I look up after nearly every sentence I type. Or at least once a minute. Assuming that I am in the neighborhood of normal, so do you. Even with your amazing (and highly unlikely) 99th percentile self-control powers, on that 100th time you look up, you will reach for that cookie. It won't matter one bit that you resisted it successfully 99 times already. You get no credit for that. You won't be one bit different from people—like my nine-year-old son—who succumb the first time they see the cookie. You will have eaten the cookie; they will have eaten the cookie. Your amazing powers of self-control—your near-perfect willpower—will have gotten you nowhere.

## SOME PEOPLE HAVE LOTS OF WILLPOWER, RIGHT?

It's not that different people don't have different aptitudes for self-control. We all fall somewhere on the spectrum between rampant self-indulgence and monk-like self-denial. To take an extreme example of the latter, people who suffer from the eating disorder anorexia nervosa, which is characterized by an obsessive desire to be thin, are able to harness near-perfect self-control. And while in this case their use of willpower is far from healthy, anorexics are nevertheless able to successfully resist temptation almost constantly. The same could be said for people who go on public hunger strikes. So it's not that self-control is an impossible feat. But for most people, when it comes to eating, having sufficient willpower matters a lot less than you would think.

Psychologists study self-control, and they often assess a person's level of self-control by having them fill out a questionnaire.[5] This assessment usually contains statements such as "People would describe me as impulsive"; "I am bad at resisting temptation"; and "I do many things on the spur of the moment." If these statements (and others) describe you very well, your score would indicate that your self-control ability is low. And perhaps it is. But your score on a self-control test doesn't provide the whole answer when it comes to willpower and food.

Many years ago, I gave the twenty research assistants in my lab a tedious task: I asked them to hunt down every study ever performed that included one of these self-control questionnaires. They found more than five hundred studies. Then I had them read each one to find the studies in which researchers not only had participants complete the self-control questionnaire, but also put the participants through an exercise in which they needed to use self-control. We found a grand total of twenty-six studies that fit the bill.

In one of the studies,[6] psychologists Malte Friese and Wilhelm Hofmann asked participants to try to resist some potato chips, and then they looked at whether subjects who got high scores for self-control on the questionnaire had been better able to resist the potato chips than subjects who scored low. They hadn't. When it came to resisting highly tempting food, it turned out that self-control ability didn't matter much.

But it's not that self-control has no impact at all on human behavior. On the contrary. A few years after we completed this research, another set of researchers tracked down more self-control studies and examined how well self-control ability correlated with the inhibition of various types of behavior.[7] When it came to things like schoolwork, grades, and even happiness and depression, self-control played a major role. Eating, however, was far less influenced by self-control ability than any other type of behavior they studied. In fact, self-control mattered only half as much for eating as it did for most other behaviors.[8]

Maybe you don't find these kinds of studies persuasive. After all, people are not necessarily willing to admit on a questionnaire that they are impulsive or that they cannot resist temptations. Some people may lack the self-awareness to admit these things to themselves, let alone write them on a psychologist's questionnaire. The truth is, psychologists have these same concerns about questionnaires, so whenever possible, we try to learn things about people without asking them about themselves.

When it comes to measuring self-control, a clever test called the "delay of gratification test" is often used.[9] For example, if you want to assess self-control in children, you're not going to get a very accurate answer by asking them questions about themselves or having them fill out a questionnaire. Instead, researchers leave them alone in a room with a marshmallow. The children are told that they will be given a second marshmallow if they can resist the first one until the researchers return. Otherwise they only get the one. The longer a child can resist the first marshmallow, the better his or her self-control.

One occupational hazard of being a psychologist is that you sometimes try these tests out on your friends and family. I made the tactical error of administering the marshmallow test to both of my sons when they were little. Each of them grabbed and ate the marshmallow before I could even get out of the room. This bodes poorly for their futures, as self-control ability is correlated with many measures of success and well-being later in life. For instance, the longer children resist the marshmallow, the better equipped they have been shown to be when it comes to dealing with stress and frustration ten years later.[10]

This measure of self-control also relates to their adult body mass index[11] thirty years later,[12] but importantly, the relationship is very small—even smaller than the correlation we found with the questionnaires.[13] So let's put the idea to bed, once and for all, that having sufficient willpower is the key to being thin. It just isn't. Self-control is an important quality to have for many things in life, but when it comes to body weight, it doesn't play that big a role.

## SELF-CONTROL DEPENDS ON YOUR CIRCUMSTANCES, NOT YOUR ABILITY

I know what you're thinking: *Yes, but then how does that explain my mother-in-law, Trudie, who eats like a rabbit and stays so thin? She obviously has amazing self-control!* I would ask you to consider that your perception of Trudie may be flawed. Sometimes it may look like people are doing an impressive job of resisting something, when really they simply aren't tempted by it. Maybe your friends who are so good at resisting cookies are just not that into cookies. People like that are, after all, alleged to exist. It doesn't count as self-control if you didn't want the thing in the first place. My collaborator Joe Redden calls this "apparent self-control,"[14] because you look like you are controlling yourself, but you either never wanted the thing, or you are sick of the thing. Joe is an expert on getting sick of things (yes, it's possible to be an expert on that). He does studies in which he has people listen to a song they love twenty times in a row, or eat seventeen of one flavor of jelly bean, so that they get sick of it, and then he makes them like it again.

Perhaps this is obvious, but food preferences and desires matter. Like many women, I have experienced what it would be like to live with an entirely different set of preferences. It's a natural part of being pregnant. When I was pregnant with my older son, I had no interest in the kinds of foods I am usually tempted by—sweets like ice cream, brownies, and marshmallows. Instead, I wanted cucumbers, salads, and most of all, apples. Normally I have no feelings whatsoever about apples. They exist. I see them in stores. I see them representing the letter *A* in picture books. But when I was pregnant, they were objects of joy and deliciousness. I bet it's no coincidence that my son absolutely adores apples. I ate *a lot* of apples during that pregnancy. If ice cream was nearby, I would not eat it. Not because I was exercising impressive self-control over my diet (which, believe me, was not something I was trying to do while pregnant), but because I had absolutely no desire for it. It was like being plopped into someone else's mind and body for nine months, and it was eye-opening. It made me understand firsthand how some people would have no trouble resisting certain foods, while for other people it would be a struggle. It would have nothing to do with their self-control ability, and everything to do with their physiologically based preferences.

## WHAT SABOTAGES WILLPOWER?

Every time I tell people that I study self-control, the first thing they do is ask for advice on how to control themselves. Actually, that's the second thing they do. The first thing they do—and tellingly, there are no exceptions to this pattern—is say something like, "Boy, I sure wish I had some more of *that*." And then they ask for advice. For years, I had no advice to offer. All I had was bad news. It slowly dawned on me that nearly every study on self-control (including most of my own, for a while) demonstrated the reasons why self-control so often fails us.

So what explains whether or not we can successfully control our behavior, if our own self-control aptitude isn't a reliable predictor? Well, there are lots of other variables that influence your ability to control yourself, and they can all be lumped into a category that I will call your *circumstances*. For example, are you distracted? Stressed? In a bad mood? In a good mood? Have you been controlling yourself all day and now you are tired? These things matter more than your self-control ability, and this is good news, because as we will soon discuss, your circumstances are things you can change.

## Distraction and Multitasking

One circumstance that causes people to fail at self-control is distraction. Regular, ordinary distraction, such as watching TV while trying to have a conversation. This doesn't sound like a big deal until you take a moment to think about how often you are distracted every day.

Multitasking is the normal state of existence for most of us, rather than the occasional hurried exception. In fact, in his book *The Shallows*,[15] Nicholas Carr argues that the Internet is slowly destroying our "capacity for concentration," by training us to quickly scan and skim small pieces of information from all over the Internet, rather than focusing deeply on any one thing. Generations of children may be paying the price for this. In recent research, psychologists have found that while studying in their homes, students from middle school to college age lasted only about six minutes before getting distracted by their phones or computers.[16] Not a lot of time for deep thinking.

Long before I started the Health and Eating Laboratory, I did a study[17] on the effect of distraction on self-control of eating. In fact, it was the first eating study I ever ran, and I did it in graduate school with my classmate and close friend, Andrew Ward. The lab rooms we were given for the study were in the dingy basement of the psychology building at Stanford. It was so gloomy down there that we weren't surprised to learn that they had previously been used as prison cells in the infamous Stanford Prison Experiment in 1971.[18]

Andrew and I had found some research that showed drinking alcohol caused dieters to overeat.[19] Since we were just out of college ourselves, we knew it wasn't unusual for college students to eat piles of some crazy food after a long night of partying. At my alma mater, the University of Virginia, there is a diner called the White Spot that is famous for serving a sandwich consisting of two glazed doughnuts slapped around a scoop of ice cream, and then fried on the grill. This was (and is) notoriously eaten late at night while drunk. Overeating while intoxicated is definitely something that happens. We wanted to know *why* it happens.

We thought that maybe alcohol clouds your thinking[20] and keeps you from noticing that you are overeating. If that were true, then perhaps dieters would overeat if we clouded their thinking in another way, say by simply distracting them. Thus, our study was born. We brought students into the lab, one at a time, and asked them to eat cookies, M&Ms, and Doritos while watching a slide show of dozens of paintings. We told them that later there would be a memory test on the paintings, and that we provided the snacks to put them in a good mood so that we could study the effects of their mood on their memory. None of this was true.

In social psychology we call that a "cover story." In the regular world we call it a "lie." We believe this to be a harmless lie, and that our participants don't much care if we are studying the effects of mood on memory or the effects of distraction on eating. This type of deception is necessary in most eating research because we can't learn about people's behavior around food if they know we're observing their eating, or if they even think we might *notice* how much they're eating. When people know they're being watched, they become self-conscious, act unnaturally, and won't eat very much. So we have to be a little sneaky. We pile their bowls extremely high with food so that they can eat quite a lot without making a noticeable dent in it. And we use a cover story to explain why there happens to be an impressive spread of food there in the first place. But with every study, we are very careful to minimize the deception, and we always explain the setup to research participants at the end of the study.[21] In twenty years of conducting eating studies, we have not had a participant who seemed to be distressed by our methods.

In this study, we were interested in how much dieters and non-dieters ate when they were distracted. We could tell how much they ate because we secretly weighed the food before we gave it to them, and then weighed it again after they were done. To make sure we distracted them enough, we had them look at the slide show of paintings while listening for a tone from the computer. They were instructed to press a button on the floor as fast as they could, with their foot, every time they heard the tone. Although this seemed somewhat odd to the participants, we put the button on the floor so that their hands would be free to do what we really cared about: grab food. For comparison, we also had dieters and non-dieters who only had to listen for the tone and then hit the floor button when they heard it, without watching the slide show. Since these students are just staring at an empty wall, they shouldn't be distracted very much at all.

What we found was that the dieters who were distracted by the slide show ate about 40 percent more of the candy and chips than dieters who didn't watch the slide show. Distraction interfered with their ability to control their eating. The non-dieters, on the other hand, ate about 30 percent *less* when they were distracted than when they weren't. Non-dieters' eating habits are pretty sensible, if you think about it. They are occupied with whatever is distracting them, so they don't have the time or inclination to focus on anything else, including food. This is a pattern that we notice time and time again, not just in our own work, but in that of other researchers, too.[22] Lots of everyday events cause dieters to overeat, but don't have the same effect on non-dieters.

It turned out that Andrew and I were correct in our hypothesis that clouding dieters' thoughts would lead them to overeat, but we were wrong about why it happened. We thought dieters would be so distracted that they would lose track of how much they had eaten and then inadvertently eat more than they intended. But at the end of the study, we asked dieters how much they had eaten, and they were perfectly accurate in their estimates. They hadn't lost track of their eating. We see this in lots of our studies. Dieters always know how much they ate. Are they worse at multitasking? Are they using the task as an excuse to eat? We still aren't quite sure why distraction causes them to overeat. We just know that it does.

## Good Moods Can Mess You Up as Much as Bad Moods

As we've discussed, stress is one cause of dieting failure, as it is linked to both physiological and psychological changes that promote weight gain. Of course, we don't need a study to tell us that stress causes people to overeat. There's even a term for it: stress eating. And people do indeed stress eat.

But what about people on diets? If diets are a source of stress, it would seem logical that dieters would be more prone to stress eating than non-dieters, and plenty of research backs that up.[23] This was first shown in 1975, in a study[24] conducted by eating research pioneers Peter Herman and Janet Polivy. They used a complicated cover story in which their participants—who were both dieters and non-dieters—were told that they were about to receive either a painful electric shock or a very mild one. The researchers never shocked them, of course. Even back in 1975, shocking one's research participants wasn't considered an acceptable method of bringing about scientific progress. But the participants believed it, and those who were told that they were about to be administered a painful shock became quite stressed. Those who were expecting to receive a mild shock did not.

To examine the effects of stress upon eating, the researchers gave participants bowls of ice cream and measured how much they ate while waiting to be shocked. The participants who were on a diet and who were told to expect a big shock ate more ice cream than the participants who were on a diet and expecting a mild shock. Clearly, stress causes overeating, but the interesting thing about this study is, only the dieters ate more when they were stressed. Non-dieters actually ate *less* when they were stressed. Yet again, a circumstance in which we find ourselves regularly—being stressed—causes dieters to overeat but does not necessarily have the same effect on non-dieters. Not only do dieters overeat when they are stressed, but they also tend to choose foods that are particularly high in calories or fat.[25]

The amount of stress that causes dieters to lose control of their eating does not have to be as extreme as the stress of waiting to receive a painful electric shock. Much milder stressors—like watching an unpleasant movie[26]—also cause dieters to overeat. In fact, just being in a run-of-the-mill bad mood is sufficient motivation for most dieters to overeat. My student Janet Tomiyama and I learned about bad moods and eating many years ago, when we[27] studied students outside of a lab setting, as they went about their daily lives. We loaned them each a Palm Pilot (remember those?) and set it to beep once every waking hour for four days. When it beeped, they had to answer questions about their current mood and eating. We were surprised to learn that bad moods triggered eating for dieters *and* for non-dieters. But get this: so did good moods! That also surprised us at first, but once we thought about it, it didn't seem so unusual. If you're in a terrible mood and having a lousy day, you might decide to treat yourself to a doughnut. Why not? A doughnut will cheer you up (or so you think). Conversely, you are in a wonderful mood and had a productive day, and so you decide to reward your hard work with a doughnut. Why not? You deserve it!

## Controlling One Thing Makes It Hard to Control Another

One reason self-control ability matters so little when it comes to eating, and circumstances matter so much, is that no matter how much willpower you may have, it is a limited resource. You can only use it for a little while before it runs out—and when that happens, it takes some time for it to replenish. Think of it like working a muscle. If you want to get strong arms and you do as many push-ups as you can, eventually your arms will start to shake and you can't go any further. That's because you have depleted the resources of those muscles. You know that you have to rest and refuel before you can use them again. Self-control isn't a muscle, but it does seem to work in much the same way. If you are relying on the strength of your willpower to control one thing, you'll be less able to exercise self-control over the next thing you encounter.

This wearing-out or depletion of self-control has been extensively documented[28] in the research literature, probably more than any other source of self-control failure. To fully appreciate it, let's consider an example.[29] Imagine you show up for a study and you are seated in a small room, with a bowl of radishes and a plate of chocolate chip cookies in front of you. The cookies are still warm and have that wonderful smell unique to freshly baked cookies. Now imagine that a researcher tells you that you are participating in an experiment about taste perception, and that you have been assigned to taste the radishes. He leaves you alone, and you have to resist the cookies and eat only radishes. This takes some self-control. Luckily, this takes only a few minutes, and with effort, you do manage to resist them for this short amount of time. This was an act of self-control. It took willpower. When the researcher comes back into the room, he takes away all of the food and asks you to help him solve a puzzle that is completely unrelated to the taste perception study. At least, that's what he says.

As you've seen in several sneaky eating studies now, things are not quite as the researcher says. Not only is this "unrelated" puzzle very much related to the study, it is also cleverly designed so that even though it looks reasonably easy, it is in fact unsolvable. Persisting at trying to solve this puzzle is an activity that requires self-control. Participants who had just resisted eating the warm cookies gave up on the puzzle very quickly, because they had just used up a large reserve of self-control. Other participants, however, had been allowed to eat the cookies during the first part of the study, so they didn't deplete their self-control resources. They persisted for longer at trying to solve the puzzle. Exercising self-control in the first task clearly reduced the subjects' ability to exercise self-control in the second task.

It is quite common to try to control two things in a row. In some sense, practically everything that you do can be considered an act of self-control, at least when it comes to the effect it has on controlling something else afterward. Hiding your emotions while watching a violent movie counts as self-control, as does trying not to think about a white bear or crossing out all the letter *e*'s in a paragraph.[30] Even such trivial (and relatively simple) acts of self-control as these led research participants to fail at controlling themselves at something else afterward.

Of course, those are not things that you do in your life (unless you happen to be a participant in one of these studies or have some very odd hobbies). But plenty of things that you do regularly engage in also mess up your ability to control something else. One of the most common of these activities is being faced with multiple choices and needing to make a decision. While nobody wants to have *no* choices in their lives, there is a downside to having too much choice.[31] My former graduate school classmate and social psychologist Sheena Iyengar conducted a study that showed that if people chose a piece of candy from a display of thirty different chocolates, they were less satisfied with the candy than if they chose from a display of only six chocolates.[32] The more choices, it seems, the greater the pressure to get it right, and the greater the possibility of feeling regret.

Making choices has been shown to deplete self-control resources, leading to worse self-control on a subsequent task.[33] This is truly unfortunate, because we make choices regularly, not just between products, but also between activities to engage in, friends to call, and recipes to make for dinner tonight. We channel-surf among 800 cable channels to select a show to watch, scroll through 1,200 songs on our smartphones to select one to listen to, and choose among millions of blogs to read and Twitter feeds to follow. Most of the time we are making a choice about something. If making a choice causes us to fail at subsequent tasks that require self-control—which it does—then we are in trouble when it comes to more than just dieting.

In fact, President Barack Obama acknowledged the burden of making choices in a 2012 *Vanity Fair*[34] interview, in which he mentioned this research and said: "You'll see I wear only gray or blue suits. I'm trying to pare down decisions. I don't want to make decisions about what I'm eating or wearing. Because I have too many other decisions to make." By limiting the number of decisions he makes, he may be helping to protect himself from making impulsive decisions. At a minimum, it keeps him from depleting his self-control resources before breakfast.

## SMART REGULATION

Although we know that self-control can become depleted quite easily, we still do not know why this happens. It could be that exercising self-control makes you tired, and once tired, you lack the energy to control something else. It could be that you just get sick of controlling things, and so after controlling one thing, you can't be bothered to try again right away. It could be that controlling one thing is distracting, and as we've discussed, distraction reduces your ability to control another thing.

Not knowing why self-control becomes depleted makes it hard to come up with solutions for enhancing it. It seems that one way in which self-control is *not* like a muscle is that we can train our muscles to get stronger and work more efficiently, but we can't really train ourselves to get better at self-control. Several researchers (and a gazillion unscientific websites) claim you can "harness" your willpower abilities or learn to control yourself through a variety of exercises. These experts[35] always cite the same handful of articles,[36] but none of them actually offers convincing evidence that you can strengthen willpower like a muscle.

Humans were simply not made to willfully resist food. We evolved through famines, hunting and gathering, eating whatever we could get, when we could get it. We evolved to keep fat on our bones by eating the foods that we see, not resisting them. It is difficult to imagine how any species could evolve to be successful at resisting the foods that keep it alive. I am not saying there are not times when you would be better off resisting food. Of course there are. I am simply saying that you will not be good at it. You were not meant to be good at it.

Think of willpower as brute strength. The amount of it you need is larger than the amount of it that you have, and the amount you have is all too easily depleted by nearly everything you do. It's foolish to rely on it. In the Netherlands they say, "if you can't be strong, you must be smart,"[37] and that is the solution to the willpower problem: using your brain to make sure you don't need any.[38]

PART TWO

# WHY YOU ARE BETTER OFF WITHOUT THE BATTLE

# CHAPTER 4

# DIETS ARE BAD FOR YOU

Is anyone going to disagree with me if I say that it sucks to be on a diet? I know this from personal experience, because I went on a diet once. In high school, with my girlfriends. None of us was overweight, but it seemed like the thing to do. We made up the rules ourselves, though what we based them on I cannot recall. Cheese was allowed, but milk wasn't. Bread was not allowed, but Ritz crackers and Wheat Thins were part of the daily menu. So were pickles and canned tuna fish with Miracle Whip. We had to stay below 1,200 calories each day, which is pretty standard for a diet and not nearly as strict as many. But it was miserable.

I hadn't thought very much about what I was eating before I went on the diet, then suddenly I was tracking every bite I ate and my mind was full of calorie counts. The world quickly divided into foods I could eat and foods I could not eat. I started craving foods that I typically ate infrequently, but were all the more enticing now that they were off-limits. Like doughnuts. While I was on the diet, my mom brought home a kind of doughnut that was new to me. I recall it vividly: a glazed buttermilk bar. I didn't eat it, but I was very aware that as long as I was on a diet, it would be off-limits.

My lifelong interest in *never dieting* started after just two weeks on that diet. I still remember that feeling of grayness, of life without the pleasing zing of color an occasional doughnut provided. I remember those urgent cravings for foods I hadn't found special before, and that feeling of being denied what other people got to have. No doubt many dieters will agree that my two weeks were pretty standard. I recall my father saying, "It's so hard. Nothing's harder," as he glumly packed his tiny can of fruit cocktail—his entire allotted lunch on his diet—into his briefcase to take to work. Of course we know that diets cause relatively minor miseries. I could understand enduring these miseries if diets were highly effective. I am not, after all, opposed to sacrifice for a good reason. But diets are not effective, and more important, they cause more than minor miseries—they can also cause serious problems. Plus obesity, as we will soon discuss, is not as good a reason as you think.

## DIETS MESS UP YOUR THINKING

The men who volunteered for Ancel Keys's semi-starvation study[1] in 1944 definitely had a good reason to "diet." As pacifists, they were conscientious objectors to fighting in World War II, and they were eager to help those who were suffering because of it. Keys planned to starve the men for six months and then test several different refeeding menus on them, so that the safest, most effective method could be recommended to the starving troops coming back from battlefields, as well as starving populations around the world. In the process, Keys was going to learn everything he possibly could about the effects of starvation on the human body and mind.

At the time, very little was known about the biological effects of starvation, and anything that was known was gleaned from observations of the unfortunate souls who happened to find themselves in that situation. Most populations of starving people are the victims of famine or war and hardly have the ability or inclination to document their experience, but there's another category of starving people who tend to chronicle their lives meticulously: explorers. Explorers didn't always find the new lands they were searching for, and sometimes they ran out of food. But they almost always kept journals. From those journals we know that while starving, explorers were preoccupied with thoughts of food and apathetic about pretty much everything else. One member of an expedition that was unexpectedly stranded in the Arctic for an entire winter wrote, "Our constant talk is about something to eat, and the different dishes we have enjoyed, or hope to enjoy on getting back to civilization."[2] He also mentioned feeling "an apathy and cloudiness impossible to shake off."[3] We also know that starving explorers were (not surprisingly) irritable. Another member of that expedition wrote, "We are all more or less unreasonable, and I only wonder that we are not all insane. All, including myself, are sullen, and at times very surly."[4]

It's hard to know what to make of this account, or any account written by an explorer. Explorers are not your average guys, and Arctic explorers . . . Well, to be fair, I am an indoor person and cannot begin to comprehend this, but to head for the Arctic in the days before Thinsulate and electric blankets (or even electricity) is walking a fine line between brave and crazy. One explorer came so close to starving to death that he ate his boots, but instead of retiring to the tropics after being rescued, opted to go back to the Arctic.[5]

Explorers tend to also be proud, as well as on the stoic side, which might lead them to play down their suffering, even in the privacy of their journals. It's likely their symptoms were worse than they reported. It's also possible that their symptoms had little to do with starvation. If explorers were anxious, perhaps it had more to do with their concern that they might encounter a polar bear or fall off an ice floe, and less to do with hunger. It is for this reason that Keys wrote "the psychology of people exposed to 'natural starvation' is as much a psychology of fear and desperation as a psychology of hunger and food deprivation."[6] It is impossible to separate the effects of starvation from the effects of whatever traumatic situation caused the starvation in the first place.

Keys wanted to study the effects of starvation in safety and comfort, and that is exactly what he did. He created a brochure depicting impoverished children with a caption that read, "Will you starve that they be better fed?" and he distributed it at the service camps where conscientious objectors were stationed during the war. From more than four hundred men who responded, Keys selected thirty-six that he deemed physically and mentally healthy enough to take part in his study. The men moved to the campus of the University of Minnesota and lived in a special dorm under the football stadium.

For the first three months, they ate 3,500 calories per day while Keys and his staff measured everything about them. Not only the size of each body part, but also the functioning of every system of the body, from respiration and circulation to endocrine function and metabolism, plus the condition of their skin and bones, their posture, muscular abilities, sensory abilities, mental abilities, and psychological state. If it was possible to measure something, Keys measured it. These were baseline measures that would be used as a comparison for the measurements taken while the men were starving. After three months of living under these baseline conditions, the men spent the next six months on a semi-starvation diet, which was composed mainly of bread, potatoes, cabbage, and rutabagas.

The experiences of these volunteers make an interesting case study of the effects of dieting, because their semi-starvation diet provided them 1,570 calories a day. To most people these days, that does not sound like starvation at all, but rather a fairly manageable diet. But things were different back then, and this was less than half as many calories as the men were used to eating. They lost 25 percent of their body weight in six months, and pictures taken at the end of the diet show emaciated men with gaunt faces.[7] You shouldn't be surprised to learn that they regained all the lost weight, plus more, within a year of the diet ending. But along the way they experienced psychological symptoms that can reasonably be considered side effects of semi-starvation, or dieting.

The most common symptom was a preoccupation with food. As you may recall from Chapter 2, during this semi-starvation study, these men did nothing but talk and think and dream about food. In fact, the announcement of Japan's surrender, which effectively ended the war, was made while the men were eating one of their small meals. "This went through the group and we kept on eating," said one of the participants, years later. "The food was the important thing. We didn't care whether the war was over or not as long as we got our food."[8]

This intense focus on food is also evident in the journals of Arctic explorers, but for explorers, a single-minded pursuit of food is a little more practical. They needed to devote all of their mental and physical energy to finding their next meal, since they weren't sure where it would come from. But being preoccupied with food made little sense for the volunteers in the semi-starvation study. They were safely living at the university and didn't have to forage for their next meal. Nevertheless, their focus on food does not surprise me, based on my brief experience of dieting. It's remarkable how quickly thoughts of food take over when you feel deprived. And lest you think this preoccupation with food is merely a harmless nuisance, it isn't. The men in the semi-starvation study reported that they were unable to concentrate for more than a brief period of time, that they were having trouble forming thoughts, that their comprehension had declined, and that they were unable to stay alert. The formal tests of "intellective functions," as Keys called them, were quite different than tests that are used today, and not particularly sensitive to cognitive difficulties. Even still, the men performed worse on many of them during starvation, compared to the baseline period beforehand.[9]

The clearest evidence that dieting causes cognitive impairment comes from a series of laboratory experiments in which researchers asked a group of dieters and a group of non-dieters to complete the same series of mentally challenging tasks.[10] These studies have shown that dieters cannot remember as many words or sentences as non-dieters, they can't focus their attention on a task as long as non-dieters, and they react more slowly to stimuli when speed matters.[11] In addition, and most important, dieters experience impaired central executive function, that all-important aspect of cognition that is necessary for impulse control. Executive function allocates your attention to competing demands,[12] and when it is limited, it interferes with your ability to plan, make decisions, and solve problems, all of which are necessary for effective self-control.

These differences in cognitive functioning are not a biological result of malnutrition or of being underweight.[13] Instead, the impairments have been linked to that preoccupation with food thoughts[14] that was common in starving explorers, the men in Keys's study, and, it turns out, most dieters. As one lifelong dieter told me, "Thinking about diets and what I am doing wrong takes up about ninety percent of my head space." And British comedian Vanessa Engle observed, "you can be reading about Syria or Egypt, and at the same time there are these trivial but revealing thoughts in your head like, 'I shouldn't have had that for breakfast.'"[15]

Focusing extensively on food and eating (and sometimes also concerns about your weight) steals valuable attention from other activities, and the more preoccupying food thoughts dieters have, the more difficulty they experience thinking about other things and handling other cognitive tasks.[16] It doesn't take much for a dieter to become preoccupied with thoughts of food. In one study, researchers tested dieters and non-dieters on their memory ability before and after having them eat a chocolate bar. Not surprisingly, dieters had more preoccupying food thoughts after eating the chocolate bar, and their memory function suffered as a result.[17] These kinds of memory and problem-solving deficits may make it difficult for dieters to successfully focus on important daily activities.

You might be tempted to conclude that dieters are not as smart as non-dieters, which is why they struggle with thinking, remembering, planning, and problem solving. This is not true. The same studies that show cognitive impairments in dieters find no differences between dieters and non-dieters in general intelligence.[18] One of the studies compared cognitive ability in people when they were dieting and when they were not dieting, and only found that cognition was impaired when the individuals were dieting.[19] So it's not that people who go on diets aren't smart, but that dieting causes people to, in essence, be less smart than they are.

One other thinking deficit that occurs when people diet is distorted time perception. Time seems to move more slowly when you are on a diet. The men in the Keys study experienced this, and it has also been documented in studies of men who lost large amounts of weight on strict diets. Their time perception changed from before to after they lost weight.[20] Research has also found that trying to control anything at all causes this same experience of time moving more slowly.[21] I've heard it said that being on a diet doesn't make your life longer; it just makes it *feel* longer.[22] There may be more truth to this than anyone would have thought.


## DIETING IS STRESSFUL

You wouldn't mind your life feeling longer if you were enjoying yourself. But time moving slowly when you're feeling bad is especially unpleasant. And when you're on a diet, you often feel bad. In particular, as Janet Tomiyama showed when she had people diet and then assayed their saliva, dieting causes a stress response, a release of the hormone cortisol into your bloodstream.[23]

In addition to making it hard to keep weight off, cortisol sets off a stream of chemical changes throughout your body. We know that cortisol's job is to get energy out of the places it's stored and make it readily accessible for you to respond to immediate stressors. In order to do that, energy gets diverted from bodily functions that aren't immediately useful for fighting or fleeing from a predator. The kinds of functions that are switched off for a bit include immune function, reproduction, growth, and energy storage. If this stress response happens every once in a while, it's no big deal. But if it happens a lot, say every time you worry about your job, your relationship, or whether you ate an inappropriate amount of marshmallow Peeps for a respectable adult, the changes it causes add up and may lead to serious physical problems.[24] Over time you become more susceptible to infections. Bone density decreases. Your blood pressure increases and blood vessels get damaged, because your heart has to work harder to divert these energy resources. The body becomes more insulin resistant and increased fat gets stored in the abdomen, which is the least healthy place to store it.

In addition to these well-documented effects of the stress response, there are some other responses to stress that scientists are only starting to get a handle on. The most exciting research on this topic, in my view, again comes from Janet and her collaborators, who have conducted studies that suggest excessive cortisol release may also harm a part of a cell responsible for aging. This part of a cell, called a telomere, is a protective cap at the end of a chromosome. Every time a cell divides, telomeres get shorter. Telomeres eventually get so short that cells can no longer divide, at which point the cells die. As this happens to more and more of your cells, the effects of aging appear—muscles weaken, skin wrinkles, eyesight and hearing fade, and thinking abilities diminish. Janet found that the more cortisol people released in response to stress, the shorter were their telomeres.[25] And other researchers have found that chronic dieters have shorter telomeres than non-dieters.[26] This work is still in its infancy, but it is possible that dieting, or the stress from dieting, may actually accelerate the aging process.

## DIETS MAKE YOU FEEL BAD

We've been talking about the physical problems that may result from the stress of dieting, but let's not forget how stress feels. For many people, the unpleasant consequences of dieting are emotional ones, such as depression, low self-esteem, or even anger.[27] The starving volunteers in Keys's study experienced "general emotional instability" and became "increasingly ineffective in their daily life," as Keys wrote,[28] and six of the thirty-six volunteers had more serious psychological responses. Their symptoms included extreme mood swings, compulsive gum chewing (of dozens of packs a day, until Keys limited gum to two packs per day), shoplifting, and bouts of unrewarding cheating on the diet by eating, for example, raw rutabagas or garbage.

One of these six men had such a severe reaction that while chopping wood for a friend, he chopped three fingers off his hand with an ax. He may have done this in a desperate attempt to get kicked out of the study. The volunteers were technically free to drop out of the study at any time, but they tended to view their participation as a badge of honor, a sign of their toughness and their willingness to sacrifice for the war effort. The pressure to be virtuous certainly raised the stakes. Sure enough, this volunteer stayed in the study and adhered to the diet while in the hospital. Was it an accident? Even the man himself isn't sure. Fifty years later he remarked to an interviewer, "I still . . . am not ready to say I did it on purpose. I am not ready to say I didn't."[29]

Overall, however, severe reactions like his were atypical. Aside from the bothersome preoccupation with food, the most common problem among the men in the starvation study was depression. Is depression a typical consequence of dieting? Well, yes and no. Many studies find high levels of depression in dieters,[30] but others show improvements in mood right after a diet.[31] It's not unusual for people to begin a diet when things aren't going well in their life, so their "before dieting" mood may look pretty grim. And if you catch people about six months after starting a diet, right around when they have taken off some weight and haven't yet started regaining it, their "after dieting" mood will look pretty good. There are lots of studies set up in this way,[32] and those are the ones that show that dieting improves your mood. On the other hand, some studies measure your moods every week while you are on a diet. Those studies find that the daily process and experience of dieting causes symptoms of depression, and for many dieters, those symptoms can be severe enough for people to be diagnosed with a clinical case of depression.[33]

Even when dieting does not lead to a serious disorder like depression, it can lead to other unpleasant feelings, because dieters tend to mix up their eating habits with the emotions of guilt and shame. In fact, breaking a diet is one of the most frequent responses people give on surveys when they are asked what makes them feel guilty.[34] Dieters are much more likely than non-dieters to say they experience feelings of guilt based on food,[35] and nearly half of the women in one study agreed that they felt guilty after eating potato chips, ice cream, or candy.[36] I once turned down the free pretzels on an airplane and the stranger sitting next to me offered some unsolicited words of comfort: "You don't have to feel bad about eating those. They're low fat." As annoying (not to mention insulting) as I found her remark, this sort of comment does not violate social conventions. We—and I would argue, women in particular—are expected to feel guilt about eating.

This needs to stop. I say this as a person, not as a scientist. There is no cause for guilt or shame about things you eat. Eating is not a moral act. Perhaps there are certain circumstances in which eating can be immoral, such as the occasional act of cannibalism, taking candy from a baby, or finishing your husband's carton of salted caramel ice cream before he gets home from work. But aside from situations like those, eating or not eating a particular food should not be a source of guilt or shame. Psychologist Deb Burgard, who works with individuals with eating disorders, has an attitude the rest of us should take note of. In response to an interviewer posing a question about her guilty pleasures, she burst out laughing and said, "I don't have much use for guilt around pleasure."[37]

To be fair, guilt has its redeeming qualities. Because guilt is a negative response to a real or perceived failure,[38] it tends to motivate people to try to repair what went wrong. On certain occasions, this can be useful. The problem is when guilt starts to morph into shame. Shame occurs when instead of feeling bad about a particular mess-up, the feeling spreads to a more general sense of messing up, causing you to feel like a bad person. Shame is more painful than guilt, and to add injury to insult, shame has been shown to lead to a release of—you guessed it—the stress hormone cortisol,[39] and another kind of cell in the immune system (called a proinflammatory cytokine), which, among other things, can promote the growth of disease.[40] In addition to these physical problems, shame is also linked to psychological problems such as depression, anxiety, low self-esteem, and eating disorders.[41]

Even without the link to shame, dieting has been implicated in the development of eating disorders, although it is not clear if dieting is truly a *cause* of these disorders. On the one hand, the eating disorder of anorexia is characterized by excessive restriction of eating, so it is not possible to have it—by definition—without dieting. But to say the diet caused anorexia is perhaps unfair. On the other hand, eating disorders that are characterized by binge eating do not, by definition, have to include dieting. And yet, it is likely that individuals with binge eating disorders (including bulimia) were on a diet first.[42] The volunteers in the Keys study were prone to binge eating after the starvation ended, and many reported feeling an insatiable hunger, regardless of how much they ate, which lasted for more than a year. The results of lab experiments on this topic, however, are inconsistent,[43] and recent evidence suggests that only certain types of diets lead to binge eating. These diets involve full-on fasting,[44] or else extreme calorie restriction or meal replacement.[45] For example, reducing your calories by 50 percent seems to lead to binge eating, but reducing by 25 percent does not.[46]

If severe calorie restriction leads to binge eating, it may have something to do with neurological responses to restriction. The longer people restrict their calories, the stronger their brain responses become to images of food and to actual food.[47] This brain activity is observed in areas responsible for reward and attention, as well as craving.[48] At the same time, activity quiets down in the prefrontal cortex, the area responsible for controlling impulses. When you combine hunger from strict dieting with extra attention to food, a more positive response to food, cravings for it, and reduced self-control, it certainly sounds like a recipe for binge eating.

## ONE LAST PROBLEM

Years ago I did a research project with women who were struggling with substance abuse problems, and one of the women earnestly told me that quitting heroin was easy—she'd done it five times. By that definition, dieting is easy, too. Many dieters lose the same ten or more pounds multiple times, and one dieter told me that if she lost all the pounds she's lost in her life at once, she would disappear from this earth. It's typical to lose weight, regain some or all of it, and then go on another diet. This is often referred to as yo-yo dieting. The official term for it is weight cycling, and it is common in dieters. In a study of more than 45,000 female nurses, 80 percent had dieted at least once in the previous four years, and more than half of those dieters had been on more than one diet during that time. Twenty-five percent of the dieters had lost more than ten pounds three or more times.[49]

There is no consensus in the medical community on whether weight cycling is unhealthy. Researchers can't even agree on what constitutes weight cycling. How much weight do you have to lose, how much of that do you have to regain, and in what time frame? How many times do you have to lose weight and regain it to count as a weight cycler?[50] The situation is further complicated because with many diseases, it is common for people to lose weight as they get sicker, and researchers don't always know whether people lost weight as part of an intentional diet, or if they unintentionally lost weight because they were ill.

There are some studies that show that weight cycling (with intentional weight loss) has no health consequences,[51] and a few that suggest that it's good for you,[52] but the majority of the evidence suggests that weight cycling is associated with an increased risk of illness and death.[53] Those studies find that you are better off maintaining a stable obese weight than starting obese, losing weight, and gaining it back. In one study, for example, researchers measured men's weight four times over fifteen years and categorized them according to whether they were weight cyclers. Then they looked at who lived and who died over the next fifteen years. They found that men who had weight cycled were more likely to die in that time period then men who were not obese,[54] whereas men who stayed obese the whole time lived just as long as their slimmer peers. And it doesn't appear to be the case that the men who weight cycled engaged in other unhealthy behaviors that would have increased their odds of dying.

## IS DIETING REALLY WORTH THE TROUBLE?

At worst, dieting can be hazardous for your mental and physical well-being. At best, it is ineffective and unpleasant. Low-carb diets, for example, are known to cause bad breath, and a side effect of the cabbage soup diet is "almost unavoidable" gas.[55] Diet pills are another can of worms entirely. I won't go there, except to mention that the website for the diet drug Xenical includes the following among its most likely side effects: "oily rectal discharge," "passing gas with oily discharge," "urgent need to have a bowel movement," and "being unable to control your bowel movements."[56]

Those are deal-breakers to me, but none of these side effects seem to stop the millions of people who go on these diets (or use these pills). Maybe the other physical and psychological miseries of dieting I discussed here don't seem particularly troublesome to you, either. Maybe they seem like they would be worth enduring for the sake of overcoming obesity and preventing all of the many diseases it causes. But there are two problems with that logic. As you've now seen, diets don't cure obesity, and as we'll discuss next, obesity is not as bad for you as you think.

......................................................

# CHAPTER 5

# OBESITY IS NOT A DEATH SENTENCE

You might be under the impression that obesity is going to kill us all. I couldn't blame you, given the headlines "Obesity bigger health crisis than hunger,"[1] or "Obesity on track as No. 1 killer."[2] You may have seen interviews with scientists who liken obesity to "a massive tsunami heading toward the United States."[3] The prevalence of obesity has increased dramatically from about 15 percent of Americans in the late 1970s to nearly 36 percent in 2010,[4] causing some scientists to suggest that the current generation of children will be the first to have shorter life spans than their parents.[5] This is scary stuff, especially coming from scientists, and you probably never thought to question it. But scientists aren't perfect and the media have a tendency to be hysterical when it comes to health headlines. So let's take a closer look at the research before we start fretting over our children's life spans.

## IS OBESITY GOING TO KILL YOU?

On the first day of my health psychology course, I try to get my students excited about the possibility that psychological factors (such as stress, or their personality, or their social status) can affect their physical health. I tell them about a strange study that shows that if you are unlucky enough to have a name in which your initials spell a word with negative connotations (like "B.A.D." or "P.I.G."), you will have worse health than someone whose initials spell something with positive connotations (like "W.I.N." or "T.O.P.").[6] This link between your initials and your health suggests that psychological processes that seem like they would have nothing to do with physical health can affect it. In this case, the psychological factors might include your self-esteem, or how much of a hassle it is every time you tell someone your name and they raise an eyebrow and say, "Your parents gave you the initials P.O.O.?" The initials study suggests that those kinds of negative interactions may add up over your lifetime and affect your health.

To do that study, researchers needed to know two pieces of information about people: their full name and their health. There are many kinds of information that researchers can use to decide how healthy people are, and each type of information has certain advantages and disadvantages. None is perfect. One often-used measure, for example, is the number of sick days people take from their job. An advantage of that measure is that it can often be easily accessed from people's work records. A disadvantage is that people often take sick days for reasons other than being sick.

Part of the reason I like to talk about the initials study on the first day of class is that the researchers used a particularly convincing measure of ill health: being dead. It's not a perfect measure, because there are plenty of people who die from an unfortunate accident but were otherwise in fine health. But in general, people who live a long time are healthier than people who do not. Plus, it is rather unlikely that death will be measured incorrectly, whereas if, for example, you have to ask people how many sick days they took last year, it is easy for them to make a mistake. In the study of initials, men with positive initials lived an average of seven years longer than men with negative initials. That's a giant effect, and I find it quite interesting, but the only reason anyone takes this odd finding at all seriously is that death is a convincing measure of health. Anything less persuasive and my students might have tried to deny that there was a relationship between initials and health. But it's hard to deny death.

I told you that long story partly to explain why I think the most important evidence regarding whether obesity causes poor health comes from studies of life and death. If obesity really is unhealthy, obese people should have shorter life spans than thinner people. Do they? This seemingly simple question has been addressed in more than a hundred studies, which, combined, included millions of participants. All of that information was compiled in one tour de force article[7] by a biostatistician name Katherine Flegal.

From each study, Flegal first calculated the risk of death (during a certain period of time) for people who were categorized as normal weight (BMI of 18.5–25) and overweight (BMI of 25–30). Then she calculated the ratio of the death rates for overweight people compared to normal-weight people.[8] If the risk of death for overweight people is the same as the risk of death for normal-weight people, then this ratio will equal 1. If the risk of death for overweight people is higher than for normal-weight people, the risk ratio will be larger than 1. The more deadly being overweight is, the larger this number should be.

Although it is a highly technical paper, the results are perfectly clear. In 93 percent of the studies, the risk ratios equaled 1, showing that overweight people were at least as healthy as normal-weight people.[9] In fact, combining the data from all 140 studies, Flegal found that overweight people had a slightly lower risk of death than normal-weight people. Being overweight appears to be even a bit healthier than being the recommended weight.

Then Flegal repeated the whole process for people who were categorized as obesity class I (BMIs from 30 to 35). In 87 percent of the studies, the risk ratios again equaled 1, showing that people in this weight category (which is the majority of obese people) were just as healthy as normal-weight people. Only when Flegal looked at people in obesity class II (BMI of 35–40) and higher (BMI>40; what you might have heard referred to as "morbid obesity") did she find risk ratios larger than 1. Even then, the majority of the studies (64 percent) had ratios equal to 1. So in two out of three studies, even the very heaviest obese individuals had the same risk of death as normal-weight people. In fact, the only group of people who had a higher overall risk of death than normal-weight people were people in obesity class II and up who were also under the age of 65. For those people, their ratio of risk compared to normal-weight people was 1.3. To help put that number in perspective, the ratio of risk for lung cancer[10] among smokers compared to nonsmokers is over 30. In the handful of articles that separates obesity class II from obesity classes III and up, it is clear that it is obesity class III and up, not class II, that is the culprit here. Only 6 percent of the U.S. population has a BMI that high.[11]

Being overweight or obese (at least classes I and II) is not going to kill you, but interestingly, being underweight (BMI<18.5) may be a problem. Although Flegal didn't include underweight people in her tour de force article, she did include it in an earlier paper. She found that people categorized as underweight had a higher risk of death than normal-weight people.[12] This was even true when she did special analyses to control for smoking status and to rule out the possibility that people were underweight because they had serious diseases that caused them to lose weight. We are told that skinny is healthy, but it just might not be.

## THE OBESITY PARADOX

The mortality evidence is important because mortality is the most straightforward and convincing measure of health. But there is more to life than not being dead, so it's also important to consider whether obese people suffer from more diseases or have a worse quality of life than thinner people.

Here again, the findings are not what you might expect. Overweight and obese people are more likely than normal-weight people to be diagnosed with several diseases, particularly diabetes, and cardiovascular diseases.[13] These are serious diseases that cause a lot of suffering, and their link to obesity is undeniable. But it's not a perfect link. You would think that rates of these diseases would have skyrocketed over the decades in which obesity rates more than doubled, but they didn't. The prevalence of diabetes went from 9 percent to 11 percent,[14] and rates of cardiovascular diseases, which are supposed to be the most serious and alarming consequence of obesity, actually decreased from 12 percent to 11 percent.[15]

Not only that, but once people have a disease, overweight and obese people may even have a better prognosis than normal-weight people. This has been shown for cardiovascular diseases (hypertension, heart failure, coronary heart disease),[16] stroke,[17] diabetes,[18] kidney disease,[19] chronic obstructive lung disease,[20] rheumatoid arthritis,[21] pneumonia,[22] and even advanced lung[23] and prostate[24] cancer. This pattern is found so often that it has a name: the obesity paradox.

This obesity paradox is surprising to the masses of people who have never thought to question the relationship between obesity and health. So far, researchers cannot explain why this happens. Some researchers have suggested that overweight and obese people may be protected from malnutrition when they have illnesses that cause significant weight loss, as in many cancers and AIDS.[25] They have also suggested that specific hormonal patterns that occur in obesity may be protective.[26] But this paradox remains unsolved, for now.

## IS IT REALLY THE CULPRIT?

Even if people who are very obese are more likely to die or develop certain illnesses than non-obese people, it still does not mean that their weight is the *cause* of those problems. To be fair, the same goes for the studies showing that obesity leads to better prognoses once people have certain diseases. Those studies do not show that obesity causes better prognoses. In fact, there are no studies that show that obesity causes health problems, and no studies that show obesity causes health benefits. The important word here is "causes." Showing that obesity is the cause of a health problem (or health benefit) is a difficult scientific problem.

Showing that one thing causes another requires a randomized controlled trial, which, as we discussed in Chapter 1, is the gold standard of scientific study design. Without randomly assigning people to be obese or not, researchers cannot draw conclusions about what obesity does or does not cause.[27] Of course, this kind of obesity study does not exist—at least not with people. It would be unethical, as well as flat-out ridiculous. Imagine signing up to be a participant in a study. You figure you can aid science and also earn a little money for your efforts. The researcher approaches you with a coin. He says that he will flip it, and that if it comes up heads, you will have to gain enough weight to become obese (if you aren't already obese), and then stay obese for, well, ever, so that he can see what diseases you get and how long you live. If it comes up tails, you will have to become normal-weight (if you aren't already), and then stay at that weight forever. Not only is this unethical, it's not even possible.

It's not possible because, as we've discussed, people can't easily gain enough weight to become obese and stay that way (or lose enough weight to become thin and stay that way). If people assigned to become obese did become obese, but then lost the weight, they would no longer be a useful test of the health effects of being obese. In addition to that, remember that a thin person who purposely gains weight is different, biologically, from a person who was obese for most of his or her life. So anything researchers learn from thin people who are assigned to get fat (or fat people who are assigned to get thin)—even if people can maintain their assigned weight for long enough—may not apply to people who have always been thin or fat.[28]

Another possibility, then, is to do the opposite kind of study: take obese people, randomly assign them to become thin or not, and then track them over the next several decades. If obesity is bad for you, then surely becoming thin would be good for you, right? The closest thing we have to studies like this are long-term diet studies[29] like those we looked at in Chapter 1. In those studies, participants were randomly assigned to diet or to not diet, and then they were studied for two or more years after that. Of course, participants didn't generally become thin, and the majority of them regained most of the weight they lost, so researchers can't say much about whether there are health benefits from no longer being obese. But still, if obesity is unhealthy, then the more weight people manage to keep off, the healthier they should get.

To see if we could find evidence that losing weight improves health, Janet Tomiyama, Britt Ahlstrom, and I dug back into each of those long-term diet studies to see if they included any measures of health. None of the studies measured death, very few measured whether people developed diseases, but many measured blood pressure, cholesterol, triglyceride, and blood glucose levels. We looked at whether those measures of health improved, when people kept the weight off. They did not. The participants' health, at least according to those outcomes, was unrelated to their weight loss.[30]

There is one study[31] that is often cited because its participants did manage to keep off a substantial amount of weight for a long period of time. It was designed to look at the long-term effects of weight loss in overweight and obese people with type 2 diabetes, and it was a highly respected and methodologically rigorous study. Nearly ten years after the study began, participants had kept off 6 percent of their starting weight. This may not seem like a lot of weight—if you started off at 200 pounds, 6 percent would be about 12 pounds—but since the government has defined "successful dieting" as keeping off 5 percent of your starting weight, this was considered to be impressive.

The health benefits from this weight loss, however, were not impressive, even to the government. The National Institutes of Health ended the fifteen-year, $15 million study two years ahead of schedule for the official reason of "futility," which means that they could already conclude that there was a "low likelihood of finding a benefit of the intervention."[32] In this case, statisticians determined that given the minimal health benefits they'd observed so far, it would be nearly impossible to show over the next two years that the diet was actually helping to prevent strokes, heart attacks, or deaths from cardiovascular disease, which is what the diet was designed to prevent.[33] There were other benefits to the diet program though. Most important, diet participants were better able to manage their diabetes without medication than control participants.[34] That's a good thing, but it wasn't good enough for the government to keep funding the study.

## OTHER DIFFERENCES BETWEEN OBESE AND NON-OBESE PEOPLE

Most studies on obesity and health[35] compare people who are already obese to people who are already non-obese, instead of randomly assigning people to be obese or not.[36] This is a problem, scientifically speaking, because already obese people are not only different from non-obese people in terms of their weight, but they are different in lots of other ways, too. For example, obese people are less likely to exercise than non-obese people,[37] so if they get sick more often, there is no way to know from this kind of study if they got sick because they weigh more, or because they exercise less. The automatic assumption of most people is that obesity is the culprit, but there is reason to believe that other factors matter just as much, or even more. Let's look closely at some of the pre-existing differences between obese and non-obese people to see if they might account for health problems that we typically blame on obesity.

## Differences in Level of Physical Fitness

Obese people are more likely to be sedentary than non-obese people,[38] and we all know that being sedentary is bad for us and that exercising is good for us.[39] Unlike studying the overall impact of obesity on health, which is not possible, it is possible to study the effects of exercise. Researchers can randomly assign some participants to exercise and some to be sedentary, and then determine if the exercise is beneficial to the participants' health, maybe not for a very long period of time, but for quite a while. There are even studies that require participants to exercise in front of researchers so that researchers can be sure the participants really did it.[40]

We know from these studies that exercise benefits your health in many ways, including reducing risk factors for type 2 diabetes[41] and improving blood sugar control among people with diabetes.[42] It has also been found to reduce mortality among patients with coronary heart disease[43] as well as to prevent cardiovascular disease,[44] raise high-density lipoprotein ("good") cholesterol, lower triglycerides, and decrease blood pressure in people with hypertension.[45] There is also suggestive evidence that exercise may protect against colon cancer[46] and breast cancer,[47] although these cancer findings were not from studies that could test causality.

We can't know for sure what role exercise plays in the health profiles of obese and non-obese people, but we do know that exercise has been shown to improve your health even when it doesn't lead to weight loss.[48] Active obese individuals have lower rates of sickness and mortality than non-obese sedentary people.[49] In one study of older men, for example, the obese men who were physically fit had lower mortality rates than men of all sizes who were not physically fit.[50] Since the health benefits of exercise do not require you to be thin, it seems plausible that your health has more to do with your fitness level than with your weight.

## Differences in Weight Cycling

We know that weight cycling—yo-yo dieting—may cause all sorts of health problems. And who is likely to have weight cycled the most? Obese people.[51] If weight cycling causes health problems, and if obese people are more likely than non-obese people to have weight cycled, then any differences in health between obese and non-obese people could be at least partially attributed to weight cycling, rather than the excess weight itself.

## Differences in Socioeconomic Status

There are enormous differences between people in this country in wealth, status, and education. The sum of these three factors is called socioeconomic status, or SES, and it is strongly correlated with health.[52] People with low SES have worse health—no matter how you measure health—than people with high SES.

They have shorter life spans[53] and are more likely to have diseases such as cardiovascular disease, diabetes, hypertension, metabolic syndrome, arthritis, and respiratory disease.[54] The relationship between SES and health is so strong that addressing it (and other health inequities) was listed as one of the four overarching goals in the ten-year health agenda the U.S. government published in 2010.[55]

There are many reasons why people with low SES are more likely to become ill than people with higher SES,[56] including reduced access to good quality health care (or perhaps any health care at all). People with low SES tend to lead more stressful lives, with concerns about job security and financial obligations, as well as access to proper shelter and sufficient healthy food. The daily stresses can add up, leading to health problems across many systems of the body.[57] People with low SES also have more dangerous jobs, live in more dangerous neighborhoods, and are more likely to be exposed to environmental toxins and carcinogens than people with higher SES.[58]

Importantly, obese people have lower SES than non-obese people,[59] and these differences may partially account for health differences between them. It's not hard to imagine. People with low SES may gain weight because they can only afford to eat junk food and may not have time or a safe place to exercise. They may also gain weight because of the increased amount of stress they experience. Gaining weight, in turn, could make it hard for them to find a job due to weight-based discrimination. This could further lower their SES, which could then lead to worse health. In sum, obesity and low SES may form a vicious cycle in which low SES makes obesity more likely and discrimination due to obesity lowers people's SES. At least some of the relationship between obesity and health is likely accounted for by differences in SES.[60]

## Differences in the Distribution of Fat on Your Body

You may have noticed an unfamiliar disease—metabolic syndrome—on the list of diseases that people with low SES are more likely to develop. Metabolic syndrome is not actually a disease, rather, it is a cluster of symptoms that tend to occur together and indicate that a person is at risk for cardiovascular disease and diabetes. People are diagnosed with metabolic syndrome if they have at least three of these five symptoms: high blood pressure, high fasting blood sugar, high triglyceride level, low HDL (good) cholesterol, and high waist circumference.[61]

Your waist circumference is a useful indication of your body composition, or how fat happens to be distributed on your body. If you have a high waist circumference, your body will likely have the apple shape: bigger belly, smaller legs. This generally means that you have increased visceral fat, which is the kind of fat that gets packed around the organs in your abdomen, and which is linked to health problems. If your waist circumference is on the lower side, your body will likely have the pear shape, with more fat distributed on your hips and thighs than in your belly. This kind of fat, called subcutaneous fat, is not related to health problems.

Waist circumference is of course related to obesity, but it is also importantly different from it. There are many obese people with a relatively low waist circumference, as well as non-obese people with a high waist circumference (imagine a skinny guy with a beer belly). Studies have carefully teased out the effects of your weight and your waist circumference on health, and they show that waist circumference is what matters. A higher waist circumference leads to a higher risk of mortality, regardless of your weight.[62] In fact, the people with the highest risk of mortality in one study were people who were at a "healthy" weight, but who had a high waist circumference. People who were obese but had a low waist circumference had the lowest death rate.[63]

So what matters is how your weight is distributed on your body, rather than how much weight there is, and it is the apple pattern that is problematic, not the pear pattern. Think about the people in your life who are apple-shaped. Notice anything they have in common? Odds are, they are mainly men. And odds are, most pear-shaped people you know are women. I can't think of any pear-shaped men that I know. And I can only bring to mind one apple-shaped woman. Even if women are obese, since they generally carry their excess weight in their hips and thighs, they have less to worry about than men with the same amount of excess weight, but carried in the belly.

## Differences in Medical Care

For many people, the hardest thing about being obese is enduring the stigma and discrimination that accompany it. In our increasingly open-minded culture, most people wouldn't discriminate (or at least admit to discriminating) against others based on their gender or ethnic group, but people are still willing to admit that they discriminate against obese people. The more discrimination people experience, the worse their health.[64] In effect, weight stigma can make you ill.[65]

One way that this discrimination can lead to illness is when it keeps people from accessing good quality medical care. If you avoid going to the doctor, you are less likely to benefit from early intervention and treatment of preventable diseases. Obese people often say that they avoid the medical system because they feel they are treated disrespectfully by doctors,[66] that doctors make inappropriate comments about their weight,[67] and that they are given unsolicited weight loss advice[68] when seeking treatment un-related to weight loss (such as for an ear infection or a broken toe).

Unfortunately, it is not the case that obese people are being paranoid or are misperceiving doctors' attitudes toward them. I wish they were. Doctors freely admit these attitudes. On one sur-vey of more than 600 physicians, at least half reported viewing obese patients as awkward, unattractive, and noncompliant, and a third rated them as weak-willed, sloppy, and lazy.[69] At a scien-tific convention on the study and treatment of obesity, fat people were rated as more lazy, stupid, and worthless than thin people by obesity researchers and doctors who care for obese patients.[70] If you specialize in obesity, shouldn't you be more understanding than this?

These negative views translate into worse care. In another study, doctors were asked to give their treatment plan for a pa-tient based on her medical chart. They were given one of several medical charts that (unbeknownst to them) were created to be identical except for the patient's weight.[71] The doctors reported less desire to help the obese patients, said that seeing them would feel more like a waste of their time, and said that they would spend less time with them. Audio recordings of outpatient visits show that doctors were less empathic and warm with obese pa-tients than non-obese patients.[72] Medical students—our future doctors—also show strong biases against obese people.[73]

Given these biases, it is not surprising that obese people are 50 percent more likely than non-obese people to have changed doctors five or more times.[74] Switching doctors disrupts the conti-nuity of care, prevents the development of a strong doctor-patient relationship, and leaves patients with periods of time in which they don't have a primary care doctor, increasing their likelihood of needing to seek treatment in the emergency room. Even more alarming, obese people are less likely than non-obese people to be screened for cervical cancer,[75] breast cancer,[76] and colorectal cancer,[77] and they are less likely to have gotten a flu vaccine.[78]

## Differences in Stress

Weight stigma can also make you sick by causing stress, leading to all of the many health problems that stress brings about. Dozens of studies show that being stigmatized based on race, gender, or other traits is linked to stress.[79] Many of these studies are able to show that stigma isn't just associated with stress, but that stigma causes stress. They can show the causal connection because in those studies, researchers randomly assigned participants to experience discrimination or not, right there in a lab. That sounds a little harsh, I know, but they keep it brief and mild and when the experiment ends clearly explain what they were up to. They might have participants write an essay, for example, and then give them sexist feedback on it. In other studies they ask people to think about events from their past in which they experienced discrimination.

In one particularly clever study, obese and non-obese women had to prepare and then give a speech about why they would be a good person to date.[80] Half of the women were instructed to give their speech on camera. The rest were audiotaped as they gave their speech. It sounds a bit horrifying either way, but for the women speaking on camera, concerns about how viewers would react to their weight would be heightened, whereas the women who were audiotaped did not have to worry about that. Sure enough, for the women who were videotaped, the more they weighed, the more their blood pressure increased while they gave their speech. This did not happen to the audiotaped women. Notice that the women did not experience any discrimination during the study, but in the videotape condition they knew there was the possibility that it could happen later.

The fact that relatively minor episodes of discrimination in the lab, reminders of past discrimination, or the possibility of future discrimination cause a physiological stress response is both remarkable and troubling. It is remarkable that subtle psychological experiences have physiological effects (though not surprising to health psychologists), and troubling because outside of the lab, obese people experience larger and more consequential forms of discrimination, and for many obese people, it happens relentlessly.[81]

## THE BOTTOM LINE

We are often warned about the health effects of becoming overweight or obese. And there are many noted health differences between obese and non-obese people. But there are also a multitude of ways in which obese and non-obese people differ from one another beyond simply how much they weigh. These differences are not a secret to obesity researchers, and yet they continue to report studies comparing the health of obese people to non-obese people, blame obesity for causing the health problems of obese people, and rarely acknowledge the potential of alternative explanations.

But variables such as exercise, weight cycling, socioeconomic status, fat distribution, and discrimination all factor into a person's overall health. And there are many other factors that may also be significant. Obese people eat more unhealthy trans fats and less healthy fiber, fruits, and vegetables than do non-obese people, and these nutrition differences may influence their health.[82] Obese people consume more artificial sweeteners (for example, in diet soda),[83] and these sweeteners have been linked to increased levels of cardiovascular disease,[84] as well as glucose intolerance, which can lead to diabetes.[85] Obese people are also more likely to use diet drugs,[86] and over the years, many of these drugs have been found to be dangerous, causing hypertension, valvular heart disease, or other cardiovascular problems.[87] In addition, obese people are more likely to be lonely or socially isolated,[88] and loneliness has been found to be associated with mortality.[89]

There are statistical techniques that can be used to minimize the extent to which these kinds of variables bias study results. They are routinely used to account for age and gender differences, but it is not routine to use them for these other potential forms of bias. I went through the list of ninety-seven studies on obesity and mortality that Katherine Flegal included in her thorough review and counted how many studies controlled for each of these factors.[90] Physical activity was the most likely to be statistically controlled for, but that was done in fewer than half of the studies. Only sixteen of the studies took socioeconomic status into account,[91] one study controlled for distribution of body fat, and none accounted for weight cycling, stigma or stress, or use of diet drugs. No study controlled for more than two of these factors, and half didn't control for any. When researchers fail to statistically control for these factors in their studies on obesity and health, they make obesity look more dangerous than it is.

Even with all of the statistical flaws in obesity studies, the actual difference in life expectancy that they find between people who are obese (class I) and people who are normal weight is one year.[92] And that difference goes away for people age sixty-five or over.[93] You know what that means? Your life expectancy is about six years shorter if you have the initials F.A.T.[94] than if you *are* fat (class I obese).

Why has the case that obesity will kill you been overstated? Partly it's because the media tends to overhype health headlines.[95] Partly it's because the medical community fears that if people don't think obesity is a death trap, they'll stop trying to eat a healthy diet and end up behaving in truly unhealthy ways. But you also have to look at which scientists are saying that obesity will kill you: Scientists with a vested interest in that being true. Scientists who are taking money from companies that sell diet drugs and other weight loss products. Scientists who sit on the boards of directors of these companies. Researchers are required to list these conflicts of interest at the end of articles they publish in medical journals,[96] and in obesity research, you could use these lists as a handy directory of companies in the weight loss industry.

Think I'm exaggerating? Consider the scientists who claimed that the current generation of children would have a shorter life expectancy than their parents,[97] which isn't close to true (and which they don't even seem to believe themselves).[98] The conflict of interest statement at the end of that paper says that one of the authors received "grants, monetary donations, donations of product, payments for consultation, contracts, honoraria or commitments thereof" from 148 companies, most of which are weight loss and pharmaceutical companies.[99] Those companies include Weight Watchers, Jenny Craig, and Slim-Fast; the makers of weight loss drugs Xenical, Meridia, and Redux; plus four companies that produced the dangerous combination diet drug fen-phen, along with the law firm that defended those companies in court. As a comparison, the biostatistician who summarized all the mortality studies and found that obesity was probably not going to kill you did not receive money from any companies at all.[100]

I hope you're not still under the impression that you have to diet or else obesity will kill you. If you exercise, eat nutritiously, avoid weight cycling, and get good quality medical care, you don't need to worry about obesity shortening your life. Especially if you shield yourself from weight stigma and the stress it causes, which we'll talk about in Part IV. But now let's talk about smart regulation strategies for living at the lower end of your set weight range. These strategies will painlessly stabilize your eating and keep your weight from yo-yoing.

# PART THREE

# HOW TO REACH YOUR LEANEST LIVABLE WEIGHT

(NO WILLPOWER REQUIRED)

..................................................

# CHAPTER 6

# LESSONS FROM A LEAN PIG

One day I got a phone call from a stranger who told me that he had lost a lot of weight on a diet and wanted to know if he was doomed to regain it. Believe it or not, I get lots of calls like this. Since I don't know these people or their individual circumstances, I tend to respond by saying that yes, the majority of people who lose weight on a diet will gain it back at some point, but that there is a small minority who successfully keep it off. I can't predict what will happen to any particular person. Usually, the conversation ends there. But this time, I stayed on the phone. The voice on the other end, Mac Nelson,[1] was a seventy-four-year-old man from rural Texas with a thick accent. He said that he had figured out the secret to keeping weight off. From his pig. Since pigs are not known for their svelte figures, I was intrigued.

He told me that when he was young, he raised a pig for the state fair. His friends did, too, and the pigs all came from the same litter. His friends fed their pigs the standard way: They left the food in a self-feeder in the pigs' pen, so the pigs had access to it all day long and could eat whenever they wanted. Mac didn't have a self-feeder for his pig, and even though his Future Farmers of America instructor told him to build one, he never got around to it. Instead, he brought out a slop bucket twice a day, and let the pig eat as much as it wanted.

When it was time to bring the pigs to the state fair for judging, Mac's pig had grown to be strong, healthy, and lean, while his friends' pigs had grown strong, healthy, and fat. Fatness is prized in pigs, so Mac's pig "got beat," as he put it. But Mac had an insight about eating that he remembered and made use of years later, when he wanted to lose weight. He realized that the longer there was food in front of him, the more he would eat. So he began eating twice a day—whatever he wanted, as much as he wanted. But that was it; he didn't eat anything else all day. Over the years, he weighed himself once a month and wrote down the number on the scale (he sent me a photograph of the piece of paper that held the tally). Mac lost 42 pounds in two years, and has kept it off for seven years and counting.

I'm not endorsing the Mac Nelson diet plan, because eating only twice a day sounds miserable (though it wasn't for Mac), but his main insight is right on the money and is the basis for the three strategies for weight management that I'll share in this chapter: If it's not there, you can't eat it, and if it is there, you will. These are smart regulation strategies, because they rely on our brains rather than the brute strength of our limited willpower to resist temptation.

Pioneering self-control researcher Walter Mischel noted that the way kids in his classic marshmallow self-control studies managed to resist eating the marshmallow was by "converting the difficult conflict from one requiring acts of self-denial and grim determination to a more playful enjoyable time."[2] Instead of staring at the marshmallow, they covered their eyes, turned their back, pretended the marshmallow was a cloud, sang songs, or played games with their hands or feet. They succeeded at self-control by changing the situation so that self-control was not needed. This is smart regulation, and you are going to use it to reach and stay at your leanest livable weight.

## SMART REGULATION STRATEGY 1: ENCOUNTER LESS TEMPTATION BY CREATING OBSTACLES

There are two different routes that I can take to the office each day. One route involves a freeway that is slow and crowded during rush hour, but speedy the rest of the time. The other involves surface streets that have a lot of annoying traffic lights, but the route is faster than the freeway during rush hour. Because of this, I generally choose my route based on the time of day. When I want a treat, however, no matter what time of day it is, I choose the surface streets. On that route, I pass my favorite bakery. My resistance to that bakery is nonexistent. Some mornings I wrestle with this decision, and frequently I lose the battle and take the bakery route. But if I am trying to limit my calorie intake, I take the freeway, regardless of what time of day it is.

There are many aspects of your day that might benefit from this strategy.[3] Where do you encounter tempting foods? How about lunchtime at work? Do you tend to go out for lunch? Most of the time you will eat a healthier, lower-calorie meal if you bring it yourself, rather than eating in a restaurant. I have a handy obstacle to going out: winter. Specifically, Minnesota winter. I can't bear to go out in the cold when it's nonessential, so in the winter, it is easy for me to avoid going out to lunch. During the other five months of the year, I arrange my day so that I am unable to go out to lunch. I schedule my meetings so that I don't have enough time between them to go out to eat. That keeps me stuck in the office, so I need to rely on whatever I have packed for myself. Another obstacle at work is that despite your careful planning, your colleagues can sabotage your best efforts—a coworker brings in a box of doughnuts on a Friday morning, or there's a party in the conference room to celebrate someone's birthday with a few dozen cupcakes. In my lab, there is near-constant temptation from leftover food hanging around from our eating studies. It's hard to resist these items when they're right in front of you, but you can make an effort to avoid encountering them by staying out of the office kitchen or skipping out on the birthday party. In my case, I try to stay in my office rather than going into the lab, where the food is kept.

Sometimes the temptation is already right there on your dinner plate, and there is nothing harder to resist than food on your own plate. In fact, in recorded history, there are no documented instances of this occurring. Okay, I made that up, but still, this is the last thing you want to have to do. It's not just difficult, but it feels bad—it makes you feel deprived if you can't eat it, or guilty if you throw it away. When you prepare your own food, don't put yourself in a situation where you have to resist some of the food that is on your plate—only serve yourself a reasonable portion that you can feel good about eating.

When we eat out, we have a lot less control over what's on our plate—and as we all know, restaurant serving sizes are completely out of control. Serving sizes of convenience foods and drinks are, too.[4] Think about the size of the drinks we buy. The bottle that Coca-Cola patented in 1916 held 6.5 ounces of soda. Now it is not uncommon to buy Coke in a cup that holds a quart (32 ounces) or half gallon (64 ounces) of soda. Newer models of cars even come with larger cup holders to accommodate these massive containers.[5]

In high school I worked part-time at a Baskin-Robbins ice cream store. In 1983, when I first started, my boss taught me the mantra, "Think 2.5 ounces," because that was the size a scoop of ice cream was supposed to be. He had me weigh every scoop until I got accustomed to what 2.5 ounces looked and felt like. A couple of years later, while I was still working there, the company introduced the 4-ounce scoop. A scoop that large was so unusual, the company had to have larger ice cream scoopers specially made.[6] Four ounces is now the standard size for ice cream scoops at most national ice cream chains, and 2.5 ounces is considered a child-size scoop, if it's offered at all. Similarly, McDonald's french fries originally came in only one portion size, and that size is now considered the small.[7] Newer editions of *The Joy of Cooking* have the same cookie recipes as the original edition, but these same quantities of butter, flour, and sugar are now described as making fewer—but larger— cookies.[8] One serving is not what it used to be.

My favorite piece of evidence about the increase in portion sizes comes from a study comparing the size of the foods in different paintings of the Last Supper from over the centuries.[9] To control for the different-sized paintings, the researchers did their comparisons by calculating a food-to-head ratio. Presumably heads have not gotten larger in that time. Over the years, however, the bread, entrees, and plates all did.[10]

There is plenty of evidence that the larger the portion, the more you eat.[11] The larger the cereal box (or any box) you serve yourself from, the more you take and the more you eat.[12] The larger the serving spoon you serve yourself with or the serving bowl you serve yourself from, the more you take and the more you eat.[13] You'll even eat more from one big chocolate bar than you would if you were given that same amount of chocolate, but in several small bars.[14]

You can easily change the portion sizes in your own home. I wouldn't suggest this if it would feel like deprivation, but there is plenty of research showing that for most people, it doesn't. This comforting evidence comes courtesy of Brian Wansink, head of Cornell's Food & Brand Lab and author of *Mindless Eating*. In one of his clever food studies he created a bottomless soup bowl: a bowl that subtly refills itself while you eat from it, so it never looks like it is emptying.[15] How'd he do that? Something complicated with tubes and pipes and pressure physics. But what he learned by having study participants unknowingly eat from this deceptive bowl is that people have no idea how much they are eating, and they decide how full they feel based on what they see, not how they feel. So if they see that their bowl of soup is full, they assume they haven't eaten much, and that they are still hungry, even though they may have eaten the equivalent of two (or more) full bowls.[16]

But we can also take advantage of this concept in reverse. If you use a smaller plate and fill it up, you think you are eating more food, because food on a small plate looks like more food than that same amount of food on a big plate.[17] This tricks you into feeling full sooner, and amazingly, it still works even when you know about it.[18] The small plate also forces you to serve yourself less food, and the less you have on your plate, the less you eat.[19] There's no need to rely on willpower to resist anything.

There is one recent phenomenon working against the portion size trend. Even though standard portion sizes are larger than they used to be, some foods are starting to come in slightly smaller packages than before. Companies are sneakily trying to hide price increases by putting less food in the package, but keeping the price the same. This is presumably more tolerable to consumers than price increases, but no consumer I know has been anything but annoyed when they noticed this subterfuge. One ice cream brand now has only 14 ounces of ice cream in what it absurdly continues to call its pint, but the price is the same as it was when it had 16 ounces in it, and the package looks the same.[20] If this continues, corporate greed may lead people to eat less without realizing it.

## No Obstacle Is Too Small

Want to know a secret to saving money on toilet paper? Just squish the roll a bit (to make it flatter) before putting it on its spindle. It won't turn as easily, so it will be incrementally harder to rip toilet paper off the roll. When that happens, people use less. This is a tiny inconvenience. I might even argue that this is the tiniest possible inconvenience. And yet it alters people's behavior enough that this tip routinely turns up as a suggestion for thriftiness in blogs about saving money.[21]

Here's why it works: People are lazy. Even the most hardworking among us are, on some level, pretty lazy. At the very least, we are constantly assessing situations for the path of least resistance—or, to put it another way, the path with the fewest obstacles.

Another, more serious example of the effectiveness of tiny obstacles was documented in the United Kingdom, after laws required acetaminophen (Tylenol) to be packaged in small blister packs instead of bottles.[22] To use the medication from a blister pack, each individual pill must be pushed out of the packaging separately from the other pills, and it is harder to grab a handful at once. That small obstacle to accessing pills was linked to a 21 percent reduction in suicides and accidental poisonings from the over-the-counter drug.

I am not suggesting that potato chips should be packaged in individual blister packs. But how snack food is packaged and presented, and where it is located, can make a big difference in whether or not you eat it. Researchers at Utrecht University did a study in which they measured how much candy people ate in relation to the proximity of the candy dish.[23] The researchers found that people ate less candy when the dish was across the room from them than when the dish was right next to them. Walking less than five feet across a room should not be an effective obstacle, but it was. Perhaps that part doesn't surprise you. Getting up from your chair and walking across the room is a real obstacle—it causes you to take a pause in your work, get up, and walk around. But it turns out that the candy doesn't even need to be that far away. Merely having to extend your arm across a table was shown to be as much of a deterrent as having to walk across the room. Why? Because people are lazy, so tiny obstacles can be formidable. You might be thinking that if you did go to all the trouble of walking across the room to get some candy, you would probably make it worth your while and take a lot. That feels to me like what I would do. The researchers wondered about that, too, so they looked at the behavior of just the people who did walk over to the dish. Those people did not take or eat more candy than the people who took candy from the closer dishes.[24] So being farther away did not have a downside.

Laziness leads to less eating in other situations, too. At salad bars, people eat less of the foods that they have to reach the slightest bit farther under the sneeze shields to get. They also eat less of foods served with tongs, which require a little more effort to operate than a spoon.[25] Similarly, if you are not particularly adept at eating with chopsticks, you will likely eat less when you use them compared to when you use a fork.[26]

In 2012, the city of New York passed a law banning restaurants, movie theaters, and sports stadiums from selling drinks in cups larger than sixteen ounces, with the goal of reducing soda consumption. The ban spawned thousands of jokes and critiques, many pointing out that people still could drink as much soda as they wanted by purchasing multiple cups, and that all the law would do was inconvenience them.[27] The inconvenience, however, is exactly why I thought the ban was a good idea, and indeed, it was the point of the ban. Having to get back in line to purchase another beverage is a much larger obstacle than, say, reaching out your arm, serving yourself tomato slices with tongs, or rotating a slightly smushed toilet paper roll. Alas, to the disappointment of public health officials, as well as to data geeks like myself, the law was overturned and we'll never know what would have happened.

But effort isn't the only effective obstacle in preventing over-eating. Other obstacles are effective because they make the food less noticeable or distract you from it. For example, in an effort to get employees to stop eating so much of the free candy that is readily available at Google's New York office, M&Ms were switched from clear containers to opaque ones. In the first seven weeks after this change, the 2,000 employees ate 3 million fewer calories from M&Ms than they had eaten in the seven weeks before the change.[28]

I've seen every member in my family use this strategy without even knowing they're doing it. My kids use it in restaurants to resist drinking their entire soda before the meal is served. We don't let them have soda very often, so this is difficult. They manage it by pushing their cups out of their line of sight and as far away from themselves as possible until the entrees arrive. Similarly, one evening in a Mexican restaurant I realized that my husband had moved the basket of tortilla chips entirely off our table and onto the windowsill to stop himself from eating them.

I take advantage of the small obstacle strategy, too, when I make a pan of Rice Krispies treats, which are pretty close to irresistible to me. There is no place in my house that is far enough away for distance to be a sufficient obstacle on its own. If I leave the pan on the counter, I go back and forth, cutting myself thin slice after thin slice, until it is mostly gone. But I find that if I cut myself a decent-sized slab, put the knife in the dishwasher, cover the pan with tin foil, and put it in the fridge, I end up eating much less than if the pan were left uncovered on the counter. The knife part is important. If I leave the knife in the pan with the Rice Krispies treats, it is too easy to cut another little slice off. But the knife in the dishwasher is another small barrier. Not only do I have to go to the effort of getting another knife, but I also have to convince myself that it is worth it to dirty another knife for this purpose. And seeing the pileup of knives also becomes an embarrassing deterrent, reminding me of how much I have been eating. The beauty of these strategies is that they help you eat a little less, but without suffering for it. When I cut myself a piece, I end up feeling like I ate a lot, since I can see the whole piece at once. Those thin slices add up to more than the one piece, but it doesn't look like it at the time, and it doesn't feel like it.

## SMART REGULATION STRATEGY 2: MAKE HEALTHY FOODS MORE ACCESSIBLE AND NOTICEABLE

Creating small obstacles can help us limit how much unhealthy food we eat, but when we want to eat *more* of a certain kind of food, we want to do the opposite: remove as many barriers as possible. For example, if you want to eat more fruits and vegetables, make them easier to access. Make them unavoidable. Have a fruit bowl (with fruit in it) on your table. Sounds obvious and too easy, doesn't it? But it works.[29] Having the fruit in ready-to-eat form helps, too. The effort of peeling an orange can be an insurmountable obstacle, no matter how good a peeler you are. Peeling bananas, on the other hand, is a no-brainer, so they are easily eaten from a fruit bowl. Grapes are even easier, because all you have to do is grab some. At dinner on campus at the University of Cambridge, I was surprised to see that the fruit bowl on the table didn't just sit there like a table centerpiece, but it got passed around from person to person. Much more fruit was eaten because of it. And not surprisingly, the smaller, more bite-sized fruits were the first ones taken. People took handfuls of grapes, dates, and adorable tiny bananas.

Fruit is easy compared to vegetables. Vegetables have a lot of obstacles to overcome, including not being as sweet as fruits. But an even bigger problem is that many of them are high maintenance. They need to be cleaned well, parts of them need to be cut off, some need to be peeled, and many require some degree of cooking or seasoning to be appealing. These are big barriers to eating vegetables, even once you've bought them and they are safely in your house. This is why you need to at least partially prepare your vegetables the moment you get them home from the store.

Prepping your vegetables ahead of time can be a pain, but it's worth it.[30] We get a weekly farm share during the summer and fall (and once, regrettably, during a Minnesota season referred to as "deep winter"). The day we pick up the multiple bags of vegetables, my husband washes and trims everything, and chops the vegetables into usable-size pieces. He roasts beets, rutabaga, celeriac, and turnips, which is the only hope those vegetables have of being eaten, at least in our house. We manage to eat our entire farm share each week (even in deep winter), and I am convinced it is because he invests time breaking down the obstacles that would otherwise keep us from eating our vegetables.

Everyone's barriers are different, so spend some time thinking about the things that consistently prevent you from eating healthy food, and then come up with creative ways to knock those barriers down. For example, if you never have healthy food in the house because you don't have time to get to the grocery store, try shopping online and have your produce delivered. Does it take you forever to chop your vegetables? Buy them prechopped. Want to add legumes to your diet but never remember to soak them overnight? Use canned beans. Need to feed your family the moment you get home from work? Try using a slow cooker once a week. I turn it on before work and dinner is ready and waiting when I get home.

## SMART REGULATION STRATEGY 3: BE ALONE WITH A VEGETABLE

I've left my favorite vegetable-eating strategy for last. The idea for this strategy comes from something I witnessed my children do as we sat in a deli in Los Angeles (they were about three and six years old). Typically, the waitress puts down a nice bowl of pickles on the table when you arrive, but this particular day they must have run out of pickles, so they brought us a large bowl of sauerkraut instead. Pickles are delicious. Sauerkraut, in my opinion, is not. Before I had a chance to express my horror, however, my kids started eating it. And they gobbled it all up.

This happened many years ago, and I have thought about it a lot since then. After much scholarly effort, I developed a highly technical theory about why they ate the sauerkraut: They ate it because it was there. And because nothing else was there. If you're hungry and a food is right there, you are bound to eat it. But if two foods are there, it's a battle between them. In a contest between a (not particularly enticing) healthy food and an unhealthy food, the unhealthy food will usually be chosen. It seems to me there is only one contest that a healthy food has a fighting chance at winning: a contest between a healthy food and no food at all.

You don't have to believe my theory just because my kids ate sauerkraut that day. You may even like sauerkraut and find my theory preposterous. But here is some real proof: my University of Minnesota colleagues[31] and I tested it in the lab and in the real world and came up with the same results.[32]

In one test, my colleague Joe Redden told participants that we were interested in their opinions of some cartoons. As you are beginning to realize with our studies, this was a lie. We did not care about their views on the cartoons. But while the participants watched cartoons, we gave them baby carrots and M&Ms to snack on. Some of the people got both snacks at once, and some got baby carrots first, followed by the M&Ms five minutes later. As we expected, people ate more baby carrots when they were alone with them for a while, rather than when they had an opportunity to choose from among vegetables and candy.

We tested the same theory as part of a project to get kids to eat more vegetables in school cafeterias. One obstacle between kids and their vegetables is that they never see healthy food all by itself in most cafeterias—there's always another less healthy and more tempting food right next to it on the tray. We figured that if we could get hungry kids alone with a vegetable, they might eat it. So instead of having kids go right through the cafeteria line when they arrived for lunch, we had them first sit down at their lunch table. Waiting for them in front of each place at their table was a little cup of baby carrots, whether they wanted it or not. We didn't tell them to eat it, or say anything about it at all. On any given day, only about 10 percent of kids at that school chose carrots from the self-serve cafeteria line. But on this day, more than 50 percent of the kids ate the baby carrots we gave them.

We tried this a few more times, partly to see if it would work with other vegetables, partly to see if it would keep working over time, and partly to see if it would work if we gave the students their little cup of vegetables while they were standing in the cafeteria line (since it's not always possible to have kids sit down at a table before they go into the cafeteria). It always worked beautifully. On a regular day in one of the studies, 36 kids ate broccoli. But when we gave them a little cup of broccoli while they waited in line, 235 kids ate broccoli. Overall, kids ate nearly four times as much broccoli when we gave it to them first compared to a regular day. We had even better luck with strips of red and yellow bell peppers. A lot of the kids were unfamiliar with these, but when we gave out cups of pepper strips in the line, five times as many kids ate some, and more than six times as much red pepper was eaten. Even better, after a few days of giving them peppers, they started eating more peppers even when we didn't provide them first. We think they learned to like them.

It shouldn't be hard to make this strategy work for you. There are a few ways you can arrange to get alone with a vegetable. One of the simplest ways to do this is to mimic our approach with the school cafeteria study: start every meal with a vegetable. Meaning, you don't eat anything else until you have eaten your vegetables. The simplest way to do this, of course, is to eat a salad before dinner. Not with your dinner, on the side of your plate—on its own salad plate, before you eat anything else. If possible, eat it before you even prepare the rest of your meal. Eating your salad before cooking the rest of your meal will satisfy some of the hunger you feel before a meal, which will keep you from snacking on the rest of your meal while you prepare it. I don't know about you, but I eat an awful lot of food while I am preparing a meal. If I am grating cheese to add to something I am cooking, even if it is going to be added to the dish in moderation, the amount of cheese I eat off the cutting board often ends up being more than what was going in the dish in the first place. But if I had eaten my salad course before starting to cook the rest of the meal, I would be less hungry while cooking, and would snack on less cheese.

This same strategy applies out of the home. If you're at a party with a spread of finger foods, load up your plate with crudités before you move on to anything else. When you go out to dinner, order an appetizer-sized salad. Ask the server to please bring out the salad first and hold off on serving the main course until you are done with your first course. You may also need to ask the server to hold the bread basket until later, or perhaps not bring it out at all.

There is no downside to eating more vegetables. At minimum they provide all kinds of additional vitamins to your diet. But ideally they will replace other foods that are less nutritious or more caloric, and you won't find yourself face-to-face with a tempting food that you are trying to resist. Take a lesson from Mac Nelson and his slender pig. If it's not there, you can't eat it. What could be easier?

# CHAPTER 7

# HOW TO TRICK YOUR FRIENDS INTO IGNORING A COOKIE

Last summer, my twelve-year-old son informed me that he would no longer wear shorts that exposed his (perfectly lovely) knees. Not too long before that, my younger son announced that he would no longer eat tomato sauce on his pasta, even though he had eaten pasta with tomato sauce about a thousand times before then. Did my older son suddenly develop fashion sense? Doubtful. Did my younger son's preferences suddenly change? Unlikely. Although both of these boys probably believe they are making fully independent choices, their behavior, like everyone's, is influenced by the people around them. The kids at school were not exposing their knees or eating tomato sauce on their pasta, so my kids weren't either.

In 1956, social psychologist Solomon Asch demonstrated that people conform to those around them when he asked research participants to reply out loud, one at a time, to a very easy multiple-choice question.[1] Although the answer was obviously choice A, the first six students gave the answer B loud and clear. They were secretly in cahoots with Dr. Asch, who had told them ahead of time to say B. But the seventh student was not in on the secret. Asch wanted to know whether this student—and others like him—would give the correct answer or go along with the group. The multiple-choice question was silly and there would not be any consequences to the group or the student if the student gave a different answer from everyone else. Not only that, but the group was made up of strangers that the student did not expect to ever see again. Nevertheless, 75 percent of the students in this situation went along with the group and gave an obviously incorrect answer.[2] The pressure to conform has a powerful influence on our behavior.

People conform to groups in many ways, including in what they eat. Another social psychologist, Muzafer Sherif, said in 1936, "We do not simply eat; we eat certain things, in certain ways, at certain places, and more or less at certain times, all prescribed within limits for a given established group."[3] The group that has the most influence, at least in terms of which foods people eat, is their cultural group or ethnic group.[4] In both Germany and Korea, for example, fermented cabbage is eaten regularly. In Korea it is an ingredient in spicy kimchee, whereas in Germany it is eaten in a different form, as sauerkraut. Nothing prevents Koreans from serving sauerkraut or Germans from serving kimchee, but they rarely do.

Every year I have the students in my Psychology of Eating class go around the room and report what they eat with their family on Thanksgiving. Although many (but not all) of their celebrations include turkey, it was also common to serve additional dishes that are typical of their culture or ethnic group, such as roast duck, adobo, tamales, noodle kugel, pierogis, homemade sausages, or curried vegetables. My family always has chopped liver and kishke at the Thanksgiving table. None of us had ever thought there was anything out of the ordinary about our own family meal, but learning what everyone else was eating demonstrated just how important a role culture plays in food choice. You learn to eat by modeling your behavior on the people around you, without necessarily realizing you are doing it. If your entire family and all of your friends eat kimchee nearly every day, you probably will, too.

In addition to which particular foods you tend to eat, the *amount* of food you eat at a given meal is also influenced by the people around you. This is not always evident, because there are many competing pressures at work when you are eating a meal. Sometimes you may be hungrier than others. Sometimes you may not like the food you are eating. Maybe you don't feel well at one meal, or are in a hurry. But still, the people around you play an important role, influencing your eating in several ways.

One way they influence your eating is by keeping you at the table longer. The longer you are at the table with food in front of you, the more you will eat. I bet you've been in a restaurant and have eaten all you want from your plate, but the waiter is nowhere to be found, so your plate stays in front of you. You invariably continue eating from the plate. By observing people eating in restaurants and recording how much they eat, researchers have shown that the more people you eat with, the longer you stay at the table, and the more you eat.[5] Not only that, but being around people is distracting, so you may pay less attention to how much you are eating, or be less likely to notice feelings of fullness, both of which tend to lead to overeating.[6]

On the other hand, there are also circumstances in which people eat less when they are with other people. This tends to happen in situations where you are highly concerned about the impression you are making, such as when you are on a first date or eating with strangers.[7] Neither situation can be turned into a useful strategy for eating less. Nobody has that many first dates. And how often do you eat with strangers? What really matters is the effect our friends have on our eating, and this is not as straightforward as the effect of strangers. In restaurants, people eat similar amounts of food to the other people in their group, and different amounts than people eating in other groups.[8] But from observing people in restaurants, you can't tell whether one person in a group set a standard that the others then follow, or if the people chose to eat together because they happen to have similar eating habits in the first place.

## SMART REGULATION STRATEGY 4: EAT WITH HEALTHY EATERS

To figure out whether friends influence each other's eating, my students and I conjured up the sneakiest study my lab has conducted to date.[9] We wanted to see how people ate around their friends (rather than strangers), but we also wanted to control the situation so that we could tell who was setting the standard and who was responding to it. So we invited groups of three friends to come to our lab for a study on how friends solve problems together. We were not remotely interested in how the friends solved problems; rather, we cared about what they ate while they were solving the problems they thought we cared about.

Before we got the groups of friends settled at a table together to work on the problem, we put them into three separate rooms so that they could have some privacy while they filled out questionnaires. That was our cover story, anyway. We didn't really need to put them in separate rooms to fill out the questionnaires, nor did we even need them to fill out questionnaires. We needed them in separate rooms so we could sneak into two of the rooms and secretly talk to two of the friends. By doing that, we were able to get two of the friends in each group to be in cahoots with us. We told them that they would be offered a variety of snacks when they were solving the problem with their friends, and that when that happened, they should eat only the vegetables. And of course they should not let on that we told them to do that.

Once the two friends understood that they were only going to eat vegetables, we put all three friends back together to work on their problem, and soon we brought in an enormous tray of assorted cheeses, meats, vegetables, and sweets. Each item was bite-size, and each had a colored toothpick in it. We worried it might seem ridiculous that we would provide students with such an incredible spread, so we told them that we had set it up for a special event with a professor and that it had just gotten canceled.

The colored toothpicks weren't just hygienic and pretty. They were also our method of figuring out what each person ate so that we wouldn't have to stay in the room with them, which might cause them to act unnaturally. Whenever anyone ate any of the foods, they would have to leave a used toothpick on their plate, and these were color-coded so that green toothpicks were in vegetables, red in sweets, blue in meats and cheeses. Everyone had a different-colored plate, too, so all we had to do was count each color toothpick from each person's plate.

We were worried that the students would see through our scheme, but that's the one problem we didn't have. In the first group we ran, the students dumped their plates (toothpicks and all) into the trash before we came back into the room. It was easy enough to prevent that from happening again by removing the garbage can. In the absence of the garbage can, one of the students in the next group picked up all the toothpicks and came out of the room to ask us where she could throw them away. We told the next group of students to stay in the room and wait for us to come back. They waited, but while they were waiting, they stacked up the plates and combined all of the toothpicks on the top plate. Since there is apparently no way to stop University of Minnesota students from tidying up a room, we started entering the room a bit before each group's time was up—before they had a chance to disrupt the separate toothpick piles.

With this elaborate setup, we could see what the other friend (the one not in cahoots with us) ate when both of her friends only ate vegetables. As we had expected, when in that situation, the other friend ate more of the vegetables and less of the sweets, meats, and cheeses, compared to participants from other groups where the friends were not restricted to vegetables. If we eat with people who eat a lot of vegetables, our study suggests that we'll eat vegetables, too.

Our eating may also be influenced by our friends when we aren't with them. Psychologists have long known that people's behavior—though not necessarily eating—is influenced by what they think everyone else is doing and by what they think they are supposed to do.[10] These standards or expectations are called "norms," and they have a strong influence on how people behave. For example, if notices are posted in hotel rooms that 75 percent of the guests in the hotel reuse their towels over several days, the guests in those rooms are more likely to reuse their towels than guests in rooms without these notices.[11]

In that example, the norm was specifically stated ("75 percent of guests reuse their towels"). Most of the time, however, norms are implied rather than explicitly stated, but even implied norms are influential. Consider a life-saving example: organ donation. In some countries you are required to sign a form to allow your organs to be donated (called "opting in"), whereas in others you have to sign a form to decline (called "opting out"). An opting-out system implies that agreeing to donate is the norm, and countries with that system have agreement rates of more than 90 percent. An opting-in system implies that *not* being a donor is the standard, and countries with that kind of system have agreement rates around 20 percent.[12]

Given the significant impact of implied norms on such an important decision, we had some reason to expect that implied norms would also affect more mundane behaviors, like eating. We thought that people's eating habits might be influenced by an eating norm their friends had recently implied, even when their friends were no longer present. This would mean they had accepted the norm as their own standard, or "internalized" it.[13] To test that, we conducted a second version of the sneaky toothpick study. This time we provided the most tempting food we could think of: freshly baked chocolate chip cookies, straight out of the oven, with their irresistible smell filling our lab and wafting down the hallway. People in the nearby labs started popping in under flimsy pretenses, suddenly quite interested in our research. As in the other study, we separated our research participants, got two of them in cahoots with us, and told them not to eat the cookies when we brought them in. We assured them that after the session was over we would give them cookies that they could eat. Then we put the three friends back together to solve their problem, and counted how many cookies the third friend (the one not in cahoots with us) ate. Just like in the first study, the friend ate fewer cookies when her friends didn't eat them (compared to groups where the friends did eat them).

The twist to this version of the study was that after the group was done solving the problem that we didn't care about, we separated them again (to complete more questionnaires that we didn't care about) and gave them more cookies to eat alone. That way we could see if the friend who was not in cahoots with us ate lots of cookies now that her friends were gone, or if she continued to resist the cookies according to the norm her friends had just set. Alone in her private room, her friends would never know if she ate any cookies. Even still, the friend continued to resist the cookies.[14]

In sum, once you have learned the norms of your friends, you tend to follow them, even when you are alone.

## How to Trick a Child into Eating a Vegetable

Because norms are influential, it is possible to take advantage of them to nudge whole groups of people to do something healthy. In many cases, though, the healthy behavior is not the norm, and this presents a problem. In a study conducted at Utrecht University, researchers explained to their participants the importance of eating fruit, and then told some of them that the majority of their classmates (73 percent) ate the recommended amount, and told others that only a minority of their classmates (27 percent) did. Over the next week, participants tracked how much fruit they ate, and most of them increased their fruit consumption during that time. The only participants who did not increase their fruit intake were those who had been told that a minority of their classmates ate enough fruit.[15] This suggests that if you want people to do something, telling them what other people are doing is only useful if the majority of people are doing it.

When the majority of people are not doing it, it may still be possible to change the norm, but these kinds of broad changes to norms may take years, or even generations. Sushi, for example, is commonplace in the United States now, but in 1985 it was so unusual that in the movie *The Breakfast Club*, one of the characters had to explain to her classmates what the odd-looking food on her plate was. In the meantime, we have to be clever when we try to influence people's behavior based on norms.

In some cases, people are incorrect about what the norm actually is, and correcting their misperception can lead to healthier behavior. For example, college students tend to overestimate campus drinking norms. At one university, students estimated that their classmates consumed more than thirteen drinks per week, when in fact, their classmates were consuming about five drinks per week.[16] Students at that school who were given accurate information about the local drinking norms drank less over the next six months than students who were not given this information.

If you are trying to get kids to eat vegetables, you would prefer they believe an inaccurate norm, because the actual norm is that most kids are not eating vegetables.[17] The tricky thing here is that we cannot misinform kids about the norm. Although we freely lie to adult research participants in our lab (and then explain it all to them afterward), we don't lie to children. It's frowned upon (except with your own children, who, if the occasion calls for it, may be told that Clementine the goldfish has gone to stay at Grandma's house). But allowing children to jump to an inaccurate conclusion is not unreasonable. And that is what we attempted to accomplish in one of our U.S. Department of Agriculture school cafeteria projects.[18]

We did something so simple, it seems to me everyone should do this. We took standard-issue plastic cafeteria trays, which were divided into different-sized sections, and we put a photograph of carrots in one little section and a photograph of green beans in another. That's it. We did not say one word to the kids about it. But we thought the pictures in the trays might give the kids the impression that other kids were using those sections of their trays for those vegetables. That impression was false. Other kids were not using those sections of their trays for vegetables. But we figured it wouldn't matter, because people are influenced by whatever they believe a norm to be, whether their assumption is right or wrong.

To see how much the kids ate when we put pictures in their cafeteria trays, we did the tedious job of pre- and post-weighing the vegetables. We weighed the vegetables on the cafeteria line before the kids showed up for lunch, and then after lunch we weighed the vegetables that were left on the kids' trays. The difference between the pre-weights and the post-weights should be the amount of vegetables that made it into the kids' bellies. Our research assistants soon realized that weighing the leftovers at the fifth-grade table was a more civilized job than having to crawl around on the floor under the kindergarten table, weighing their scraps. (It should be clear at this point why we chose to do this study with carrots and green beans instead of peas and corn.)

All this effort paid off, because we found that the kids who used the trays with the pictures ate three times as much of those vegetables as they ate on a regular day without those pictures.[19] So simple! When this article was published, I got lots of calls from administrators at school districts across the country asking where they could get this kind of tray. But we just used the regular school trays and placed pictures on them. We printed the pictures with a color printer, cut them out, and laid them in the tray compartments. We didn't even glue them down. It didn't take long to do, and any school could do this every once in a while. And every once in a while is how often I think this would work. I don't think this would work if the trays looked like that forever. Then the pictures would fade into the background of stuff you never notice anymore—like the pictures on coins, or the details of your watch face.[20] But every once in a while this could be a useful little boost to get kids eating more vegetables.

## SMART REGULATION STRATEGY 5: GET SOMEONE (OR HEY, WHY NOT EVERYONE?) IN YOUR HOUSEHOLD TO CHANGE THEIR EATING HABITS, TOO

We've been talking about how people's eating is influenced by their culture, by the norms among their peers, by their friends,

and even by strangers, but we haven't mentioned the people that
we eat with most often: our family members and romantic partners. Sometimes our family members have an unspoken influence
on our eating. When I am sneaking thin slice after thin slice of
Rice Krispies treats from a pan on my counter, I eat a precisely
calibrated amount. I eat until right before so much is gone that
the people in my household will kill me if I take any more. But
unlike cultural factors or norms, which influence us passively, our
family members and partners often actively and explicitly try to
change our eating habits by, for example, urging us to diet or
the opposite—encouraging us to indulge with them. When we
instigate changes to our eating habits ourselves, the response of
partners and family members can have a large effect on whether
we succeed. Being supportive of someone who is trying to change
their behavior is not an easy job. Whether that support is effective
depends on the partner's motive for helping, the tone of the partner's help, and the type of help that is offered.

There are times when you have a personal goal, and it comes
to take on great importance to other people in your life for their
own reasons, rather than for your reasons. They want you to succeed not simply because they know it matters to you, but because
it matters to them. You might have a friend whose husband wants
her to lose weight—not because the husband knows this matters
to your friend—but because the husband wants to have a thinner
wife. I'm going to go on the record right now saying that I don't
like this husband. But aside from that, research shows that people
get less effective support—and are less successful in achieving
their goals—if their partner's motives are self-focused like this.[21]

If you are trying to change your eating habits, it is helpful if
your partner offers encouragement and shows some understanding that these changes are important to you. If your partner (or
other family member) nags you, tries to force you to eat (or not

eat) certain things, questions or criticizes the food choices you make, or expresses irritation about your choices, you will have a harder time succeeding at your changes.[22] In addition to that, it may become a source of stress and tension in the relationship. It is probably best not to have your partner or family members become your eating police. You may be tempted to ask them to take on this role, but I urge you to resist that temptation. It invariably leads to battles and hurt feelings, and might even compel you to sneak around in your own home or to eat in secret.

The most useful type of help that family members can provide is to change their behavior with you.[23] This is likely to lead to support that has a less nagging, critical, or irritated tone. They won't have to tiptoe through the minefield between being encouraging and acting as the food police. People have a bit more leeway in the kinds of things they can say without offending you if it is clear that they are saying it to themselves as well as to you. I would slug my husband if he were to tell me that I was not exercising enough. But I wouldn't have a problem with him saying that we weren't exercising enough (if he really meant both of us, and wasn't using "we" in that condescending way people sometimes do when they really mean "you"). You don't feel bossed around if your family members are also trying to change their own behavior. Psychologist Maryhope Howland calls this "invisible support" because it does not appear condescending or judgmental, or even like support at all, even though it is incredibly supportive.[24]

It's not only the *tone* of the support that will improve if others in your household are trying to change their behavior along with you. The *type* of support will also be more useful. Imagine you are trying to eat more vegetables by having a salad as your first course at dinner every night. If your family is also making this change, they can help prepare the vegetables, they won't mind waiting for the other parts of the meal, and you won't have to prepare separate foods for them and for you. If you are trying to avoid eating unhealthy foods by keeping them out of sight, it's a lot easier if you don't have to cook those foods for your family. If you are going to use smaller plates to help you eat smaller portions, it is easier if the entire family uses smaller plates instead of you having a different plate from everyone else.

All of the strategies in this book will work better if everyone in your household does them together. And since I am not suggesting that people restrict their eating, but simply aim to live at the low end of their set range, there is no reason why everyone couldn't make these healthy changes. Plus, helping other people—being the giver of social support—improves your mood, and when support is a two-way street, with each person helping the other, your mood improves even more.[25] So instead of causing household strife with just one person making changes, if everyone helps each other do these sensible things, the entire family will be healthier and happier.

.............................................................

# CHAPTER 8

# DON'T CALL THAT APPLE HEALTHY

I've never really understood the classic TV show *The Three Stooges*. Well, I understand the show—the plotline isn't exactly complex. I just don't get why people like it. Seeing someone get whacked over the head with a frying pan makes me cringe, not laugh. I watch the same images that so many of its fans do, but my reaction differs from theirs. This is a very simple example of an idea that forms the backbone of modern social psychology. It's not the particular event we experience that affects how we feel, but rather, it is *how we interpret* the event that matters.[1] That's why two people can experience the same thing, but have a completely different emotional response to it. They interpreted it—thought about it—differently.

Similarly, the way you perceive certain foods affects how you react to them. Food manufacturers know this. If I encounter a tub of vanilla ice cream named Tahitian Vanilla Bean, I am a lot more likely to buy it than if it were simply labeled "vanilla." Is this ice cream really made with vanilla beans from Tahiti? No idea. Is it good to make ice cream with vanilla beans from Tahiti? Who knows? For all I know, all the world's vanilla beans might come from Tahiti. It doesn't matter. Descriptive labels, even when they don't provide any meaningful information, still influence how we think about foods.

To test how people react to different types of food labels, researchers changed the names of several foods in a college cafeteria for a few days. When dishes were given descriptive labels such as Homestyle Chicken Parmesan (instead of Chicken Parmesan), or Grandma's Zucchini Cookies (instead of Zucchini Cookies), students found them more appealing to look at, said they tasted better, and thought they had more calories than those same foods without the fancy descriptions. They also felt somewhat more satisfied and full after eating the fancier versions.[2] You might think the names wouldn't matter since the foods were identical, but they did. They led people to have different kinds of thoughts about the foods, and those thoughts led to differences in their perceptions of the foods, and how they felt after eating them.

Your thoughts about food impact more than your mood—they also affect you on a chemical level. In a convincing demonstration of this, researchers placed intravenous catheters in participants' arms and collected blood samples before, during, and after the participants drank a milkshake.[3] The subjects were given shakes on two separate occasions. On one occasion the milkshake was described to them as decadent, indulgent, and containing 640 calories; on the second occasion it was described as nonfat, guilt-free, and containing 140 calories. Unbeknownst to the participants, they were given the same milkshake each time. But the perceived differences in how they thought about the milkshake triggered a chemical reaction that was evident in the participants' blood. When they thought the milkshake was indulgent and high calorie, levels of the hormone ghrelin—which signals hunger—decreased steeply after they drank it. But when people thought the milkshake was sensible and low calorie, their ghrelin level stayed about the same, signaling that they weren't fully satisfied with the "light" version and remained hungry.[4]

There is of course a biological reason why we have ghrelin—it is there to signal our *actual* state of hunger or satiety, so that we know when to eat and when to stop eating. But this study shows the power our thoughts can have over our biology—the participants' ghrelin levels were influenced not by how hungry they actually were, but by how hungry they thought they were. Thoughts matter. Changing your thoughts can lead to changes in your emotions, your behavior, and as this milkshake study found, even physiological responses in your body. Because thoughts matter, the strategies that follow are all based on the idea of altering them. If we can change the way we think about healthy foods, we may be more likely to choose them. And if we can change the way we think about tempting foods, we may have an easier time resisting them.

## CALORIE AND HEALTH LABELS: USEFUL, USELESS, OR WORSE?

If I told you that one slice of pecan pie contains 670 calories—about 50 percent more calories than a slice of pumpkin pie—it might cause you to choose a different kind of pie at your next Thanksgiving dinner.[5] Or it might not have any effect on your pie choice, except that you would feel guilty the next time you ate pecan pie. Or, for some of us, it would just make us want pecan pie even more. The same information changes different people's emotions and behaviors in different ways. For this reason, even though it's generally assumed that providing calorie information on menus will lead people to make healthier choices, it may not.

Since 2010, chain restaurants with at least twenty locations have been required by law to provide calorie information on their menus.[6] It is a sensible-sounding idea, and I firmly believe this information should be available to consumers so they can make informed choices. But dozens of studies have analyzed consumer behavior since this law went into effect, and the weight of the evidence suggests that posting calorie counts has little to no effect on what people order.[7] One particularly rigorous study found no change in the calorie content of orders at McDonald's and Burger King restaurants in Philadelphia when calorie information was added to the menu board, even though customers said they did notice it.[8] At that same time, customers' fast-food orders at the same chains in Baltimore, where calorie information was not provided on the menu, were no different than those in Philadelphia.

Nutrition labels on the back of food packages have not been resoundingly successful in leading to healthier choices, either.[9] Studies have found that consumers may not look at the nutrition information at all, or they look at it without processing it, don't understand it, or are unable to use it to make comparisons among products.[10] Because of these problems, current efforts to make food labels more useful focus on simplifying the information and putting it on the front of packages, where it is more noticeable.[11] Public health organizations, food companies, and researchers have experimented with different kinds of information and formats for displaying it, including, for example, the heart healthy symbol that the American Heart Association[12] has used, or stoplight symbols that are colored green, yellow, or red to indicate the levels of fats or sugars in foods.[13] In Australia and New Zealand they have a system called "Pick the Tick," in which products that are low in fat, added sugar, and sodium are labeled with a tick mark.[14] In the Netherlands, a similar type of label is officially authorized by the government.[15]

The Food and Drug Administration is currently developing a front-of-package label system for the United States based on recommendations from the National Research Council.[16] If the FDA follows these recommendations, the system will provide calorie information plus an overall health score based on levels of fats, sodium, and added sugars. Not surprisingly, there is heated debate between food industry leaders and public health officials over what levels of these substances will be considered unhealthy. The food industry has already spent $1.5 billion lobbying against using a traffic light system, and it strongly opposes putting a red light—indicating a food is too high in fat, sugar, or sodium—on any product, presumably fearing that doing so would negatively impact sales.[17]

Before the FDA settled on a label format, lobbying groups for food producers and food sellers joined together to create their own labeling program, called Facts Up Front,[18] which has been accused of being unduly confusing and not science based.[19] In a head-to-head test, consumers found this format harder to understand and more confusing than traffic light symbols, and were more likely to underestimate the amounts of fats, sugars, and sodium in products that had the Facts Up Front labels on them. Forgive my cynicism, but this may be just what the food industry intended.[20] Regardless of which system the FDA ultimately chooses to adopt, you can expect to hear a lot of screaming from food companies whose products score poorly.

## SMART REGULATION STRATEGY 6: DON'T EAT HEALTHY FOOD BECAUSE IT'S HEALTHY

Perhaps the easiest kind of label to understand would consist solely of the word "healthy." But while people do want to know if their food is healthy, the problem with labeling it that way (aside from getting competing interests to agree on which items qualify) is that for many people, the word "healthy" is strongly associated with tasting bad or remaining hungry.[21] In one study, for example, customers at a grocery store were given a cereal bar that was described as healthy or as tasty, and those who were told it was healthy said they felt hungrier after eating it than did customers who were told it was tasty.[22]

Although these results suggest that labeling foods as healthy might prompt people to avoid them, it's also possible that asking people how they feel after eating may not be the ideal way to measure the success of this labeling. The customers might have felt like they were supposed to say they were still hungry after eating the "healthy" bar, or that they shouldn't admit if they actually were hungry after eating the "tasty" bar. We also wondered if the label would matter for foods that people already know are healthy, because much of the time people do already know whether the foods they plan to eat are healthy. So we decided to test the effect of different types of healthy food labels, and to do so without directly asking people how they felt.

We took advantage of a convenient pool of unwitting participants: psychologists from all over the country who were coming to Minneapolis for a social psychology conference. My department was the host for the conference, and as part of our hosting duties, we were providing small hospitality gifts at the conference registration desk. Conferences often give away mugs (which are tough to pack in a carry-on), or tote bags (which nobody needs any more of), or pencils engraved with the name of the conference (okay, fine, these are handy). I surprised none of my colleagues by suggesting that we offer food instead.[23] So when people came up to the registration desk at the conference, we offered them some of our favorite Minnesota-made foods. One was the Nut Goodie candy bar, which is made of nuts and nougat and chocolate and is quite delicious. The second was a source of much local pride, as it was developed at the University of Minnesota itself: the Honeycrisp apple. (At U of M, people often talk about this apple variety with the same reverence as another local invention: the pacemaker.) The third gift item was a bag of coffee beans from a

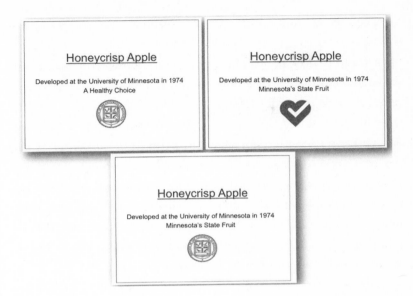

FIGURE 2. Sign with the word "healthy" (top left), the image implying healthy (top right), or neither (bottom).

company called Peace Coffee, which is a local roaster that delivers coffee beans by bike, even in the dead of winter.

To test the effects of food labeling, we put signs on each of the baskets of food. For the baskets of Nut Goodies and Peace Coffee, the signs had nothing to do with health, and we left them there throughout the study. But for the basket of Honeycrisp apples, we rotated through three different signs over the course of the conference registration. One of the signs used the word "healthy" (Figure 2, top left). It read: "Honeycrisp Apples. Developed at the University of Minnesota in 1974. A Healthy Choice." On the second sign, in place of the phrase "A Healthy Choice," we inserted the American Heart Association's heart healthy symbol (Figure 2, top right).[24] The third sign contained neither the word "healthy" nor the heart healthy symbol, and it was used for a comparison (Figure 2, bottom).

Then we stationed our research assistants unobtrusively near the registration desk, and they recorded what each social psychologist took as they registered for the conference, and also wrote down any comments they made about the foods. Social psychologists use deception in their research frequently, so it makes them (myself included) a little suspicious. We were worried that everyone would see right through our little ploy, but as far as the research assistants could tell from people's comments, only one person did. For the most part, people's comments had nothing to do with the foods, although one person said, "I can't eat that. I'm going to eat a steak as big as my head later," and someone else said, "This is the best conference because it has apples." People don't say that about tote bags too often, I would guess.

Although everyone that I talked to once the study ended swore up and down that the signs had no effect on their choices, classic social psychology research shows that people are awful at pinpointing the causes of their own behavior,[25] and whether or not they realized it, the signs did influence them. Calling the apple healthy did not lead more people to take it, but using the heart healthy symbol did. About 50 percent more people took an apple when it had the symbol sign than when it had the sign that said "healthy."[26] We don't know for sure why the symbol for healthy worked but the word "healthy" didn't. We don't think the word "healthy" made people think the apple would taste any different from any other apple they've ever eaten. Everyone knows how apples taste, and everyone knows that apples are healthy. They are practically the definition of healthy. It may be that seeing the word "healthy" on the sign makes people feel like they are being told what to do, whereas a more subtle symbol doesn't. People don't like being told what to do, and they sometimes react to that by doing exactly the opposite of what they were told (or think they were told) to do.[27]

We were pleased to find something (the symbol) that did increase people's likelihood of taking an apple and we decided to do another study to confirm that, and to see if we could find anything else that would persuade people to choose a healthy food over an unhealthy one. The conference registration setup had been so convenient that we decided to do the second study at another conference on campus. It was a medical conference predicted to attract more than a thousand scientists. We contacted the conference organizers and offered to provide snacks for all of the conference attendees if they would let us hang around and test different signs and record how many people took each snack. This arrangement was win-win. We got to collect our data and they got to look like very nice hosts.

It was no longer apple season, so we used individual bags of baby carrots as the healthy food, and a local brand of potato chips (Old Dutch) as the unhealthy one. We rotated through a lot of different signs on the carrots over the seventeen hours of conference registration. And we gave away a lot of food. A group of very dedicated research assistants[28] hung out at the registration desks discreetly rotating signs and even more discreetly recording what people took. It's efficient and exciting to collect data on such a large group of people in a two-day period, but it is intense. In particular, the day before the conference, our carrot supplier failed to supply our carrots, and we were left with one afternoon to find and transport seven hundred bags of baby carrots to the conference location. Most stores do not carry hundreds of bags of baby carrots, so my students[29] and I raced from store to store having crazy conversations with produce sellers:

Us: Do you sell bags of baby carrots?
Seller: Yes, how many would you like?
Us: All of 'em.

By going to a dozen stores, we were able to buy enough carrots and disaster was averted. In fact, we had a lot of carrots left over because we mistakenly thought people would take carrots in the same proportions as they had taken apples in the first study. We were way off. About 50 percent of the participants in the first study took an apple, but only about 20 percent of participants in the second study took carrots. Despite that, we still confirmed what we found in the apple study: labeling carrots as healthy didn't encourage people to take them. The healthy sign had no more impact on people's decision to take carrots than a sign that simply said "Carrots: A Snack." But putting that heart healthy symbol on the sign once again led to 50 percent more people taking them. We also tested out signs with other messages, such as "Carrots: An Energizing Snack," or "Carrots: A Snack to Keep You Focused," or "Carrots: A Quick Snack," and people took more carrots when they saw those signs, too. What we learned from people's reaction to these other signs is that labeling a healthy food as pretty much anything other than "healthy" encourages more people to eat it than if you label it as "healthy."

The results of these studies led us to one clear conclusion, which is the basis of Strategy 6. If you want someone to eat something healthy, even something that they already know is healthy, do not explicitly label it as healthy.[30] If you generally regard fruits and vegetables as "health foods" and you tend to avoid them when given a choice between, say, an apple and a bag of chips, try to change your perception of an apple. It is indeed a quick snack, and an energizing snack. Maybe eating one a day really will keep the doctor away—who knows? The important thing is that you come up with reasons that are compelling to you. Maybe you will choose a cucumber because you planted it yourself, or a salad because it has lots of variety, or an apple because it is crunchy and convenient. What we've learned from these studies is that if you reframe the way you look at "healthy" foods you are much more likely to actually eat them.

## Health Halos or Healthy Trade-offs?

Not only is labeling or thinking of food as healthy unhelpful, but it can actually backfire. Sometimes the mere presence of a healthy option licenses people to indulge in other ways. In one study, participants tasted bread that was labeled as either healthy or tasty, and then were brought into a different room for an "unrelated study" where pretzels just happened to be available. Participants ate more pretzels after eating the bread that was labeled "healthy" than after eating the "tasty" bread.[31] In another study participants were given either a healthy sandwich from Subway or an unhealthy McDonald's Big Mac, and were then asked to select the rest of their meal from a menu. Participants who were given the healthy sandwich were less likely to order a diet beverage and were more likely to order dessert. In the end, their full meal was less healthy than the meals of people who had been given the unhealthy sandwich.[32]

Researchers refer to this phenomenon as the health halo effect. But it's important to note that there's a fine line between the health halo effect— which leads to overeating when you think you are being healthy—and making sensible trade-offs that allow you to have some balance in your life. If you know you want ice cream for dessert, it makes sense to have a salad as your main course so you can indulge a little after dinner. The trick is getting the balance right so that you don't feel so deprived by your healthy meal that you are tempted to reward yourself in ways that cause you to overindulge. The same is true when people make these kinds of trade-offs with exercise. Exercise doesn't license you to overindulge.

For decades researchers didn't think people could engage in healthy compensation. They conducted studies where they required dieters to consume a milkshake in the lab, thereby breaking their diet, and then asked them to taste-test several flavors of ice cream, which were provided in large quantities. Participants were told that after tasting each flavor, they could eat as much of the remaining ice cream as they wanted. The dieters who had already had a milkshake ate more ice cream than the dieters who hadn't had the shake.[33] It was thought of as a "what the hell" effect. "I already broke my diet for today, so what the hell, I'll have a bunch of ice cream, too."[34]

My students[35] and I thought that study was fascinating, but we wondered if it was realistic. How often are people stuck alone in a room and asked to taste multiple flavors of ice cream from large containers? In their dreams, maybe. But in real life, it would be a very odd situation in which to find oneself, and not many dieters would choose to subject themselves to such circumstances. We also wondered what happened to the participants after they left the lab. Did they continue with their "what the hell" attitude, or did they compensate for eating the ice cream by following their diets more closely?

After years of wondering about this, we conducted our own study to see how dieters would behave in real-life circumstances.[36] We told dieters that we were testing new software for tracking calories, and asked them to use it to report what they ate every day for a week. While we were showing them how to use the software, we were interrupted by a graduate student who was desperately trying to get a few more people to participate in her dissertation study. The graduate student asked the dieter if she would be willing to come back during the week to be in her study. Most of our participants agreed to come back to do this other, "unrelated" study. And of course the other study was not unrelated, nor was it a dissertation study, nor was the desperate graduate student a graduate student at all. She was one of our research assistants, and the other study was our way of getting the dieter to come into the lab and unexpectedly drink a milkshake while she was tracking her calories. That way we could see if she compensated for the milkshake later in the day, or if she fell victim to the "what the hell" effect and continued to overindulge after she left the lab.

Unlike the participants in the classic lab studies, our participants successfully compensated for drinking the milkshake by consuming fewer calories for the rest of the day. When they were free to do whatever they wanted after leaving the lab, they managed to avoid situations that would have required them to be alone in a room with unlimited quantities of ice cream. They tended to have a light dinner and no more indulgences. Our study showed that what many researchers believed to be true for years was missing an important part of the story. When given a choice, people do generally attempt to make trade-offs to balance their indulgences, either by balancing high-calorie foods with lower-calorie foods or with exercise.[37]

## SMART REGULATION STRATEGY 7: CHANGE HOW YOU THINK ABOUT TEMPTING FOODS

So far we've discussed how to reframe the way we think about healthy foods so that we are more inclined to eat them. But you may be concerned about the reverse: how can we change the way we think about unhealthy foods so that we are less inclined to eat them? After all, no matter how much we try to avoid temptation, sometimes we find ourselves face-to-face with a doughnut anyway. It's a tough situation, and if we are stuck staring at the doughnut for long enough, the odds of successfully resisting it are slim. But if the situation won't last too long, say if a coworker is walking around offering doughnuts to people and you just need to say one quick no, changing your perception of the doughnut may be enough to successfully resist.

There are many ways to think about a doughnut, and it can mean different things to different people in different contexts. In the present, this doughnut is a burst of deliciousness, but in the future, this doughnut is what may keep you from getting near the low end of your set weight range. Thinking about the long-term consequences of eating the doughnut makes it easier to resist, so think about it that way, instead of thinking about its immediate charms.[38] Not only that, but just thinking about the future *in general* (not even about what eating a particular food will mean to you in the future) can also help people resist temptation. When researchers asked dieters to focus on the future by having them imagine positive events that could possibly happen (such as getting a promotion or attending a party), and then provided them with a meal, the participants ate fewer calories at the meal than dieters who had imagined past events described in a travel blog before eating.[39]

Sometimes your thoughts about a doughnut are specific and detailed rather than abstract or general. It's this particular doughnut, a chocolate-frosted glazed doughnut, a magical combination of fluffy and crispy that will melt in your mouth and leave sugary frosting on your fingers for you to discreetly lick off. Those details are what destroy your resolve. An abstract idea of a doughnut has none of the sensory features that make thoughts of a specific doughnut so tempting. So you should try to think about specific temptations in an abstract way.[40] When your coworker walks by with the doughnuts, instead of thinking about their taste and smell, think about their size, shape, or color. Instead of thinking about that specific glazed doughnut with chocolate icing, think of it as a generic dessert, or even just as one of many breakfast foods. Thinking about the general category makes it easier to resist, at least for a moment, which may be all you need before your coworker walks by. Just as Homestyle Chicken Parmesan is more tempting than regular old Chicken Parmesan,[41] the more you think about the specific features of a tempting food, the more tempting it becomes.

A perfect example of this comes from the classic study of self-control in which children were given a single marshmallow and told that if they could resist it for a little while, then they could have two marshmallows. The researchers trained the kids to think about the marshmallow in several different ways.[42] Kids were more successful at resisting the marshmallow when they were told to think of it abstractly, in terms of its size, shape, or color (for example, "it's a puffy white cloud"), rather than thinking specifically about its taste or smell (for example, it's a sweet, yummy marshmallow).

Not only does focusing on the abstract aspects of a temptation help you resist it, but thinking at an abstract level in general— even if it has nothing to do with any temptations—also helps you resist temptations. It doesn't seem like it should work, but Ohio State psychologist Ken Fujita[43] quite cleverly showed that it does.[44] To get people to think at a more abstract level, he gave a group of participants a list of forty words (such as "dog") and asked them to name a category under which each word could be listed (such as "animals" or "mammals" or "fluffy creatures"). Since a category is more general or abstract than a particular item, naming categories for all forty items on his list put people into an abstract frame of mind.

To get the participants to think at a more specific level, he gave them the same list of items, but asked them to name examples for each one. So for dog, instead of providing the overarching category ("animal"), they would list a specific type of dog (for example, "collie" or "terrier"). After getting his participants to think at these different levels by naming categories or examples for the items on his list, he gave them a choice of an apple or a cookie as a snack. The people that he put into the more abstract mindset were 50 percent more likely to choose an apple than people he put into the specific mindset.[45] Thinking abstractly helped them resist temptation. I'm not saying you should necessarily categorize everything you see the next time a doughnut stares you down, but trying to think more abstractly about doughnuts just might do the trick.

Of course, there will be times when this doesn't work. When changing your thoughts isn't enough to prevent you from eating unhealthy foods, sometimes the best thing to do is stop thinking altogether. In the next chapter, we'll look at some smart regulation strategies that help make healthy eating automatic, so that you do it without even thinking about it.

....................................................................

# CHAPTER 9

# KNOW WHEN TO TURN OFF YOUR BRAIN

I f you happen to find yourself walking around Paris, you need to be constantly vigilant or you will find, at some point, that you have stepped in dog poop. It is almost unavoidable, because it is everywhere. The problem is so extreme that every year about 650 people are hospitalized for dog-poop-related injuries,[1] and it is the source of the majority of complaints Parisians make to city hall.[2] In New York, however, this a much less frequent occurrence, even though picking up after one's dog is the law in both cities; the fine for failing to do so is similar in both cities; and both cities have publicized these laws extensively. I have trouble believing that New Yorkers are generally tidier than Parisians, or that they have more delicate senses of smell than Parisians, and I would bet a fairly large sum of money that Parisians don't leave cat poop around their apartments longer than New Yorkers do. So why do Parisians fail so miserably to clean up after their pups?

One possible explanation, if you don't mind me making some broad cultural generalizations, is that the Parisian lifestyle does not make it likely that poop scooping will become a habit, whereas the New York lifestyle does. By "habit" I mean a behavior that is paired with a specific cue in your surroundings enough times that they become linked in your mind, or, in fancy lingo, a mental association forms between the two.[3] Once that association forms, you'll do that behavior whenever you are in those surroundings, without having to think about it or make a conscious decision to do it. It becomes automatic.[4]

In New York, dogs usually stay at home while their owners go to work, so people walk their dogs before and after work, generally in the same place each day. With that lifestyle, scooping can become a habit, because people repeatedly scoop in the same surroundings. In Paris, however, it is not unusual for people to bring their dogs with them nearly everywhere they go, as there are very few places dogs are not allowed.[5] Because of this, they are less likely to take their dogs on walks for the sole purpose of relieving themselves. Cleaning up after a dog cannot easily become a habit with that kind of lifestyle, because the ever-changing poop location makes it difficult to form a link between scooping and a specific location. Without that all-important link, every time your dog visits *la toilette* in Paris, you have to make a snap decision about whether to bother scooping it. And snap decisions are subject to all sorts of interference from your current situation, regardless of your intentions. If you see a cop, or if you notice that the owner of the lawn your dog just used as a bathroom sees you, you will almost certainly scoop it. But if nobody's around, or if you don't see a trash can nearby, you may skip it.

You might also skip it if you think about it too much. Most of us are brilliant at talking ourselves out of doing the things we intend to do[6] (which is why so many gym memberships go unused), so sometimes the best strategy is to prevent ourselves from thinking at all. The strategies in this chapter are all geared toward helping you to behave in certain ways automatically, without conscious consideration or effort. This is smart regulation, because if you do things automatically, you do not have to consciously confront temptation.

## SMART REGULATION STRATEGY 8: TURN HEALTHY CHOICES INTO HABITS

One way to make behaviors automatic is to turn them into habits. You probably already have lots of healthy habits. Consider one of the most important things you can do for your health: wear a seat belt. For many of us, every time we get into our car, we automatically reach over and put on our seat belt. We don't have an internal decision-making process. We don't weigh the pros and cons of seat belt wearing four times a day. We just put the thing on. Wearing a seat belt is a healthy habit.

You can create healthy habits around eating in the same way. You can make a habit of ordering a salad in certain restaurants. Once it's a habit, it won't be a decision you grapple with each time you visit one of those restaurants; it will just be something you do automatically. You can make a habit of choosing fruit when you pick up a snack at the grocery store, or of walking through the grocery store without going down the candy aisle. You can make a habit of serving yourself a reasonable portion of food at dinner and then putting the rest away so that you are not tempted to take more later. You can make it a habit to drive a route to work that doesn't pass a bakery, or to walk a route through town that does pass a fruit stand. And you can make it a habit to always buy fruit when you encounter a fruit stand. Once these habits are established, you will consciously face temptation less often.

To create a habit, you need to pair the behavior (say, ordering a salad) with a cue in your environment (such as a certain restaurant). Once you order a salad in that restaurant often enough, the behavior will become automatic. How often is often enough? One study found that once you pair a behavior and a cue repeatedly for two months, it tends to become automatic, and you won't need to think about it.[7] But that's just one study, and as far as I know, no others have come close to quantifying this process. I wouldn't consider two months to be a hard-and-fast rule, and there is great variability between people, and between habits. All we can safely say is that the more times you pair the behavior with the cue, the more you reinforce the connection between the two.

You can also strengthen the link between the behavior and the cue by visualizing the performance of that behavior in that context. I do not mean the hokey kind of visualizing that is popular in self-help books, in which you imagine yourself holding the keys to your brand-new car or successfully achieving some other lofty goal. In fact, that kind of visualizing has been found to make people less likely to achieve their goals, partly by sapping their energy and enthusiasm about trying.[8] There is evidence, however, that if you visualize the *process* of getting to that successful point, including the specific steps involved in accomplishing it, then you are more likely to succeed.[9] That kind of visualizing helps you anticipate and plan for obstacles that may come up, and that is the kind of visualization that may help in habit formation. You might envision serving yourself a reasonable portion of food, wrapping up the rest and putting it in the fridge, and only then sitting down to eat your meal. This won't make it happen, but it may alert you to some obstacles that you will need to overcome, such as needing to find lids for your Tupperware, or having to contend with family members who might want a second helping. It may also help you remember to do the behavior when the situation arises.

Once you have created a habit by pairing a healthy behavior with a cue, you want to make sure you routinely encounter that cue. Now that you always order salad in that restaurant, you should go there often, and now that you always buy fruit when you pass a fruit stand, you should make a point of passing fruit stands regularly. You can also increase how many times you encounter your cue if you choose another, already established habit, as your cue. For example, if you already have the automatic habit of taking a walk at lunchtime, why not create the new habit of walking by the farmers' market? By linking your new habit to your existing habit, you will be more likely to solidify the new behavior.[10]

In addition to forming new healthy habits, you may have some unhealthy habits that you want to get rid of. It's never easy to break a habit (especially a bad one),[11] but one way to fight the "bad" automatic behavior is to consciously avoid the cues that you know are linked to it.[12] For example, if you have a habit of buying candy in the checkout lane every time you go to the grocery store, you may be able to outwit that habit by changing the store you go to, or even by grocery shopping online. If your habit is snacking on the extraordinarily unhealthy[13] popcorn at movie theaters every time you see a movie, you could change this behavior by avoiding the cue—movie theaters. In other settings, people are less likely to eat popcorn, even when it is there. When students were given a box of popcorn in a campus meeting room, they ate only half as much as they ate when they were given a similar box of popcorn in a movie theater.[14] Of course, it would be ridiculous to deny yourself the pleasure of seeing movies in theaters just to reduce your popcorn-eating habit, so instead of changing how often you go to movie theaters, you may be better off trying to link a new behavior to that cue by bringing your own food to the movies.[15] Nearly any food you bring will be better for you than the popcorn there.

The easiest time to make changes to a habit is when you have a big change in your overall environment, such as when you move to a different city. You can link new habits to cues in that city, and you won't have to worry about old habits being cued there.[16] One study found that when college students switched universities, they were able to change their exercise, TV watching, and newspaper reading habits.[17] I have many healthy habits linked to cues in my home, but when I go on vacation, those cues are gone and my healthy habits go out the window.[18] If your habits at home are unhealthy, on the other hand, then vacations may be a time to try to establish healthier ones.

## SMART REGULATION STRATEGY 9: CREATE AN AUTOMATIC PLAN FOR ANTICIPATED PROBLEMS

Some behaviors that you would love to turn into habits don't happen very often, so it's tough to create a strong link between the behavior and a cue. For example, most people don't ride in taxis all that often (unless you live in New York City), so there aren't many opportunities to make a habit out of wearing a seat belt in a taxi. Because of that, on the occasions when you do ride in a taxi, you are probably less likely to wear a seat belt than if you were driving your own car. Given the way some taxi drivers drive, if there is one place that you definitely should wear a seat belt, it's in a taxi, so it would be helpful to make that behavior automatic.

Luckily there is an easy way to make behavior automatic even for situations that we don't find ourselves in every day. In fact, it's so easy that you are not going to believe that it works. But it does. All you have to do is create something called an "implementation intention," which is a jargony way of saying a specific plan of action for a situation that you expect to encounter.[19] (It's so jargony that I'll call them i-intentions from here on in.) Suppose you are going to your friend's wedding, and it is going to be a big formal event. There will be a cocktail hour before dinner with roaming waiters offering tempting platters of finger foods. You can easily eat a dozen of these little bites before noticing how much you've eaten. Unless you get invited to a lot of fancy cocktail parties, this situation probably doesn't come up often enough for you to form healthy habits for dealing with it.

I-intentions are the perfect solution. They take the form of an if-then statement that specifies where, when, and how you will handle a particular situation. For example, "If I am at a fancy cocktail party, then I will keep a drink in one hand and a napkin in the other." That will keep your hands occupied and make it difficult for you to grab mini sliders or crab puffs when they are offered. I like this i-intention because it doesn't say you can't have any appetizers, but it makes it just hard enough that you are likely to eat them in moderation. (Remember, humans are lazy. The more obstacles you can put between you and an unhealthy behavior, the better.) No extreme rules and painful denial. Enjoy some appetizers. Just not too many. Here's another i-intention that may be useful in that situation: "If waiters offer me appetizers, then I will eat only one of each kind offered."

To make this strategy work, you need to think of your i-intention before the event, and then simply repeat it to yourself a few times. That's all it should take to make it work automatically during the event. Instead of having to decide what to do on the spot, your decision has already been made. It sounds magical, I know. That's how I felt when I first read about i-intentions. But the efficacy of setting i-intentions is well documented. There are more than a hundred studies that offer evidence that i-intentions work for a variety of behaviors, including things like practicing daily exercise or engaging in safe sex.[20] There is also a lot of evidence that they can help you make healthy food choices.[21] In one study where people were asked to create i-intentions for their meals on a particular day, researchers found that the participants ate more healthy food over the next five days than people who were not asked to set i-intentions for a meal.[22] There is no research on this issue, nor do I intend to conduct any myself, but I bet if Parisian dog owners set i-intentions, the sidewalks of Paris would be a lot cleaner.

The reason i-intentions work is that they help us avoid the common obstacles that get in the way of what we want to do versus what we actually do. For example, one common obstacle is distraction. We tend not to make choices that are in line with our goals when engaged in an absorbing activity (such as watching TV) or when we are distracted in some way. Since i-intentions make a behavior automatic, you should be able to do it even when you are distracted. The father of i-intention research, psychologist Peter Gollwitzer, compares the way i-intentions habitualize behavior to the way you automatically start driving when a traffic light changes from red to green. You don't consciously intend to do it. You just do it.[23] At the cocktail party, even though you are distracted by your friends, you will still be able to stick to your i-intention of keeping your hands occupied, because that behavior is now automatic.

Another common problem that prevents people from acting on their goals is that they don't notice opportunities to do so, or they don't know what an alternative behavior might be in a given situation. When you set an i-intention, you specify the situations you might encounter and what you want to do in those situations. So not only do you have a plan in mind when the time comes, but you are more likely to notice the opportunity when the situation arises.[24] If you hadn't formed the i-intention of keeping your hands occupied at a cocktail party, you might have just written off your health goals while attending it, because you assumed there was no alternative. And even if you did want to make healthier choices at the party, you wouldn't have a plan to make it happen.

Not just any old i-intention will work. Research shows that i-intentions are most effective when they are specific.[25] Instead of "if I go out, then I will eat healthy food," you are much better off with "if I am in a restaurant, then I will order a salad." Researchers have also shown that i-intentions work even better if you first imagine the specific obstacles that stand in the way of achieving your goal, and then devise the i-intention to directly overcome those obstacles. It works just like visualizing your habits, by helping you identify potential stumbling blocks and then devising solutions.

Certain forms of i-intention are ineffective, or can even backfire. For instance, setting a goal to *not* do something rarely works. People ate more unhealthy snacks after creating an i-intention of "If I am bored and I want to have a snack, then I will not eat chocolate!" compared to "If I am bored and want to have a snack, then I will eat an apple."[26] The problem with the negative form of i-intention is that the thing you are *not* supposed to do is put into the forefront of your mind, without a replacement behavior. In this case, being bored puts the thought of chocolate front and center, and does not help you think of any alternatives to chocolate. Because of the ineffectiveness of these "if this, then not that" types of i-intentions, it is not surprising that i-intentions to reduce unhealthy snacking do not work quite as well as those to increase healthy snacking.[27]

All you need is one strong i-intention. In her clever dissertation studies,[28] Charlotte Vinkers showed that even having a "plan B" for a situation is not effective. She had some participants make an i-intention for a situation, starting with "if I see chocolate and feel like having a snack, then I will . . ." She had other participants use that same beginning, but come up with two different endings to it. You might think having two solutions to this problem would be better than just having one, but Charlotte found that the participants who came up with two solutions ate nearly 50 percent more calories' worth of chocolate than people who came up with one solution. She reasoned that the strength of the association between the situation and the solutions got split between the two solutions. If i-intentions work by creating a strong link between the situation and the solution, then having two solutions, each weakly linked to the situation, would be less effective than having just one solution that was strongly linked to it. The bottom line is that you are better off creating one strong i-intention for a particular situation than two weak ones.

## SMART REGULATION STRATEGY 10: PRE-COMMIT TO A PENALTY FOR INDULGING

There's one other way to prevent your sneaky, rationalizing thoughts from derailing your best-laid plans. In addition to making things automatic so that you don't have to think at all when the time comes, you can also change *when* you think. When the temptation is at a safe distance in the future, you can pre-commit yourself to a costly or unpleasant penalty that will be imposed automatically if you succumb to temptation later. You won't be able to wiggle out of it in the heat of the moment.

This approach can be useful when you are unable to arrange your day so that you entirely avoid temptations. Instead, if you know you are going to be tempted at some point—say, a coworker's birthday party celebration with cupcakes, or your kid's parent-teacher night with free doughnuts—you can pre-commit to some cost that kicks in automatically if you end up indulging. For example, I briefly used a computer program that was set up to start deleting paragraphs of this very manuscript if I didn't write enough words each day. It was highly effective (until I outsmarted it by repeatedly typing "please don't eat me please don't eat me" until I reached the required word count).

There are many examples of people successfully using this kind of strategy in their daily lives. To force themselves to save, people sometimes choose to put their money in savings accounts that have large fines for early withdrawal, even if those accounts don't have other benefits (like more favorable interest rates).[29] To prevent procrastination, students in one study voluntarily pre-committed to earlier deadlines for their school assignments than their classmates, along with locked-in grade penalties for missing their deadline.[30] In another study, people who were scheduling unpleasant medical tests (and who feared they'd chicken out of showing up) opted to set up a fine ahead of time that they would have to pay if they didn't show up for it.[31]

This strategy was also shown to be successful with families that were trying to eat more vegetables. The families agreed to buy a certain amount of vegetables each month, or else they would have to pay considerably higher prices for all of their groceries the next month. These families purchased more vegetables than families that either didn't agree to be locked into this situation, or that were not given the option to do so.[32] People are willing to lock themselves into penalties for future self-control failures because they know it is good for them, but also because they tend to over-estimate their ability to resist temptations in the future.[33] They don't think the penalty will need to be imposed, so they don't mind pre-committing to it.

Once you get the hang of creating habits, i-intentions, or pre-committing to certain courses of action, you will realize that you can use these techniques to make the other strategies in this book even more effective. For example, you can use each of these techniques to help you get alone with a vegetable. You can make it a habit by repeatedly starting dinners in your own kitchen with a vegetable course. You can make an if-then plan about it, such as "If I am eating in a restaurant, then I will ask the waiter to bring my salad before the rest of the meal." Or you can lock yourself into eating a vegetable by packing in the morning only a salad for lunch. It's easier to stick to your goal of healthy eating when the healthy eating is happening later, rather than now. When lunch-time comes, you will be stuck with either eating the salad or being hungry.

You can make most of the smart regulation strategies in this book automatic, and that makes them smarter than they already were, because you won't have to consciously resist a temptation, even if you do happen to get caught face-to-face-with it. It'll hap-pen automatically, even if your mind is elsewhere.

· · · · · · · · · · · · · · · · · · · · · · · · · · · · · · · · · · · · · · · · · · · · · ·

# CHAPTER 10

# HOW TO COMFORT AN ASTRONAUT

For most people, losing weight is a struggle, but there is one known group of perfectly healthy people who are able to lose weight without trying: astronauts. When they spend an extended amount of time in space (at the International Space Station), most astronauts tend to accidentally lose weight. This phenomenon has very little to do with the effects of zero-gravity conditions—being weightless and floating around in a rocket. Astronauts lose weight in space because they don't eat enough,[1] partly because space food isn't the most enticing food on any planet. Many foods are dehydrated before they are sent into space so that they weigh less and stay fresh longer. Those foods have to be rehydrated in space, and while astronauts generally find them palatable, they're nothing to write home about.[2]

There are plenty of space foods that are identical to what we eat down here, but they may still be less enjoyable in space because being weightless causes nasal passages to swell,[3] which makes it more difficult to smell things. This is useful for dealing with space toilets, but it's not ideal when it comes to eating, because food doesn't taste as good when you can't smell it.[4] Even if it did taste as good, you may still get sick of it if you eat it often, which is likely to happen when you are somewhere as isolating as outer space.

Another reason astronauts don't eat enough when they're on a mission is that they're under a lot of stress.[5] They don't like to admit it and they would never complain about it, but they generally have a lot of work to do and not always enough time to do it and meet the high expectations of the people on the ground. Plus there's that nontrivial matter of their lives being in danger, which likely adds to their overall stress levels. As we've discussed, studies have shown that dieters tend to overeat when they are stressed,[6] but astronauts—or at least the nearly two hundred astronauts NASA has studied in recent years—undereat, perhaps because they don't want to take time away from what they are doing.

You might be thinking that this sounds like an added perk of being an astronaut, but it is actually somewhat problematic. While losing five or six pounds over the course of three months spent on the International Space Station is not a big deal, over a longer mission, that rate of weight loss could become unhealthy. And NASA is thinking about a much longer mission: Mars. It takes nine months to get to Mars, and after traveling that far you don't just stay for a long weekend. A Mars mission is expected to last for three years,[7] and NASA is researching all sorts of problems that must be solved before it can even be considered. How do you get enough food and oxygen to Mars? What does three years of weightlessness do to your body? Where do you dump waste? What sorts of people are best suited to handle the isolation and the long journey?

When my colleagues[8] and I heard that NASA was looking for scientists to study stress and eating among astronauts, we jumped at the chance. The idea of helping with the Mars effort was exciting to all of us. Plus, after years of studying people's failed attempts to eat less, I loved the idea of finding ways to help people eat *more*. For several years now, we've been testing ways to reduce astronauts' stress levels and get them to eat more. We thought if we gave astronauts comfort food, maybe we could kill two birds with one stone—they would eat more and get a mental lift.

When you work with NASA, the first step in the research is

creating what NASA calls "ground studies." Ground studies involve only non-astronaut people (who I will, from here forward, refer to as "people"). If the ground studies work, we can then go to the second step, "flight studies." The participants in those studies are the astronauts at the International Space Station.

At first we scoffed at the idea of doing ground studies of comfort food, because everyone already knows that eating comfort food makes you feel better. But when we searched for studies that supported this idea, we found that it was so widely accepted that nobody had ever bothered to test it scientifically.[9] This is exactly the kind of experiment we like to conduct in my lab—one that questions a "fact" that everyone assumes to be true.

To test whether comfort food could fix people's moods, we first had to ruin people's moods. You can't just start with people already in a bad mood, because the bad moods will differ in so many ways that it will be very hard to isolate the effects of comfort food. So we put everyone in the same bad mood by having them watch an eighteen-minute compilation of movie scenes that were carefully chosen to induce strong feelings of sadness, anger, and anxiety. We went through a long, unpleasant process of having our research assistants nominate scenes from movies that they thought caused any of these emotions. If they "worked" on the rest of us, we tested them on students from the Introduction to Psychology class.

Creating these videos was easily the least pleasant task my team has ever done. The process went on for almost a year—and people were routinely crying in what is typically a cheerful lab. We warned the participants before showing them the clips that they might find them to be disturbing, and we always made sure to cheer them up afterward by showing them a series of funny and happy film clips. Plus we always sent them home with the classic American comfort food: a Hershey bar.[10] Nevertheless, it was a gloomy time.

Once we created two mood-killing sets of film clips, we could finally conduct our study. The plan was to show the clips to participants, and then offer them either a food that they considered to be their "comfort food" or some other food. In order to have participants' comfort foods on hand, we had them complete an online survey a couple of weeks ahead of time. We asked them to list three foods they would eat to make themselves feel better if they were feeling bad, and to be very specific about the brands and flavors, because (unbeknownst to them at this point) we wanted to provide their exact comfort food. We thought it might be disappointing to receive something similar to one's comfort food, but not quite right. I would not be delighted to receive Häagen-Dazs Rocky Road ice cream instead of Ben & Jerry's Marsha Marsha Marshmallow, for example, even though both flavors are chocolate with a marshmallow swirl. One has graham cracker bits and the perfect amount (lots) of toasted marshmallow, and the other has almonds and (not enough) raw marshmallow.

We didn't want our participants to know that the sole point of the survey was for us to figure out what their comfort food was, so we also included a lot of other food questions that were designed to throw them off track. We had them list foods they would eat if they were watching a movie (since that's what they would be doing in the lab), or in a hurry, and in a bunch of other circumstances. Our hope was that by the time they came to the lab for the study, they would have forgotten the details of the survey.

From their list of three comfort foods, we selected one to give them during the study. We couldn't always acquire their first choice. It was not possible for us to provide one participant with her mother's homemade apple pie, for example, or to provide another with a cake that was decorated with a picture of himself. But we[11] managed to get everyone one of their three choices. We also made sure that the food we gave them wouldn't seem absurd to have on hand as a snack after watching a film in the lab. We thought it would seem perfectly reasonable to offer them a piece of cake, or a cookie, or potato chips, for example, but we thought it would seem odd to say, "Please enjoy this bowl of mashed potatoes as a thank-you for taking part in our study."

All of our participants did the study twice (and were shown different unpleasant film clips each time). One time we gave them their comfort food after the film, and the other time we gave them a food that they liked as much as their comfort food, but that they didn't think provided them comfort. If comfort food is really a special thing, then it should do more for your mood than any other food. But it didn't.[12] Comfort food did help people's moods improve some. But the other food improved their moods just as much as the comfort foods did.[13]

This surprised us. We thought comfort food was special. We considered the possibility that only certain kinds of comfort foods would have special powers to improve people's moods. But no kind of food was special. Sweet items, like candy or cookies, did not have special powers. Neither did savory items, like chips. Even chocolate was found to have no special powers.[14]

At this point in the research, we started to feel foolish for comparing comfort food to other foods people liked so much. It seemed like a ridiculously tough test of the power of comfort food, and we couldn't believe we had ever thought it was a good idea to design our study that way. We decided to do the study again, but instead of comparing comfort food to another well-liked food, we compared it to a neutral food: granola bars. We conducted some food opinion surveys and found that granola bars tended to occupy a middle point in people's preferences. They aren't disliked, but they also aren't something people get excited about. Surely comfort food would be more comforting than a granola bar? Nope.[15] As we found with the first study, participants reported that both foods made them feel a little better after watching the film, but comfort food didn't make people feel any better than the granola bar.

We really wanted to be able to tell NASA that our ground studies had worked, and that we were ready to begin flight studies. In our desperation, we conducted one more version of our study, but this time we chose the easiest possible test of whether comfort food comforts. We compared comfort food to *no food at all*. And again, we found that comfort foods provided no special comfort. Participants reported being in the same general mood whether they had eaten after the film or not.

While NASA researchers were also surprised by these results, they still wanted us to test comfort food with the astronauts in space—which, at the time this book was written, we were in the process of doing. A year before the astronauts head out on their missions, they fill out a survey for us that asks questions about foods they like and stressful tasks that they have to do in space. NASA sends them up to the space station with their comfort foods and neutral comparison foods, and then when the astronauts do the stressful tasks they mentioned, sometimes they are given a comfort food, and other times they get a neutral food or no food. The astronauts are asked to rate their moods at certain times and to report how much they eat, so we can see if comfort food brightens their mood more than other foods or no food, and if it leads them to eat more. I hope it does. I hope our contribution to the Mars effort is that the rocket must be stocked with all the chocolate pudding[16] it can carry.

## SMART REGULATION STRATEGY 11: DON'T EAT UNHEALTHY FOOD FOR COMFORT

Whether or not pudding has special powers in space remains to be seen—but, down here on the ground, where most of us spend the majority of our time, comfort food does not provide more comfort than other foods, or no food at all. But because it does provide some comfort, we tend to believe it is special. We don't think, "I would have felt better even if I didn't eat that," because our minds don't automatically look for scientific control groups. And since we don't expect other foods—say, eggplant—to make us feel better, if we do happen to feel better after eating an eggplant, we don't give it the credit. This is probably why everyone believes in the power of comfort food and why they seek it out when they feel bad. And they do seek it out.[17] When people are in a bad mood, they are more likely to choose unhealthy foods,[18] which most (but not all) comfort foods are. Researchers looked at people's eating patterns the day after their local NFL team played a game. People ate more high-fat and high-calorie foods the day after their team lost (when they were presumably in a bad mood) than on a day after their team won.[19]

We all tell ourselves that we need—even deserve—unhealthy treats when we have endured something unpleasant, or are stressed, sad, or angry. But as our research shows, this is a flawed justification, and it is the basis of Strategy 11: Don't eat unhealthy comfort food when you need comfort. It isn't doing anything special for you. Other, healthier foods you enjoy can provide the same effect. So should foods that are just "meh." Or no food at all. Even if you've believed in the power of comfort food your whole life, it's time to let it go. Comfort food is nothing more than a food you happen to want when you feel bad. So try this next time you feel bad: instead of reaching for the cookies, remind yourself that they will not improve your mood beyond what would happen if you didn't eat anything. Remind yourself that comfort food is a myth. And in fact, by eating something that may make you feel guilty later, you are actually doing the opposite of comforting yourself.

## SMART REGULATION STRATEGY 12: SAVOR (NEARLY) EVERYTHING

Even though we know that comfort food doesn't make us feel any better than other foods do, we will probably still eat them sometimes. When you do eat these treats, slow down and take the time to savor them so you don't mindlessly overeat. Pay attention to all of the food's features, noticing its taste, smell, and texture.[20] In fact, why not savor most foods?

I recently had the opportunity to sample lemon meringue pie from a much-buzzed-about patisserie in Paris. I looked forward to it for days beforehand. I ate it slowly and paid attention to every bite. I noticed the soft, pillowy meringue, tart lemony custard, and crumbly crust, and how the ratio of these perfect parts turned the overall pie into something sublime. It was the most glorious dessert I have ever had, and I savored every bite. That pie is more of a special-occasion food than an everyday comfort food, but the point is the same: when you succumb to temptation and eat something you had been trying to avoid, slow down to enjoy it. Sometimes, because you are a human being, you will eat foods that you were trying not to eat, and on balance, I would say it is better to be a human, and occasionally succumb to temptation, than to not be one. But when you eat something unhealthy and delicious that is too indulgent to eat frequently, savor it.

Not only does savoring lead to more enjoyment of the food you eat, but there is some evidence that if you savor your food, you may be satisfied with a smaller portion of it.[21] Remember, part of savoring is eating slowly, so you may feel full before you finish the whole thing. When I was savoring my lemon meringue pie, I did not finish the entire piece (though, to be fair, it was quite a substantial piece). I ate it slowly, noticed that I was filling up, and stopped when I felt satisfied. I didn't want to experience the uncomfortable feeling my son refers to as "being stuffed to the outside."

Another reason savoring may lead you to eat less than you might normally eat is that when you savor, you are focused on your food instead of distracted from it, and distraction leads to overeating.[22] When you are distracted, flavors taste less intense, so people may overeat while distracted because they are compensating for the mild flavor—they need to eat more of the food in order to fully taste it.[23]

In recent years, many experts have espoused the benefits of mindful or intuitive eating, which teaches people to savor food and to pay attention to feelings of fullness and hunger while they eat.[24] There is some evidence that mindful eating may help people lose weight,[25] maintain a stable weight rather than gain weight,[26] or eat a healthier diet.[27] In fact, one of my students conducted a study that found that people who are intuitive eaters eat a more balanced diet (according to USDA guidelines) than people who go on specific diets.[28] Mindful-eating training has also shown promise in helping people with eating disorders reduce their binge eating, and may be a useful tool in helping them recover.[29]

Nothing bad comes from savoring the food we eat, and yet most of us don't do this often enough. Americans, in particular, aren't known for savoring their food[30] (although you wouldn't know it from watching how people eat on TV commercials, with closed eyes and ecstatic expressions on their faces).[31] We eat quickly, often while watching TV, standing over a counter, or driving. French people are known for savoring their food. They eat more slowly than we do,[32] and are more likely to associate food with pleasure than with health.[33] Americans tend to focus on the consequences of eating—what it will do to our bodies—rather than on the pleasant experience of eating.[34]

Interestingly, the Americans who seem to be least likely to savor their food are those who are wealthiest, at least according to one study.[35] And regardless of one's own income, the same study found that simply being reminded of wealth made people savor a piece of chocolate less and reduced their enjoyment of it.[36] Small pleasures—such as delicious meals—may not seem worth savoring when compared to larger, more extravagant ones, and it's possible that people who can have the very best may start to take lesser things for granted.

In addition, there seems to be a trend among the super-wealthy to take healthy, environmentally sound eating habits to the extreme[37] and only consume foods that are some combination of organically grown, locally sourced, small-batch, gluten-free, nondairy, nitrate-free, air-chilled, grass-fed, and free-range. I am in favor of most of those things, but satisfying a long list of food restrictions doesn't leave you with much to savor. And a world in which we can't savor our food sounds pretty grim to me.

# PART FOUR

# YOUR WEIGHT IS REALLY NOT THE POINT

# CHAPTER 11

# WHY TO STOP OBSESSING AND BE OKAY WITH YOUR BODY

Imagine applying for a desk job and being told you are too fat for it, being threatened with deportation because of your weight,[1] or being denied the right to adopt a baby until you lost weight.[2] These are all very real examples of weight stigma or discrimination. The far-reaching consequences of weight stigma include lost educational and employment opportunities, poor medical treatment, and even unfair jury decisions. Taken together, these injustices are far more damaging to obese people than is their weight.

Weight stigma results from negative stereotypes about obesity. Common stereotypes of obese people include being lazy, lacking self-control, and being less conscientious than thin people.[3] There is no truth to these stereotypes,[4] but they do exist, and are endorsed in our weight-obsessed culture.[5] Although most people would never openly admit to being racist or sexist, people do admit to holding anti-fat beliefs.[6] The existence of these beliefs is not only detectable through their outward actions—it can even be observed in their brain activity. For example, in one study, when participants were shown a video of an obese person in pain, researchers observed less neural activity in areas of their brain indicating an emotional response compared to when they watched videos of a non-obese person in pain.[7] Even when we may not be consciously aware of it, prejudice may exist.


## DISCRIMINATION

Stereotypes may sound like harmless (though unkind) beliefs, but they become harmful when they are put into action. Discrimination is defined as unfair treatment based on stereotypes or stigma, and weight discrimination is real, pervasive,[8] and has serious consequences, particularly for women.[9] In this day and age, it's hard to imagine being less likely to get into college because of your religion or having to pay more for your employer's health insurance because of your ethnicity—but these forms of discrimination regularly happen to people who are obese.[10] Unlike religion, gender, and ethnicity, which are protected by the law, there is no federal law prohibiting weight discrimination, and only one state (Michigan) and a handful of cities have passed laws that prohibit it.[11] Because of that, victims of weight-based bias have few options for fighting discrimination.

Education is one area in which obese people face discrimination. It is, of course, entirely possible to simultaneously be obese and get good grades in school, yet obese people are less likely to go to college than non-obese people with the same scores on intelligence tests.[12] It's hard to definitively prove that the difference is due solely to weight discrimination, but studies are beginning to show a clear link. For example, one study found that obese people were less likely than non-obese people to be admitted to graduate school if the application process included an in-person interview, even if they had similar GRE scores and grades.[13] If the application process did not include an interview, obese people were just as likely to be admitted as non-obese people.

With very few exceptions, being obese does not detract from a person's ability to do his or her job, but obese people are also less likely to be employed than non-obese people,[14] and the more obese, the lower the likelihood.[15] This pattern is found even when obese people are compared to non-obese people who have the same level of education and job experience. Dozens of studies have been conducted in which participants are shown resumes of job applicants and asked to make hiring decisions. Some of the resumes include a photograph of a fat applicant and others include a photograph of a thin applicant, but the content of the resumes is otherwise identical. These studies have found that the obese applicants are less likely to be offered jobs, even when they have the same qualifications as the non-obese applicants.[16] In one of the studies, an obese applicant and a non-obese applicant were even the same person, just before and after losing weight from bariatric surgery. But participants were still less likely to select the obese applicant for the job, ranking them at or near the bottom of six candidates they evaluated.[17]

A typical reason given for not selecting obese applicants is the expectation that they will have health problems that could interfere with their job performance, but this concern has been shown to be unfounded. Studies that compare obese and non-obese people with similar health still find the obese people less likely to be hired.[18] Some employers don't even pretend that obese people wouldn't be able to do the job, and instead suggest that having obese employees sends the wrong message to their customers. One medical center in Texas refused to hire obese people because they said it set a bad example for their patients, all of whom were presumably slender and in perfect health (aside from being in the hospital).[19]

Obese people are especially likely to be discriminated against when it comes to jobs in sales,[20] and managers have argued that customers don't like to make purchases from obese people.[21] Whether or not that is true, this is no justification for failing to hire qualified obese people. If a company wouldn't hire African-American salespeople because its customers didn't like to buy from people of color, everyone would agree the company's policies (not to mention its customers) were racist.[22]

Job discrimination doesn't end for obese people once they are hired. They also get paid less than non-obese people for the same-level jobs. This has been shown to be true in multiple studies, and like most outcomes of weight discrimination, women are hit hardest.[23] In one survey, for example, the fattest female participants earned about $29,000 less per year than the thinnest female participants, even when the job level and amount of job experience was equal among the thinner and fatter women.[24] And like the hiring statistics reported above, these comparisons statistically control for health differences that may prevent obese people from performing their jobs. So at equal levels of health, obese people still get paid less than non-obese people.[25]

Discrimination against obese people in education and job opportunities ultimately influences how far they can advance in their career, so it is not surprising that they are underrepresented in positions of power and prestige. Only 5 percent of the CEOs from the 1,000 highest-earning companies in the United States are obese, even though 35 percent of their same-age peers are obese.[26] Obese people are also less likely to be elected to government office. In the 2008 and 2012 elections for the U.S. Senate, there were no obese female candidates, and only 4 percent of the male candidates were obese. On average, the winning candidates weighed less than the losing candidates, and the bigger the size difference between the candidates, the more likely was the heavier candidate to lose.[27]

Finally, although there are no statistics available from actual court cases, a study of hypothetical jury decisions concluded that obese women were more likely than thin women to be found guilty of crimes.[28] Participants acting as jurors saw a mug shot of either an obese or non-obese defendant, and then read a description of their alleged crime. Although the guilt or innocence of the defendant was ambiguous from the description, male "jurors" were more likely to find obese women guilty than they were non-obese women (although they were not more likely to find obese men guilty). Clearly sexism is playing a part here as well. Obese male defendants were not more likely to be found guilty than non-obese males, and female jurors did not discriminate based on weight.

## THE EFFECTS OF EVERYDAY WEIGHT STIGMA

In addition to institutionalized discrimination, many obese people are treated with heartbreaking cruelty on a regular basis. In just one week of recording stigmatizing experiences, more than 70 percent of overweight and obese women reported receiving nasty comments about their weight, being stared at, or being subject to negative assumptions.[29] One of the women said that teenagers made mooing sounds outside of a store she was in, and another said that someone told her she must be a bad mother because she couldn't possibly set limits with a child if she couldn't control herself.[30]

Even in the media, obese people are often treated with a level of disrespect that would be considered inappropriate for thin people. For example, a 2013 *Time* magazine cover story about the Republican governor of New Jersey, Chris Christie, offered the double entendre headline, "The Elephant in the Room,"[31] next to an unflattering picture of the obese governor. Christie is well known for poking fun at his own weight, and sadly, laughing along with your tormenters seems to be the socially acceptable response to weight stigma. Nearly 80 percent of obese people in one survey reported using humor in response to stigmatizing experiences,[32] but that doesn't mean they find it funny, and it doesn't mean that this constant assault doesn't take a serious mental health toll.

It is not unusual for obese people to be approached by strangers who inform them they need to lose weight or who offer unsolicited health or fashion advice.[33] Sometimes people are even bold (and thoughtless) enough to remove items from an obese person's cart at the grocery store.[34] Obese people do not need tough love from strangers any more than bald men need strangers sneaking Rogaine into their shopping carts. I probably don't need to tell you this, since it's common sense—but science supports it as well. There is no evidence that bullying fat people leads them to lose weight. Unfortunately, the media[35] and even the academic community seem to think it does, and continue to[36] increase the stigma of obesity in a misguided effort to make America "healthier." For example, a columnist for the *Spectator*, a respected weekly newsmagazine in England, wrote that it is acceptable and helpful to call obese children "hideous lard-buckets," and that "if we don't stigmatize fat people, there'll be lots more of them."[37]

Not only does stigmatizing fat people *not* encourage them to diet, it may actually have the reverse effect. Female college students in one study were asked to read a news article about policies that either discriminated against obese people, or, as a comparison, that discriminated against smokers.[38] Soon after, the students were given a break to watch a film and were provided with candy and crackers as a snack. Of course the students hardly needed a break after the exertion of reading a brief article, but the researchers were interested in how much they ate. They found that overweight participants who read the article about obesity discrimination ate more of the unhealthy snack food than overweight participants who read the article about smoker discrimination. The same group of participants also reported feeling less confident that they could control their eating, or stick to a diet.[39]

Weight stigma does not motivate obese people to exercise, either. Instead, it makes them feel uncomfortable going to a gym and embarrassed to exercise in public.[40] When researchers subtly brought up the idea of weight stigma in one study, overweight women reported feeling less capable of exercising and reduced their intentions to exercise.[41] Among children, being teased about their weight—a common form of weight stigma— makes them less likely to exercise.[42]

Weight stigma can also lead to a physiological stress response. In one study, obese participants who watched a video in which overweight and obese people were stigmatized experienced a spike in cortisol levels.[43] The video was compiled of clips from comedy shows that showed obese people being laughed at, struggling to exercise, and overeating. Since this is how obese people are typically portrayed in the media (if they are portrayed at all),[44] it's fair to conclude that as seemingly harmless an act as watching television can cause this type of stress response for obese people. And don't forget that stress can cause weight gain. So considering diet, exercise, and stress, it's not surprising that weight stigma generally leads obese people to gain weight over time, not lose it.[45]

Sadly, weight stigma is not going away. Even though rates of obesity are rising[46] so that more people know someone who is obese or are obese themselves, the percentage of obese people who experience weight discrimination is also on the rise.[47] With other stigmatized groups, prejudice tends to decrease as more people come into contact with members of that group.[48] But the heavier we become, the less tolerant we seem to be getting of obese people. Even obese people buy into the negative stereotypes about obesity, internalizing the anti-fat attitudes that are common in our culture.[49] It's hard to rise up against your tormenters if you believe them.

As long as we think of excess weight as the enemy, we are all complicit in perpetuating weight stigma, and we all suffer for it, obese or not. Sensationalized reporting of the "deadly" obesity epidemic makes us view extra pounds as a personal medical crisis, while misinformation about diets assures us we could have perfect control over our weight if we would just make an effort. We berate ourselves if we can't keep weight off and judge others just as harshly if they can't. We feel threatened by people who are heavier than us, and—thanks to our society's body type ideal, which is unattainable for most people—jealous of those who are thinner. It doesn't take a psychologist to see why we are obsessed with thinness and insecure about our ability to become—or stay—thin enough.

This is a tough situation to change, but maybe the first step toward ending weight stigma is to take some of the pressure off ourselves. If we became a little less obsessed with our own weight, maybe we wouldn't feel the need to concern ourselves with everyone else's.

## BE OKAY WITH YOUR BODY

Allow me to suggest a revolutionary action: Let's try to be okay with our bodies. I am not saying you have to *love* your body. I can't help but notice that this goal is frequently pushed on women, but never men, and if men don't need to love their bodies, it seems to me that women can get by without it, too. For a long time I bought into all the talk about learning to love your body, but I've come to think it's a somewhat misguided goal. Not because it's impossible (though it's difficult for most), but because it's unnecessary. Perhaps loving your body is something to strive for, but all we really need to do is respect our bodies, appreciate them, and be generally okay with them.[50] Body okayness doesn't mean letting ourselves go, binge eating, or not being physically active. It just means not letting our bodies become our primary life projects.

Historian Joan Jacobs Brumberg researched the diaries of young women around the turn of the century and found that the girls' primary concerns for self-improvement in the 1890s focused on character.[51] They wrote about striving to be kinder and more concerned for others, working harder in school, and rejecting frivolity. One hundred years later, Brumberg found, the same age group focused its self-improvement on physical appearance, and that the means by which to achieve it almost always involved buying things.[52]

A lot of industries are profiting from our insecurity about our weight and our inaccurate beliefs about how to lose it. It's not just the diet industry. The $27 billion fitness industry (including gym memberships, exercise equipment, and workout programs, among others) is profiting from our ignorance, too.[53] Fitness fads—some more effective than others but none of them free—come and go just as diet fads do. Remember the Bowflex? The Thighmaster? How about Tae Bo? The methods differ but the promised results are the same: we are told that anyone can reshape any part of his or her body. Exercise does many wonderful things, as we'll talk about in the next chapter, but it can't change your build, bone structure, or genetic limits on the amount of muscle mass your body can achieve.[54] If we fail to get the promised result, we end up more anxious and insecure, and eventually move on to buy more and more products.

It doesn't have to be this way. As *New York Times* columnist Frank Bruni wrote in an editorial, "We're so much more than these wretched vessels that we sprint or swagger or lurch or limp around in," and we need to keep that in mind when we resolve to improve ourselves, "foolishly defining those selves in terms of what's measurable from the outside, instead of what glimmers within."[55]

If we take the focus off the outside, maybe we can put a stop to the endless cycle of misguided body improvement efforts and their disheartening and unhealthy aftermath. And if we can take care of ourselves without drama, maybe we can also look dispassionately on other people, without insecurity or judgment. Collectively, as a society, we'd be a whole lot healthier, both mentally and physically.

# CHAPTER 12

# THE REAL REASONS TO EXERCISE AND STRATEGIES FOR STICKING WITH IT

If you've ever stuck with an exercise program for a while, you probably noticed all sorts of perks. You likely had more energy, were in a better mood, looked great in your clothes, slept more soundly, and perhaps even learned that your resting heart rate or blood pressure had lowered. Exercise offers all of these benefits and many more. You may also have noticed, with some frustration, that you didn't lose a huge amount of weight. You may have thought you were somehow doing it wrong, and that exercise was making everyone rail thin except for you. Despite the weight loss reality shows you see on TV and the infomercials for fitness DVDs that run at all hours of the night, the truth is, exercise doesn't typically lead to dramatic weight loss. Exercise can help you lose weight (especially if you are watching what you eat as well), but the kind of exercise that most of us do doesn't lead to as much weight loss as we would like it to, and certainly not as much as we are told it will.[1] What exercise can do, though, is help you get to the low end of your set range—to your leanest livable weight—and stay there.[2]

One reason exercise doesn't often result in major weight loss is that you have to exercise *a lot* to burn off even one indulgent treat. For example, my standard run takes about thirty minutes. At my (admittedly slow) pace, that run burns about 300 calories—which is fewer than the number of calories in one four-ounce scoop of my favorite ice cream. It's not quite as simple as that, of course. Muscle cells burn more calories than fat cells, so the more muscle you build, the more calories you will burn.[3] But even accounting for that, people may end up consuming more calories than they burn off because they feel hungrier after exercise, or because they tend to allow themselves an extra indulgence on days they exercise.[4] One study found that merely thinking about exercising led people to serve themselves larger portions of food.[5] Even if they don't, it still takes a lot of intense exercise to lead to a lot of weight loss.[6] But that doesn't mean there aren't other good reasons to exercise.

## REASON 1: IT REALLY DOES MAKE YOU HEALTHIER

I can't tell you that exercise leads quickly to lots of weight loss, but I can offer better news. The best news, actually. Exercise prevents death. Not forever, of course, but it does increase your life span. Even moderate exercise, including walking (briskly) to work, active gardening, and some kinds of housework, lowers your risk of death.[7] In one study, diabetes patients who walked two or more hours per week had a 39 percent lower death rate than inactive patients.[8] The benefits are evident for exercising just 75 minutes per week, and exercising more often than that, or more vigorously than that, leads to greater benefits.[9]

Even more exciting, perhaps, is the news that exercise works as well as drugs in preventing death among people with heart disease, stroke, or prediabetes, according to a review of 305 randomized clinical trials.[10] The authors of this review compared the effects of fifteen different classes of drugs (such as statins and beta blockers) with the effects of exercise, and they found that exercise and drugs had the same benefits, with just three exceptions. Only one of these exceptions was a drug that worked better than exercise: diuretics for heart failure. The other two exceptions were cases where exercise worked better than drugs (both in preventing death from strokes).[11]

Exercise also lowers your chances of developing major diseases[12] including heart disease,[13] stroke,[14] diabetes,[15] and possibly even colon and breast cancer.[16] Among people who already have risk factors for heart disease, stroke, and diabetes, exercise lowers blood pressure and triglycerides and raises the good kind of cholesterol (high-density lipoprotein cholesterol).[17] And after even a short exercise session, people who suffer from chronic pain are able to tolerate more pain.[18]

Lest you worry that it is too late for you to benefit from exercise, it isn't. One study looked at people who hadn't exercised much before middle age. If they increased their level of exercise and kept at it, they cut their mortality rate in half, ultimately getting the same life span benefits—about two extra years of life—as people their same weight who had been exercising all along.[19] To put the size of that benefit in perspective, increasing exercise in middle age reduced mortality rates just as much as quitting smoking in middle age.

## Exercise Helps Even if You Don't Lose Weight

At this point you may be confused. I said that exercise doesn't necessarily lead to much weight loss. If that's the case, then how does it make you healthier? In fact, significant weight loss isn't necessary to reap the health benefits of exercise. This tends to come as a surprise to people, but the evidence is clear. For example, in one weight loss study, researchers were initially disappointed to discover that not all participants lost weight during twelve weeks of intense exercising. A few even gained four or five pounds (and this was not necessarily muscle mass—some had increases in fat mass as well). These differences in weight change didn't occur because some participants exercised vigorously and others slacked off. They all exercised in the researchers' lab, five days per week, for as long as it took them to burn off 500 calories. But when it came to assessing the participants' health, it turned out that weight loss didn't matter—the only thing that mattered was that they exercised. All of the participants showed improvements in heart rate, blood pressure, and fitness levels, regardless of whether they had lost or even gained weight.[20]

The funny thing is, this important news—which I think is headline material—was buried deep within the research article, which was titled "Exercise Alone Is Not Enough."[21] The researchers seemed to be so focused on weight loss that they didn't fully appreciate what was staring them in the face: exercise improves your health whether you lose weight or not.[22] In another study that even more clearly demonstrates this same good news, women were assigned to either exercise or diet for six weeks, and only the women who exercised experienced health improvements, even though they didn't lose weight.[23] The women who dieted did lose weight, but their health did not improve.

## REASON 2: IT REALLY DOES MAKE YOU FEEL BETTER

One of the most important reasons to exercise is to help control your stress. I don't know how much stress you have in your life, but I do know you have some. I know this because everybody has stress—especially Americans. We rank 33rd out of 36 developed countries in the amount of time we spend each day on leisure, sleeping, and eating. And unlike our European counterparts, our employers are not legally required to give us at least four weeks of paid vacation each year.[24] In fact, U.S. employers are not required to provide any paid vacation days at all.[25]

Whether the source of your stress comes from your job, your family, your relationship, school, work, money, or your weight, it's important to learn how to manage it, because stress is dangerous for your health.[26] In response to stress, the body's sympathetic nervous system releases the hormone epinephrine (among other chemicals) and raises your heart rate and blood pressure.[27] As we've discussed, this response was helpful when humans needed to flee immediate physical threats, but it's not very handy when you are stressed about a work deadline or an issue in your marriage. Over time, constant activation of the sympathetic nervous system can damage your heart and blood vessels, increasing your risk of hypertension, strokes, and other cardiovascular problems.[28]

And while stress kicks your sympathetic nervous system into high gear, it has the opposite effect on your parasympathetic nervous system, which controls functions like growth, digestion, reproduction, and energy storage.[29] Constantly stopping or slowing those functions can lead to digestive problems (such as irritable bowel syndrome and colitis), and makes it harder for your body to defend against ulcers.[30] Suppression of the parasympathetic nervous system can also lead to fatigue due to depleted energy stores, and since reproductive processes are slowed down, impotence.[31]

Stress also initiates a response that leads to the release of steroid hormones, including cortisol.[32] As we know, cortisol is no friend to weight loss, as it can lead to elevated blood sugar levels and prompts our body to store fat in the abdomen.[33] Cortisol can also suppress the activity of your immune system,[34] making you more susceptible to colds and other immune-related illnesses,[35] slow the healing of wounds,[36] and maybe even speed up the aging process.[37]

Given how dangerous chronic stress is to the body, reducing and managing it is important for our health, not to mention our quality of life. Exercise can help with this, so don't skip your workout when you are stressed—that's when you need it most! At minimum, engaging in exercise can distract people from their worries, and the rhythm and repetition of some forms of exercise, such as running or swimming, can help relax the mind. In addition, people may also have a decreased physiological response to stress after they exercise. In one study, for example, after riding an exercise bicycle for twenty minutes, participants had a smaller sympathetic nervous system response when they gave a stressful speech afterward, compared to giving the speech without exercising first.[38] This appears to work in the long term, too. People who exercise regularly may be less sensitive to stress overall, not just immediately following a workout.[39]

Most people who exercise have noticed that it makes them feel good, and this anecdotal evidence is backed by research showing that even a single session of exercise—as short as ten minutes[40]—improves overall mood,[41] provided it is not a lot more intense than what you are used to.[42] It not only works as an immediate pick-me-up, but it can also change your tendency to feel bad. For example, after being on an exercise program for ten weeks, people report feeling less anxious in general, not just right after exercising. This was even true for people who were chronically anxious,[43] as well as people with panic disorders.[44] Exercise has been shown to be an effective treatment for mild to moderate depression,[45] to prevent depression in older adults,[46] and to reduce symptoms of depression in cancer patients who are completing their treatment.[47]

## REASON 3: EXERCISE HELPS YOU THINK, SLEEP, AND AGE GRACEFULLY

Having a regular aerobic exercise program provides long-term cognitive benefits, particularly in memory and executive function,[48] and even a single exercise session can provide a small memory boost.[49] A single exercise session also has immediate effects on creativity.[50] In a series of studies, students were able to come up with more creative solutions to a puzzle while walking—either outdoors or on a treadmill—compared to standing still.

Regular exercise also improves the quality of your sleep, as long as you exercise in the morning rather than the evening.[51] After just four months of regular moderate-intensity exercise, sedentary older adults were able to routinely fall asleep faster and sleep better and longer than their peers who remained sedentary.[52]

The benefits of exercise are particularly evident among older people, even if they had previously been sedentary. Becoming active relatively late in life leads to healthier aging, in terms of preventing chronic disease, depression, disability, and memory impairments.[53] As people age, their muscle mass and muscle strength decline, but strength training exercise can reverse this.[54] Similarly, exercise can also prevent the cognitive decline—in memory and executive function— that tends to occur with age.[55]

## MOST OF US DON'T EXERCISE ENOUGH

For a person to get the health benefits of exercise, the U.S. government recommends 150 minutes of moderate-intensity—or 75 minutes of high-intensity—aerobic exercise per week, along with two sessions of muscle strengthening exercises.[56] Moderate intensity exercise is defined as exercise that gets your heart rate up to between 64 and 76 percent of your maximum heart rate (which is based partly on your age and weight).[57] This is more intense than people realize,[58] so it's worth using a heart rate monitor to make sure you are working out hard enough. You can divide the 150 minutes into thirty minutes of exercise, five days a week, or if you prefer, you can divide it into more manageable ten-minute chunks of time. You'll get the same benefits.[59] We've turned the treadmill in my lab into a desk that we can use while walking or jogging. It's too bouncy for writing, but works well for reading, and is a good way to get a couple of ten-minute bursts of exercise into a busy day.

In the 1950s (and earlier), we didn't have to worry about squeezing these bursts of exercise into our day, because without even trying we got more physical activity than we do now.[60] Technology is great, but it has also made our lives too easy. We drive instead of walk, throw our clothes into washers and dryers instead of washing them by hand and hanging them out to dry, and we accomplish a lot of our work without leaving our desks. The proportion of workers in jobs that require very little physical activity has doubled since the 1950s,[61] and jobs that have always been low activity, like my own, have gotten even lower in activity. In graduate school I used to have to walk across campus to the library and schlep heavy volumes off shelves if I wanted to read articles in journals. Now it rarely takes more than a mouse click to access an article.

We haven't made up for this decrease in physical activity from regular daily exertion by increasing the amount of exercise we do in our leisure time.[62] In the 1980s, only 19 percent of women and 11 percent of men in a nationally representative survey reported engaging in *no* leisure time exercise, whereas in 2010 those numbers had risen to 52 percent of women and 43 percent of men.[63] Instead, leisure time is occupied more and more by sedentary activities, particularly, "screen time." Kids used to have to bike to friends' houses to see them, but now they are more likely to connect via their phones or online. Exercise is this miracle treatment, recommended by the American Medical Association, American Heart Association, World Health Organization, and nearly every other medical group you can think of,[64] and yet, people don't take advantage of it.

Well, if you ask people how much they exercise, it seems that they do take advantage of it, but this may be misleading. According to one national survey, about 43 percent of adults met the recommended 150 minutes per week of moderate aerobic activity.[65] In another survey, 60 percent of adults reported meeting the recommendation (with an overall average of 324 minutes of exercise per week).[66] However, when the researchers from this second survey had the same people wear accelerometers for a week to measure their physical activity, it turned out that only about 8 percent met the recommendation (and the overall average was about 45 minutes of activity a week).[67] It's hardly surprising that people overestimate how much they exercise, but I would not have expected such a large gulf between what they said and what the accelerometer measured. No matter which estimate we use (and the truth is almost certainly somewhere in between),[68] there is plenty of room for improvement.

## Why Don't We Exercise More?

It's not that people don't want to exercise, or don't intend to exercise. The problem is the gap between what we plan to do, and what we end up doing (and not just with exercise, of course). Across ten studies of people's plans to exercise, about 36 percent of the participants said they intended to exercise but didn't.[69] We join gyms, but then rarely go to them. In fact, 67 percent of people with gym memberships never use them.[70] We buy yoga pants, but end up wearing them around our homes.[71] Why is it so hard to do what we intend to do?

There are so many things that come between our intentions to exercise and our actions that sometimes I think it's kind of amazing that anyone ever exercises at all. For example, some people (I'm thinking especially of new moms) may not have enough time in their daily routine to even schedule a workout. Or they have it on their schedule but something comes up at work, or their kid misses the bus and needs to be picked up, or they forget their exercise clothes, catch a cold, or have an injury from a previous workout. People may not have anywhere safe to exercise, may not be able to afford the equipment, or may not have anywhere to exercise indoors when the weather doesn't allow for outdoor exercise. These are all examples of external barriers—things outside of ourselves that prevent us from exercising.[72]

There are also internal barriers that keep us from exercising.[73] We might be less motivated to bother because we don't feel like we're any good at it, or that it will "work." We may have noticed we aren't losing weight or getting better at the activity itself, or suspect that we aren't getting healthier. Or maybe we can tell that we are getting healthier, but what we really care about is getting thinner. Maybe we don't really think of ourselves as the exercising type, so it's easy to let other things—things that are more central to how we think about ourselves—get in the way of it. Perhaps the people we care about are not fully on board with our fitness plans or don't think exercise should be a priority for us. It may be the case that certain moods keep us from exercising, or make us more likely to exercise.

Some people simply just don't enjoy exercising. It's hard to make yourself do things you don't enjoy doing. Some people love exercise and feel antsy when they aren't able to work out for a few days. It can be hard to like those people, but we shouldn't hold it against them personally, because studies with twins suggest that inherited biological factors may partly explain our motivation to exercise.[74] Although we don't know exactly what those biological factors are in humans, there are some intriguing clues from studies with mice. Researchers took mice that voluntarily did a lot of wheel running and bred them with each other for many generations to create a breed of mouse that is highly motivated to exercise.[75] When they compared those mice to regular, somewhat lazy mice, they found that the fitness buffs had a different neural response to exercise in parts of the brain associated with reward and pleasure. When those mice were prevented from running on their wheel, their neural activity was very similar to that of mice denied morphine (once addicted to it).[76] So for some mice, exercise is extremely reinforcing—perhaps even addictive.

## HOW TO STOP WIGGLING OUT OF WORKING OUT

For those of us who aren't that kind of mouse, it can be hard to stick to our exercise plans. Believe me, nobody is better or craftier than I am at finding a reason to skip a workout. Most of the time, though, I am able to keep my lazy side in check by using the same strategies we've discussed for changing our behavior around food. For instance, just like I don't drive to work on a route that passes a bakery when I know I shouldn't stop there, sometimes I change my daily routine so I'm not tempted to skip a workout. If, like me, you tend to be tired later in the day and therefore less likely to make it to your exercise session, schedule it for the morning or lunchtime instead. And just like setting out a bowl filled with fruit makes healthy foods more visible, you can make an effort to keep your exercise gear in your face by packing your gym bag and leaving it by the door. I know someone who actually sleeps in her workout clothes so that she's ready to go first thing in the morning. If you keep your bike easily accessible, you'll be more likely to use it instead of your car for errands. I hate dragging my bike from the shed behind our house, so when I really want to make sure I use it, I lock it up out front instead. Maybe it sounds ridiculous, but tiny obstacles like these matter a lot (remember the smushed toilet paper roll from Chapter 6?).

For many of us, exercise loses the popularity contest for what we want to do in our free time. This is why exercise cannot be entered into that contest. As with eating vegetables first so that they are never in a head-to-head competition with other foods, you can't say, "Tonight I will either go to the gym or go to the movies," or, "This weekend I will either go for a bike ride or go shopping." Your exercise time should be set aside only for exercise. If you don't make it to the gym, then use that time to run errands or do another task or chore you're not particularly looking forward to.

## Find a Way to Make Exercise Rewarding

The alternative to punishing yourself for missing a workout is to reward yourself for completing one. For a reward to work, though, it needs to be immediate.[77] If future incentives worked, we'd be fit and healthy already, because we all want the long-term benefits of exercise. Unfortunately, the future benefits do not get us to the gym on a regular basis. We need to be rewarded right away, and often.

For her dissertation study, one of my students[78] gave people a very nice reward for walking 10,000 steps per day: money. The money was indeed a motivating reward for the first week, but once it was no longer being offered, the student participants resumed their normal walking patterns, even though they wanted to stay fit and were continuing to track their steps for the study.[79] The point is: unless you have limitless financial means, tangible rewards are probably not the way to go.

What about if exercise itself were the reward? Just like an apple labeled as "healthy" is less appealing than an apple with a neutral label, thinking of exercise as simply an investment in your health is unlikely to be incentive enough to do it. We need to enjoy exercise. For most of my life, whenever people said this to me, I wanted to bop them on the head and tell them the entire problem was that I did not enjoy exercise. But the best way to stick to an exercise plan is to find a form of exercise that you actually enjoy. This sometimes happens when you least expect it—maybe a friend invites you to try a rock climbing wall with her, or to go to a Spinning class. After a session or two, you find that you're hooked.

Being active without having the specific goal of health or weight loss in mind may actually enable you to enjoy exercising more. When I was under a lot of stress and having trouble adapting to the Minnesota winter, a neighbor suggested I try power yoga. The flowing movements of yoga in a hot room and the soothing words of the instructors helped improve my moods and reduce the chill of the winter. For a while I went mainly for the stress relief, which is a great reinforcer of most kinds of exercise (and a very good reason to not skip your workout when you are stressed). But then something else happened: I began making progress. I started out knowing very little, and practically each session I picked up a new skill—a new pose I could twist myself into, hold longer, or do without agony. It was intoxicating.[80]

You might not love yoga, but the crucial lesson here is that the exercise itself needs to be rewarding, because weight loss comes slowly, if it happens at all.[81] Changes in fitness levels or skills, however, can happen fairly quickly. With yoga, those changes are very noticeable, whether you look for them or not. You couldn't do the crow pose before, but now you can. With other forms of exercise, you might not see changes unless you make a point of measuring a few things. Maybe you will steadily improve how many push-ups you can do, the amount of weight that you can lift, or how far or fast you can run, bike, or swim. Or maybe your resting heart rate will get lower and lower. I highly recommend measuring and tracking your fitness level in as many ways as you can manage.

Another perk of making exercise a reward in itself is that doing so may make you less likely to use unhealthy food as a reward for completing your workout. In two different studies, participants were sent on a walk either for exercise or for the pleasure of listening to music or sightseeing.[82] Even though everyone exerted the same amount of energy on the walk, the people who thought they were walking for exercise ate more unhealthy food afterward than the people who believed they were walking for pleasure. When you change your perception of exercise so that it is something pleasurable, you are less likely to feel the need to reward yourself in other, less healthy ways.

One final way to make exercise rewarding is to make it social—enjoy it with someone else. It's been shown that as with eating habits, other people's fitness habits can rub off on you.[83] If your friends or family members are regular exercisers, you may get swept up in their plans to go hiking, play tennis, or train for a 5K. Research also indicates that the social pressure that you internalize may help keep you on track.[84] For example, if my husband runs a few times when I don't, I feel some pressure to get back out there. Not because he says something. The man's no fool—he wouldn't dare. But his good habits have helped me internalize good habits of my own.

## Make Exercise Automatic

The bottom line with exercise, of course, is that we need to make it a habit. We can do that using some of the strategies we used to make healthy eating into a habit. To create a habit we need to repeatedly pair a healthy behavior with a particular setting or cue, and this can be helpful when it comes to your regular daily activities. You may be able to create habits to use stairs instead of elevators in certain buildings, or to walk to certain locations instead of drive. For planned workout sessions, the problem isn't usually pairing the workout with a setting. The problem is getting to one of those settings in the first place. Once you are there, you are pretty much home free.

One way to get yourself to the gym is by creating one of those if-then plans (which we called i-intentions earlier) in anticipation of situations in which you will be tempted to break your plan to exercise. So you might say, for example, "If I am tempted to skip working out because I feel too tired, then I will exercise at a lower intensity that day." This plan is useful because once you start your workout, odds are you will exercise at your normal intensity (and even if you don't, lower-intensity exercise is better than no exercise). The trick is to get yourself to start.

There is solid research showing that creating i-intentions for exercise helps people stick to their exercise plans.[85] In one study, participants were asked to form an i-intention about when and where they planned to exercise that week, to read a pamphlet about the importance of exercise for their health, or to do neither of those things.[86] Reading the pamphlet was no more effective than doing nothing. Only about 35 percent of the participants in each of those groups exercised that week. But 90 percent of the participants who had formed an i-intention exercised.[87] This makes sense, because the problem isn't that people don't believe in the importance of exercise. The problem is getting people to *act* on their intentions to exercise.[88]

In my view, the ideal way to overcome obstacles to exercise is to get locked into a plan. This is harder to do than you might think, since we are, after all, autonomous adults. When people put up the large sum of money for a health club membership, they often think that investment will force them into going. Unfortunately, as is clear from the large percent of people who join fitness clubs and either never go to the gym, or go infrequently, this doesn't work very well, or for very long.[89] The financial investment gradually fades from our mind or we grudgingly accept that it was wasted.

The problem there is that the penalty was paid in the past, so it doesn't motivate us for the future. What may work better is committing to some future penalty now, at a time when your intentions are strong, and then if you violate your plan later, when your resolve is weaker, the penalty automatically kicks in. This is an excellent idea, in theory, and it can work for eating,[90] but it is not easy to find a way to put this into practice when it comes to exercise.

The most effectively I have ever been locked into future workouts was as a member of a novice rowing team. All eight rowers on a crew must show up or nobody can go rowing, so each person is fully accountable to the group. You sign up for workouts ahead of time, when the workout is safely in the vague future and everyone is full of good intentions about exercising. When that alarm clock goes off before the sun rises, rolling over and going back to sleep is not an option, because the seven people who did drag themselves out of bed will kill you. You can't be more locked in than that.

The social nature of that penalty makes it particularly potent. You don't want to ruin things for other people, and you really don't want to make a lot of people furious at you. This is another reason why it can be helpful to have a workout partner. You'll be more likely to show up, and you'll work out at a higher intensity with your pal than if you work out alone.[91] To get that added bonus of feeling locked into the workout plan, you might choose a form of exercise that cannot be done unless both people are there, such as playing tennis. Or maybe your partner can only exercise if you drive her to the gym. That may help lock you into going.

The benefits of exercise simply cannot be denied. Regular exercise can increase your life span, prevent disease, reduce pain, make you less sensitive to stress, improve your mood, aid creativity, help you sleep better, and allow you to age more gracefully. These benefits are more easily attained than dramatic weight loss, and can be yours even if you don't lose a pound. So find a form of exercise you like, and pick a strategy or two that work for you. It really is worth it.

# FINAL WORDS: DIET SCHMIET

Someday soon, I'm sure, the diet industry will announce that it has finally found "the diet"—the one eating plan or pill or potion that is easy and pleasant, that makes the pounds melt away, and most important, keeps them off forever. When that day comes, I hope you will calmly observe the hoopla, but keep your wallet closed. A diet like that simply isn't possible, at least not with the current evolutionary state of the human body, the fragility of willpower, and our culture of ubiquitous temptations. Maybe you can lose the pounds relatively easily, but keeping them off would have to become your life's work. And your life is much too valuable to spend that way.

So diets don't work. Big deal. You don't need them to work. You need to not go on them. Should you binge eat, become a glutton, or never eat another vegetable? Of course not. Giving up dieting means eating in a sensible way most of the time, without extensive rules or restrictions. It's a perfectly reasonable thing to do, and nothing bad will happen if you do it. You won't gain a bunch of weight, because your genes will keep you in your general set weight range, and dieting wouldn't get you out of that range anyway. At least not for long.

You can be happy without dieting. And you should. Because dieting isn't merely ineffective. It is also harmful. Not just in the inevitable daily miseries that come with dieting, but in bigger ways, too.

Diets interfere with your thinking ability, lead to obsessive food thoughts, and cause stress, which leads to increases in your levels of the stress hormone cortisol. In high doses, cortisol can cause a multitude of problems, as well as lead to weight regain.[1] By not dieting, you will remove that source of stress from your life.

You can be healthy without dieting. Despite what you hear in the media, obesity will not kill you. Doing healthy things, like exercising, eating nutritious foods, and minimizing stress, will make (or keep) you healthy, even if they don't necessarily turn you into a skinny person.

Here's a perfectly sensible goal: reach your leanest livable weight, that comfortable weight at the low end of your set range. You'll have no trouble reaching it if you exercise regularly and use some of the smart regulation strategies in this book to create reasonable eating habits. The strategies will help you get to that weight and stay at that weight, without expending a lot of effort, without having to endure a life of self-denial, and without having to rely on willpower. Willpower, while quite useful in other parts of your life, is highly fallible, easy to deplete, and simply isn't potent enough to handle the onslaught of tempting foods that you are faced with on a daily basis. The smart regulation strategies don't require you to harness your willpower because again, despite what you may have heard, that has never been shown to be possible. Instead, the strategies just make sure you don't need it.

I urge you to get to your leanest livable weight and then, whatever it is, decide that it's okay. Because your weight is not the point. You were not put on this earth to mold yourself into a perfect physical specimen. As writer Glennon Melton says, "Your body is not your masterpiece—your *life* is."[2] So stop worrying about loving your body and get to work creating your masterpiece.

# ACKNOWLEDGMENTS

This book was written during my sabbatical at the University of Cambridge. I am grateful to Theresa Marteau for hosting my visit and for allowing me time to focus on this book. Thank you to Monica Luciana and the Department of Psychology at the University of Minnesota for granting this leave, for being so supportive of my unorthodox work, and for providing financial support for my lab. Thank you also to the departmental staff (especially Liz Gates and Terry Klosterman), and to my social area colleagues (led by Marti Gonzales) for really, truly, letting me off the hook on area duties this year. I'm back on now, I promise.

Gillian Sandstrom, it was wonderful getting to know you and celebrating finishing each chapter with you. I will miss you terribly when I go back home. Thank you to Sara Russo and everyone from the Clare Hall Boat Club for your patience with me; to cox extraordinaire Wilfred Wu for preventing what I was pretty sure was certain death; and to Corinne Benedek for the coffee and conversation, which was often the best part. Thanks also to Gabi Wojczuk at Café Aristo for the motivation to run when I didn't feel like it.

I am grateful to my classmates and professors at Stanford University, where some of the research I describe in this book was conducted, as well as the support I received from the National Science Foundation at the time. Thank you also to the other financial supporters of my work: the National Institutes of Health, NASA, the USDA, the Behavioral Economics and Nutrition

Center at Cornell University, and UCLA. The views in this book are mine, not theirs.

I didn't suffer as much as one is supposed to as an assistant professor thanks to the wonderful environment in the Psychology Department at UCLA. I particularly appreciated the kindness and support of my senior health psych colleagues, especially the women, who were incredible (if intimidating) role models: Chris Dunkel Schetter, Margaret Kemeny, Annette Stanton, and Shelley Taylor (who informed me that as an assistant professor I was done doing housework). And of course, my girls, Yuen Huo, Anna Lau, and Shelly Gable: I still miss you after all this time.

My lab would simply not function without my lab managers: Daniella Pallafacchina, Rachel Shasha, Ashley Moskovich, Jeff Hunger, Anna Larson, Toni Gabrielli, Britt Ahlstrom, Erin Hamilton, and Samantha Cinnick. Thank you for collaborating on this research, and for never making me feel stupid for not knowing how to do expense forms.

To the hundreds of undergraduate research assistants who worked so hard in my lab, running participants through our studies and somehow acting as if I was doing *you* a favor by giving you the opportunity to do so, I am forever indebted.

My graduate students have always been my favorite collaborators, and I have been just plain lucky to work with each of you. Thank you for taking a chance on me, on Minnesota, or both: Kelli Garcia, Erika Westling, David Creswell, Kathleen Hoffman Lambird, Ann-Marie Lew, Janet Tomiyama, Rachel Burns, Heather Scherschel, Mary Panos, and Lisa Auster-Gussman. And welcome to the family, Richie Lenne.

I am deeply grateful to the additional collaborators on the research in this book, including Zata Vickers, Joe Redden, Marla Reicks, Denise De Ridder, Ken Fujita, Elton Mykerezi, Lisa Comer, Katie Osdoba, Barbra Samuels, Jason Chatman, Nikki

Miller, Stephanie Elsbernd, Megan Spanjers, Hallie Espel, Kate Haltom, and Tiffany Ju. I know how much I owe you all, and I tried not to take too much credit here for our collaborative work (though they made me move most names to the endnotes). I sing your praises constantly out in the real world.

To Maryhope Howland Rutherford, dear friend and collaborator, I'm not sure I would have survived my first seven years in Minnesota without your support and friendship. It remains to be seen if I shall survive without you.

To Andrew Ward, my first and longest-running collaborator, people think I am joking when I say that it's fun writing grants, but it *is* fun when I write them with you. I am grateful for your sense of humor and am delighted to battle all reviewers and journal editors with you, plus Godzilla, the Smog Monster, and Lyle Brenner (thanks, Lyle, for comforting me with Bayesian stats), at least until we emerge from obscurity. So there's plenty of time.

Janet Tomiyama, former student, inspiration, and friend: I did not lie or exaggerate at your wedding. I say this without hyperbole: You are a superhero. I shudder to think what my career would have been like had I not opened my office door when you knocked on it. Watching your career has been one of the great joys of mine.

Thank you to the team of experts who kept me from making scientifically dubious claims in this book: Andrew Ward, Hallie Espel, Rob Low, David Creswell, David Sherman, Heather Scherschel, Mary Panos, Jeff Hunger, Janet Tomiyama, and Maryhope Howland Rutherford. Any errors that remain are mine. Special thanks to Britt Ahlstrom, who gave tons of extremely useful feedback on five chapters. Izzy Mann and Corral Johns also gave helpful feedback early in the process.

Two people read every word of this book, chapter by chapter, as I wrote it, and I could not be more grateful. Sabrina Lux, you are a goddess. How you can be so kind, so capable, and so good at literally everything, is beyond me. I am deeply appreciative of the comments you gave me on each chapter, despite being a very busy working mom. Laurie Abkemeier, I feel incredibly lucky that you agreed to represent me. Your willingness to read this as I wrote it, and your sensible feedback and support, have been incredibly helpful to me. You are a rockstar at your job. Thank you also to Julie Will at HarperWave for the insightful, thoughtful, and thorough editing despite being in the midst of wedding planning, and for being on the same wavelength as me about the point and goals of the book.

Like all working moms, I could not manage without outstanding child care. Thank you to the Infant Development Program at UCLA, and our many after-school nannies, including Bambi Laing, Minina Armstrong, Julia Krivi, and Sarah Eckholm. I firmly believe it takes a village, and in Edina, our village includes the clans of Chapdelaine, Huss, Johns, Ruppert, Burbach, and Orzoff, to name just a few. Thank you all, especially for your many kindnesses when my mother was ill.

I am grateful for the three women who have been motherlike to me since I lost my own: Aunt Fran Manushkin, who also gave helpful inside advice about the publishing world; my stepmom, Izzy Mann; and my mom-in-law, Trudie Engel. Also thank you to my extended family. There are too many of you to name, but this includes folks named Mann, Manushkin, Rosen, Levy, Levinson, Adler, Jacobson, Buzil, Krugman, Moos, Novak, Engel, Michels, Banton, and Kanfer, among others. That's right, we're Jews. And while we're on the subject, thank you to everyone at Shir Tikvah, the most progressive, radically hospitable community in the Twin Cities.

A special mention goes to my cousin Sally Rosen, who makes home still feel like home; my grandfather, Arnold Rosen, who turned one hundred while I wrote this and is an inspiring example of grace in adversity; and my brother, Barry Mann, who is a constant cheerleader, solid rock of the family, and just a general mensch. I'll sign any document you send me, without reading a word. And to my dad, who has made me feel special my whole life. I love you and the first copy off the presses is for you.

My husband, Steve Engel, has been ridiculously supportive throughout my career, and especially while I wrote this book. I'm pretty sure I didn't cook a single meal this entire year, and yet he (almost) never pointed that out or complained about it, despite also dealing with his own highly demanding job. He is the best writer and funniest person I know, and I'm pretty sure this book would have been better if he wrote it (but it would have taken a lot longer, so there's that). Plus, for twenty-three years and counting, he has an unblemished record of not tolerating fat talk.

Thanks to our sons, who are charming, interesting, hilarious, and infuriating. To Ben, my favorite partner in slothfulness, sushi eating, and concertgoing: Your laugh is still the best sound in the world, and your horn is a close second. Except when you make that loud elephant sound in my ear with it, which you are doing *right now*. And to Jonah: I never get tired of seeing the unique and fascinating ways your mind works. You are right and the whole world is wrong: watched pots do boil. I have just one question for you. Okay, a million questions. Starting with the most important one of all: cup or cone?

# NOTES

## CHAPTER 1: DIETS DON'T WORK

1. Many articles review the mass of short-term diet studies. These are only a sample. Albert Stunkard and Mavis McLaren-Hume, "The Results of Treatment for Obesity: A Review of the Literature and Report of a Series," *Archives of Internal Medicine* 103, no. 1 (1959): 79–85; William Bennett, "Dietary Treatments of Obesity," *Annals of the New York Academy of Sciences* 499 (June 1987): 250–63; Jeanine Cogan and Esther Rothblum, "Outcomes of Weight-Loss Programs," *Genetic, Social, and General Psychology Monographs* 118, no. 4 (1993): 385–415; M. G. Perri and P. R. Fuller, "Success and Failure in the Treatment of Obesity: Where Do We Go from Here?," *Medicine, Exercise, Nutrition and Health* 4 (1995): 255–72; Alain J. Nordmann et al., "Effects of Low-Carbohydrate vs. Low-Fat Diets on Weight Loss and Cardiovascular Risk Factors: A Meta-Analysis of Randomized Controlled Trials," *Archives of Internal Medicine* 166, no. 3 (February 13, 2006): 285–93, doi:10.1001/archinte.166.3.285.

2. For a history of diets, see Wayne C. Miller, "How Effective Are Traditional Dietary and Exercise Interventions for Weight Loss?," *Medicine & Science in Sports & Exercise* 31, no. 8 (August 1, 1999): 1129–34, doi:10.1097/00005768 199908000-00008.

3. Michael L. Dansinger et al., "Comparison of the Atkins, Ornish, Weight Watchers, and Zone Diets for Weight Loss and Heart Disease Risk Reduction: A Randomized Trial," *JAMA* 293, no. 1 (January 5, 2005): 43–53, doi:10.1001/jama.293.1.43.

4. According to the fatbet.net website.

5. Paul N. Chugay and Nikolas V. Chugay, "Weight Loss Tongue Patch: An Alternative Nonsurgical Method to Aid in Weight Loss in Obese Patients," *American Journal of Cosmetic Surgery* 31, no. 1 (April 1, 2014): 26–33.

6. The formula for BMI is (weight in kilograms)/(height in meters)$^2$.

7. K. J. Rothman, "BMI-Related Errors in the Measurement of Obesity," *International Journal of Obesity* 32, no. Suppl. 3 (August 2008): S56–9, doi:10.1038/ijo.2008.87.

8. World Health Organization, "BMI Classification," 2012.

9. The term "normal weight" is a misnomer. Those weights are not the norm, statistically speaking, and the term implies that all other weights are abnormal. I avoid it as much as possible in this book.

10.  For example, see Thomas R. Knapp, "A Methodological Critique of the 'Ideal Weight' Concept," *JAMA* 250, no. 4 (July 22, 1983): 506, doi:10.1001/jama.1983.03340040046030. A long discussion of this issue can be found in Glenn Alan Gaesser, *Big Fat Lies: The Truth about Your Weight and Your Health* (Carlsbad, CA: Gürze, 2002).

11.  Data come from the Metropolitan Life Insurance Company Tables, published in 1983.

12.  Stunkard and McLaren-Hume, "The Results of Treatment for Obesity."

13.  For example: R. R. Wing and R. W. Jeffery, "Outpatient Treatments of Obesity: A Comparison of Methodology and Clinical Results," *International Journal of Obesity* 3, no. 3 (1979): 261–79.

14.  Rena R. Wing and Suzanne Phelan, "Long-Term Weight Loss Maintenance," *American Journal of Clinical Nutrition* 82, no. 1 Suppl. (July 2005): 222S–225S.

15.  Institute of Medicine, "The Nature and Problem of Obesity," in *Weighing the Options: Criteria for Evaluating Weight-Management Programs*, ed. P. R. Thomas (Washington, DC: National Academy Press, 1995), 55–58.

16.  Robert W. Jeffery, Rena R. Wing, and Randall R. Mayer, "Are Smaller Weight Losses or More Achievable Weight Loss Goals Better in the Long Term for Obese Patients?," *Journal of Consulting and Clinical Psychology* 66, no. 4 (1998): 641–45.

17.  G. D. Foster et al., "What Is a Reasonable Weight Loss? Patients' Expectations and Evaluations of Obesity Treatment Outcomes," *Journal of Consulting and Clinical Psychology* 65, no. 1 (February 1997): 79–85.

18.  Weight Watchers has claimed to be more effective than other diets, but studies that compare different types of diets to each other do not support that. For example, see Marion J Franz et al., "Weight-Loss Outcomes: A Systematic Review and Meta-Analysis of Weight-Loss Clinical Trials with a Minimum 1-Year Follow-up." *Journal of the American Dietetic Association* 107, no. 10 (October 2007): 1755–67, doi:10.1016/j.jada.2007.07.017; Dansinger et al., "Comparison of the Atkins, Ornish, Weight Watchers, and Zone Diets for Weight Loss and Heart Disease Risk Reduction: A Randomized Trial.," *JAMA* 293, no. 1 (January 5, 2005): 43–53, doi:10.1001/jama.293.1.43; Bradley C. Johnston et al., "Comparison of Weight Loss among Named Diet Programs in Overweight and Obese Adults," *JAMA* 312, no. 9 (September 03, 2014): 923, doi:10.1001/jama.2014.10397.

19.  R. Cleland et al., "Commercial Weight Loss Products and Programs: What Consumers Stand to Gain and Lose. A Public Conference on the Information Consumers Need to Evaluate Weight Loss Products and Programs," *Critical Reviews in Food Science and Nutrition* 41, no. 1 (January 2001): 45–70, doi:10.1080/20014091091733.

20.  Ibid.

21.  Transcribed from "The Men Who Made Us Thin," series 1. The link was available on YouTube in August 2013: http://www.youtube.com/watch?v=I-_LoAm_etU

22.  This 16 percent success rate is higher than anything I've seen in the scientific literature, but it's the number the interviewer used in his question.

23.  Lucy Wallis, "Do Slimming Clubs Work?," *BBC News Magazine*, 2013, http://www.bbc.co.uk/news/magazine-23463006.

24.  Weight Watchers International, *Business Plan*, 2001.

25.  C. Ayyad and T. Andersen, "Long-Term Efficacy of Dietary Treatment of Obesity: A Systematic Review of Studies Published between 1931 and 1999," *Obesity Reviews* 1, no. 2 (2000): 113–19.

26.  David W. Swanson and Frank A. Dinello, "Follow-up of Patients Starved for Obesity," *Psychosomatic Medicine* 32, no. 2 (March 1, 1970): 209–14.

27.  Two examples are: D. D. Hensrud et al., "A Prospective Study of Weight Maintenance in Obese Subjects Reduced to Normal Body Weight Without Weight-Loss Training," *American Journal of Clinical Nutrition* 60, no. 5 (November 1, 1994): 688–94; F. M. Kramer et al., "Long-Term Follow-up of Behavioral Treatment for Obesity: Patterns of Weight Regain among Men and Women," *International Journal of Obesity* 13, no. 2 (1989): 123–36.

28.  That is why financial and other conflicts of interest must be reported at the end of papers. See Frank Davidoff, "Sponsorship, Authorship, and Accountability," *JAMA* 286, no. 10 (September 12, 2001): 1232, doi:10.1001/jama.286.10.1232.

29.  We review these studies in two papers: Traci Mann et al., "Medicare's Search for Effective Obesity Treatments: Diets Are Not the Answer," *American Psychologist* 62, no. 3 (April 2007): 220–33, doi:10.1037/0003-066X.62.3.220; Traci Mann, A. Janet Tomiyama, and Britt Ahlstrom, "Long-Term Effects of Dieting: Is Weight Loss Related to Health?," *Social and Personality Psychology Compass* 7, no. 12 (December 2013), 861–77.

30.  When we did these calculations, we statistically adjusted the means to account for the number of participants in each study. This is standard practice when some studies are huge and others are tiny. That prevents tiny studies from counting as much as larger ones.

31.  As earlier, these means are statistically weighted by the sample sizes.

32.  One researcher noted that "greater methodological rigor seems to be associated with poorer results." That is, if your study has none of these problems, it will likely show that most dieters regain the weight they lose. Kramer et al., "Long-Term Follow-up of Behavioral Treatment for Obesity," p. 126.

33.  An example is M. Hanefeld et al., "Diabetes Intervention Study: Multi-Intervention Trial in Newly Diagnosed NIDDM," *Diabetes Care* 14, no. 4 (1991): 308–17. Nineteen percent of potential participants were excluded before the study began because they had not been able to control their diabetes with their diet for the previous six weeks.

34.  Ranging from 5 percent in one study to 43 percent in another. Author's data.

35.  Francine Grodstein, "Three-Year Follow-up of Participants in a Commercial Weight Loss Program: Can You Keep It Off?," *Archives of Internal Medicine* 156, no. 12 (June 24, 1996): 1302, doi:10.1001/archinte.1996.00440110068009; C. Holzapfel et al., "The Challenge of a 2-Year Follow-up after Interven-

tion for Weight Loss in Primary Care," *International Journal of Obesity* (September 13, 2013), doi:10.1038/ijo.2013.180.

36.   M. F. Hovell et al., "Long-Term Weight Loss Maintenance: Assessment of a Behavioral and Supplemented Fasting Regimen," *American Journal of Public Health* 78, no. 6 (June 1, 1988): 663–66.

37.   Robert L. Bowman and Janice L. DeLucia, "Accuracy of Self-Reported Weight: A Meta-Analysis," *Behavior Therapy* 23, no. 4 (1992): 637–55.

38.   G. D. Foster et al., "Psychological Effects of Weight Loss and Regain: A Prospective Evaluation," *Journal of Consulting and Clinical Psychology* 64, no. 4 (1996): 752–57.

39.   T. A. Wadden et al., "Treatment of Obesity by Very Low Calorie Diet, Behavior Therapy, and Their Combination: A Five-Year Perspective," *International Journal of Obesity* 13 Suppl 2 (January 1, 1989): 39–46.

40.   This was corroborated in a survey of dieters. Sixty percent had weighed more than their starting weight at some point since the diet ended, even though only 40 percent did on the day of the survey. Grodstein, "Three-Year Follow-up of Participants in a Commercial Weight Loss Program."lol

41.   David M. Garner and Susan C. Wooley, "Confronting the Failure of Behavioral and Dietary Treatments for Obesity," *Clinical Psychology Review* 11, no. 6 (1991): 729–80, doi:10.1016/0272-7358(91)90128-h.

42.   K. D. Brownell, "Obesity: Understanding and Treating a Serious, Prevalent, and Refractory Disorder," *Journal of Consulting and Clinical Psychology* 50, no. 6 (December 1982): 820–40.

## CHAPTER 2: WHY DIETS DON'T WORK: BIOLOGY, STRESS, AND FORBIDDEN FRUIT

1.    Although many studies do show genes that are involved in obesity. For example: Eleanor Wheeler et al., "Genome-Wide SNP and CNV Analysis Identifies Common and Low-Frequency Variants Associated with Severe Early-Onset Obesity," *Nature Genetics* 45, no. 5 (May 2013): 513–17, doi:10.1038/ng.2607.

2.    Albert J. Stunkard et al., "An Adoption Study of Human Obesity," *New England Journal of Medicine* 314, no. 4 (January 23, 1986): 193–98, doi:10.1056/NEJM198601233140401.

3.    T. Bouchard et al., "Sources of Human Psychological Differences: The Minnesota Study of Twins Reared Apart," *Science* 250, no. 4978 (October 12, 1990): 223–28, doi:10.1126/science.2218526.

4.    There are many twin studies of body weight, but this one is the classic: Albert J. Stunkard et al., "The Bodymass Index of Twins Who Have Been Reared Apart," *New England Journal of Medicine* 322 (1990): 1483–87.

5.    Karri Silventoinen et al., "Heritability of Adult Body Height: A Comparative Study of Twin Cohorts in Eight Countries," *Twin Research: The Official Journal of the International Society for Twin Studies* 6, no. 5 (October 2003): 399–408, doi:10.1375/136905203770326402.

6.   Krista Casazza et al., "Myths, Presumptions, and Facts about Obesity," *New England Journal of Medicine* 368, no. 5 (January 30, 2013): 446–54, doi:10.1056/NEJMsa1208051. In this thorough scientific analysis of diet myths and truths, researchers concluded that people's weight (in relation to their height) tends to stay in the same general range over their life span, and that this is primarily based on their genes, rather than on eating habits they learned as a child. One piece of evidence they cited was T. D. Brisbois, A. P. Farmer, and L. J. McCargar, "Early Markers of Adult Obesity: A Review," *Obesity Reviews* 13, no. 4 (April 1, 2012): 347–67, doi:10.1111/j.1467 789X.2011.00965.x.

7.   The researcher summarizes his own studies in: E. A. Sims, "Experimental Obesity, Dietary-Induced Thermogenesis, and Their Clinical Implications," *Clinics in Endocrinology and Metabolism* 5, no. 2 (July 1976): 377–95. A wonderful overall summary of this kind of work is in Gina Kolata, *Rethinking Thin: The New Science of Weight Loss—and the Myths and Realities of Dieting* (New York: Picador, 2008).

8.   Sims, "Experimental Obesity, Dietary-Induced Thermogenesis, and Their Clinical Implications."

9.   Claude Bouchard et al., "The Response to Long-Term Overfeeding in Identical Twins," *New England Journal of Medicine* 322, no. 21 (May 24, 1990): 1477–82, doi:10.1056/NEJM199005243222101. Additional evidence appears in A. Tremblay et al., "Overfeeding and Energy Expenditure in Humans," *American Journal of Clinical Nutrition* 56, no. 5 (November 1, 1992): 857–62.

10.  This is not because the different pairs of twins engaged in different amounts of exercise. Other studies have held exercise constant and still found large differences in how much weight different people gained from overeating the same amount of calories. James A. Levine, Norman L. Eberhardt, and Michael D. Jensen, "Role of Nonexercise Activity Thermogenesis in Resistance to Fat Gain in Humans," *Science* 283, no. 5399 (January 8, 1999): 212–14, doi:10.1126/science.283.5399.212.

11.  A good summary appears in Jeffrey M. Friedman, "A War on Obesity, Not the Obese," *Science* 299, no. 5608 (February 7, 2003): 856–58, doi:10.1126/science.1079856.

12.  Eric Stice, Kyle Burger, and Sonja Yokum, "Caloric Deprivation Increases Responsivity of Attention and Reward Brain Regions to Intake, Anticipated Intake, and Images of Palatable Foods," *NeuroImage* 67 (2013): 322–30.

13.  Kathleen A. Page et al., "Circulating Glucose Levels Modulate Neural Control of Desire for High-Calorie Foods in Humans," *Journal of Clinical Investigation* 121, no. 10 (October 3, 2011): 4161–69, doi:10.1172/JCI57873.

14.  Stice, Burger, and Yokum, "Caloric Deprivation Increases Responsivity of Attention and Reward Brain Regions to Intake, Anticipated Intake, and Images of Palatable Foods."

15.  Jules Hirsch, "Obesity: Matter over Mind," *Cerebrum* 5, no. 1 (2003): 7–18.

16.  Erin E. Kershaw and Jeffrey S. Flier, "Adipose Tissue as an Endocrine Or-

gan," *Journal of Clinical Endocrinology and Metabolism* 89, no. 6 (June 2004): 2548–56, doi:10.1210/jc.2004-0395.

17.    Priya Sumithran et al., "Long-Term Persistence of Hormonal Adaptations to Weight Loss," *New England Journal of Medicine* 365, no. 17 (October 27, 2011): 1597–1604, doi:10.1056/NEJMoa1105816.

18.    Ibid.

19.    P. A. Tataranni and E. Ravussin, "Energy Metabolism and Obesity," in *Handbook of Obesity Treatment*, ed. T. A. Wadden and A. J. Stunkard (New York: Guilford Press, 2004), 42–72.

20.    A. G. Dulloo and L. Girardier, "Adaptive Changes in Energy Expenditure during Refeeding Following Low-Calorie Intake: Evidence for a Specific Metabolic Component Favoring Fat Storage," *American Journal of Clinical Nutrition* 52, no. 3 (September 1, 1990): 415–20.

21.    Rudolph L. Leibel and Jules Hirsch, "Diminished Energy Requirements in Reduced-Obese Patients," *Metabolism* 33, no. 2 (February 1984): 164–70, doi:10.1016/0026-0495(84)90130-6. Also see: R. L. Leibel, M. Rosenbaum, and J. Hirsch, "Changes in Energy Expenditure Resulting from Altered Body Weight," *New England Journal of Medicine* 332, no. 10 (March 9, 1995).

22.    Leibel and Hirsch, "Diminished Energy Requirements in Reduced-Obese Patients."

23.    Ancel Keys et al., *The Biology of Human Starvation*, vols. 1 and 2 (Minneapolis: University of Minnesota Press, 1950).

24.    Ibid.

25.    The collaborator was Andrew Ward.

26.    T. Mann and A. Ward, "Forbidden Fruit: Does Thinking about a Prohibited Food Lead to Its Consumption?," *International Journal of Eating Disorders* 29, no. 3 (April 2001): 319–27; Plus a study with kids finds they eat more of a food that was forbidden for just five minutes. Esther Jansen et al., "From the Garden of Eden to the Land of Plenty," *Appetite* 51, no. 3 (2008): 570–75.

27.    Shelley Taylor, *Health Psychology*, 8th ed. (New York: McGraw-Hill, 2011).

28.    Everything I say about stress in this paragraph and the next one comes from Robert Sapolsky's brilliant book, *Why Zebras Don't Get Ulcers*, 3rd ed. (New York: Holt Paperbacks, 2004).

29.    Pamela M. Peeke and George P. Chrousos, "Hypercortisolism and Obesity," *Annals of the New York Academy of Sciences* 771, no. 1 (December 1, 1995): 665–76, doi:10.1111/j.1749-6632.1995.tb44719.x; P. Björntorp, "Do Stress Reactions Cause Abdominal Obesity and Comorbidities?," *Obesity Reviews* 2, no. 2 (May 1, 2001): 73–86, doi:10.1046/j.1467-789x.2001.00027.x.

30.    C. Greeno and R. Wing, "Stress-Induced Eating," *Psychological Bulletin* 115 (1994): 444.

31.    Stephanie M. Greer, Andrea N. Goldstein, and Matthew P. Walker, "The Impact of Sleep Deprivation on Food Desire in the Human Brain," *Nature Communications* 4 (August 6, 2013): 2259, doi:10.1038/ncomms3259.

32.    Rachel R Markwald et al., "Impact of Insufficient Sleep on Total Daily Energy Expenditure, Food Intake, and Weight Gain," *Proceedings of the Na-*

*tional Academy of Sciences of the United States of America* 110, no. 14 (April 2, 2013): 5695–5700, doi:10.1073/pnas.1216951110.

33.   A. Janet Tomiyama et al., "Low Calorie Dieting Increases Cortisol," *Psychosomatic Medicine* 72, no. 4 (May 2010): 357–64, doi:10.1097/PSY.0b013e3181d9523c.

34.   Ibid.

35.   Diana E. Pankevich et al., "Caloric Restriction Experience Reprograms Stress and Orexigenic Pathways and Promotes Binge Eating," *Journal of Neuroscience{dec63}* 30, no. 48 (December 1, 2010): 16399–407, doi:10.1523/JNEUROSCI.1955-10.2010.

36.   Jeffrey Friedman, cited on page 125 of Kolata, *Rethinking Thin.*

## CHAPTER 3: THE MYTH OF WILLPOWER

1.   Sorbet is usually lower in sugars and carbohydrates than ice cream but just a little bit lower, so if you are trying to reduce those, sorbet might not be the most helpful choice for you.

2.   K. D. Brownell and K. B. Horgen, *Food Fight: The Inside Story of the Food Industry, America's Obesity Crisis, and What We Can Do About It* (Chicago: Contemporary Books, 2004). Brownell refers to this environment as a "toxic food environment."

3.   For the argument that fats and sugars cause cravings for more fats and sugars, and that the food industry has taken advantage of this, see D. A. Kessler, *The End of Overeating: Taking Control of the Insatiable American Appetite* (Emmaus, PA: Rodale, 2009).

4.   John P. Foreyt and G. Ken Goodrick, *Living Without Dieting* (New York: Grand Central, 1994).

5.   The most commonly used questionnaire for measuring self-control can be found in J. Tangney, R. Baumeister, and A. Boone, "High Self-Control Predicts Good Adjustment, Less Pathology, Better Grades, and Interpersonal Success," *Journal of Personality* 72, no. 2 (2004): 271–324.

6.   M. Friese and W. Hofmann, "Control Me or I Will Control You: Impulses, Trait Self-Control, and the Guidance of Behavior," *Journal of Research in Personality* (2009).

7.   They did a much better job than we did, which is why our study was never published, but theirs was: Denise T. D. de Ridder et al., "Taking Stock of Self-Control: A Meta-Analysis of How Trait Self-Control Relates to a Wide Range of Behaviors," *Personality and Social Psychology Review* 16, no. 1 (February 1, 2012): 76–99, doi:10.1177/1088868311418749.

8.   Brandon J. Schmeichel and Anne Zell, "Trait Self-Control Predicts Performance on Behavioral Tests of Self-Control," *Journal of Personality* 75, no. 4 (August 2007): 743–55, doi:10.1111/j.1467-6494.2007.00455.x.

9.   Walter Mischel and Ebbe Ebbesen, "Attention in Delay of Gratification," *Journal of Personality and Social Psychology* 16, no. 2 (1970): 329–37.

10.   The stress and frustration findings are in W. Mischel, Y. Shoda, and P. K.

Peake, "The Nature of Adolescent Competencies Predicted by Preschool Delay of Gratification," *Journal of Personality and Social Psychology* 54, no. 4 (April 1988): 687–96. A review of many findings from that line of research is in W. Mischel, Y. Shoda, and M. Rodriguez, "Delay of Gratification in Children," *Choice over Time* (New York: Russell Sage Foundation, 1992), 147–64.

11.  Body mass index is a measure of weight that takes height into account.

12.  Tanya R. Schlam et al., "Preschoolers' Delay of Gratification Predicts Their Body Mass 30 Years Later," *Journal of Pediatrics* 162, no. 1 (January 2013): 90–93, doi:10.1016/j.jpeds.2012.06.049. The fact that there is any relationship whatsoever to behavior that occurs thirty years later is remarkable, but the delay of gratification test explains only about 4 percent of the differences between people's weights, leaving the other 96 percent to be accounted for by other things.

13.  Other studies have used that same kind of test and found similarly small relationships, and once researchers control for common confounding factors, they tend to disappear. For example, see the following studies for, in order, a similar small relationship, an even smaller one, and no relationship at all. Lori A. Francis and Elizabeth J. Susman, "Self-Regulation and Rapid Weight Gain in Children from Age 3 to 12 Years," *Archives of Pediatrics & Adolescent Medicine* 163, no. 4 (April 6, 2009): 297–302, doi:10.1001/ archpediatrics.2008.579; Angela L. Duckworth, Eli Tsukayama, and Andrew B. Geier, "Self-Controlled Children Stay Leaner in the Transition to Adolescence," *Appetite* 54, no. 2 (2010): 304–8; Desiree M Seeyave et al., "Ability to Delay Gratification at Age 4 Years and Risk of Overweight at Age 11 Years," *Archives of Pediatrics & Adolescent Medicine* 163, no. 4 (April 6, 2009): 303–8, doi:10.1001/archpediatrics.2009.12.

14.  Joseph P. Redden and Kelly Haws, "Healthy Satiation: The Role of Decreasing Desire in Effective Self-Control" (October 25, 2012).

15.  Nicholas Carr, *The Shallows: What the Internet Is Doing to Our Brains* (New York: Norton, 2011).

16.  Larry D. Rosen, L. Mark Carrier, and Nancy A. Cheever, "Facebook and Texting Made Me Do It: Media-Induced Task-Switching While Studying," *Computers in Human Behavior* 29, no. 3 (May 2013): 948–58, doi:10.1016/j .chb.2012.12.001.

17.  Andrew Ward and Traci Mann, "Don't Mind If I Do: Disinhibited Eating under Cognitive Load," *Journal of Personality and Social Psychology* 78, no. 4 (April 1, 2000): 753–63, doi:10.1037//0022-3514.78.4.753.

18.  Philip G. Zimbardo, "On the Ethics of Intervention in Human Psychological Research: With Special Reference to the Stanford Prison Experiment," *Cognition* 2, no. 2 (January 1973): 243–56.

19.  J. Polivy and C. P. Herman, "Effects of Alcohol on Eating Behavior: Influence of Mood and Perceived Intoxication," *Journal of Abnormal Psychology* 85, no. 6 (December 1976): 601–6.

20.  This idea comes from our professor Claude Steele's work on alcohol my-

opia, described in C. M. Steele and R. A. Josephs, "Alcohol Myopia: Its Prized and Dangerous Effects," *American Psychologist* 45, no. 8 (August 1990): 921–33.

21.   Plus we have to justify to the university's Institutional Review Board why we are using deception, and show that we are using as little of it as possible.

22.   This is the classic example: C. Peter Herman and Deborah Mack, "Restrained and Unrestrained Eating," *Journal of Personality* 43, no. 4 (December 1975): 647–60, doi:10.1111/j.1467-6494.1975.tb00727.x.

23.   Seven studies of this are shown in Greeno and Wing, "Stress-Induced Eating." And there have been many more since then.

24.   C. Peter Herman and Janet Polivy, "Anxiety, Restraint, and Eating Behavior," *Journal of Abnormal Psychology* 84, no. 6 (1975): 666–72, doi:10.1037/0021 843X.84.6.666.

25.   Two examples: Elissa Epel et al., "Stress May Add Bite to Appetite in Women: A Laboratory Study of Stress-Induced Cortisol and Eating Behavior," *Psychoneuroendocrinology* 26, no. 1 (January 2001): 37–49, doi:10.1016/S0306-4530(00)00035-4; Summar Habhab, Jane P. Sheldon, and Roger C. Loeb, "The Relationship between Stress, Dietary Restraint, and Food Preferences in Women," *Appetite* 52, no. 2 (April 2009): 437–44, doi:10.1016/j .appet.2008.12.006.

26.   J. Cools, D. E. Schotte, and R. J. McNally, "Emotional Arousal and Overeating in Restrained Eaters," *Journal of Abnormal Psychology* 101, no. 2 (May 1992): 348–51.

27.   A. Janet Tomiyama, Traci Mann, and Lisa Comer, "Triggers of Eating in Everyday Life," *Appetite* 52, no. 1 (2009): 72–82.

28.   Eighty-three separate studies are cited in Martin S. Hagger et al., "Ego Depletion and the Strength Model of Self-Control: A Meta-Analysis," *Psychological Bulletin* 136, no. 4 (July 2010): 495–525, doi:10.1037/a0019486.

29.   This is the original study of this phenomenon: Roy F. Baumeister et al., "Ego Depletion: Is the Active Self a Limited Resource?," *Journal of Personality and Social Psychology* 74, no. 5 (1998): 1252–65, doi:10.1037/002 2-3514.74.5.1252.

30.   All of these are cited in Hagger et al., "Ego Depletion and the Strength Model of Self-Control: A Meta-Analysis."

31.   The many downsides of having too much choice are covered beautifully in Barry Schwartz, *The Paradox of Choice*, (New York: Ecco, 2003).

32.   S. S. Iyengar and M. R. Lepper, "When Choice Is Demotivating: Can One Desire Too Much of a Good Thing?," *Journal of Personality and Social Psychology* 79, no. 6 (December 2000): 995–1006.

33.   Kathleen D. Vohs et al., "Making Choices Impairs Subsequent Self-Control: A Limited-Resource Account of Decision Making, Self-Regulation, and Active Initiative," *Journal of Personality and Social Psychology* 94, no. 5 (May 2008): 883–98, doi:10.1037/0022-3514.94.5.883.

34.   Michael Lewis, "Obama's Way," *Vanity Fair*, 2012.

35.   See, for example, Roy F. Baumeister and John Tierney, *Willpower: Rediscov-*

*ering the Greatest Human Strength* (New York: Penguin Books, 2012).

36.  These articles seem a bit peripheral to the issue. Instead of teaching self-regulation, they have participants do things like control their posture or engage in an exercise program, and then show that they can control *something else* better. In addition, they are riddled with methodological problems that would keep a research methods class busy for hours. M. Muraven, R. F. Baumeister, and D. M. Tice, "Longitudinal Improvement of Self-Regulation Through Practice: Building Self-Control Strength Through Repeated Exercise," *Journal of Social Psychology* 139, no. 4 (August 1999): 446–57, doi:10.1080/00224549909598404; Megan Oaten and Ken Cheng, "Improved Self-Control: The Benefits of a Regular Program of Academic Study," *Basic and Applied Social Psychology* 28, no. 1 (April 2006): 1–16, doi:10.1207/s15324834basp2801_1; Megan Oaten and Ken Cheng, "Longitudinal Gains in Self-Regulation from Regular Physical Exercise," *British Journal of Health Psychology* 11, Pt. 4 (November 2006): 717–33, doi:10.1348/135910706X96481.

37.  Dutch self-control researcher Denise De Ridder introduced me to this saying. It is also common in Gaelic.

38.  See, for example, Wilhelm Hofmann et al., "Everyday Temptations: An Experience Sampling Study of Desire, Conflict, and Self-Control," *Journal of Personality and Social Psychology* 102, no. 6 (June 2012): 1318–35, doi:10.1037/a0026545.

## CHAPTER 4: DIETS ARE BAD FOR YOU

1.  All information about the study comes from Keys et al., *The Biology of Human Starvation*, vols. 1 and 2.

2.  Ibid., p. 810. Keys attributes it to A. W. Greely, *Three Years of Arctic Service*: *An Account of the Lady Franklin Bay Expedition of 1881–1884 and the Attainment of the Farthest North* (New York: Scribner, 1886).

3.  Keys et al., *The Biology of Human Starvation*, vols. 1 and 2, p. 811. Keys also attributes this to Greely.

4.  Ibid.

5.  The man was John Franklin, and it did not end well for him the next time. Anthony Brandt, *The Man Who Ate His Boots*: *The Tragic History of the Search for the Northwest Passage* (New York: Knopf, 2010).

6.  Keys et al., *The Biology of Human Starvation*, vols. 1 and 2, p. 776. The quote is from Keys, but he is paraphrasing a work in Czech, which I cannot access (or read): J. Stavel, *Hlad*: *Prispevek K Analyse Pudu* (Bratislava: Philosophy Faculty, Comenius University, 1936).

7.  For this reason, some people consider the experience of these men to be more similar to the eating disorder of anorexia than to mere dieting.

8.  Stephen Smith, "Battles of Belief in World War II," *American Radioworks*, 2013, http://americanradioworks.publicradio.org/features/wwii/transcript.html.

9.  The exception is the set of tests that the men were trained on extensively

before starvation. They continued to do fine on those even during starvation, suggesting that you might not see impairments on well-learned processes.

10. Michael W. Green and Nicola A. Elliman, "Are Dieting-Related Cognitive Impairments a Function of Iron Status?," *British Journal of Nutrition* 109, no. 1 (January 14, 2013): 184–92, doi:10.1017/S0007114512000864.

11. M. W. Green et al., "Impairment of Cognitive Performance Associated with Dieting and High Levels of Dietary Restraint," *Physiology & Behavior* 55, no. 3 (March 1994): 447–52; Michael W. Green and Peter J. Rogers, "Impairments in Working Memory Associated with Spontaneous Dieting Behaviour," *Psychological Medicine* 28, no. 5 (September 1, 1998): 1063–70; Jacqueline Shaw and Marika Tiggemann, "Dieting and Working Memory: Preoccupying Cognitions and the Role of the Articulatory Control Process," *British Journal of Health Psychology* 9, Pt. 2 (May 2004): 175–85, doi:10.1348/135910704773891032; Louise Vreugdenburg, Janet Bryan, and Eva Kemps, "The Effect of Self-Initiated Weight-Loss Dieting on Working Memory: The Role of Preoccupying Cognitions," *Appetite* 41, no. 3 (2003): 291–300; P. J. Rogers and M. W. Green, "Dieting, Dietary Restraint and Cognitive Performance," *British Journal of Clinical Psychology* 32, Pt. 1 (February 1993): 113–16.

12. Green and Rogers, "Impairments in Working Memory Associated with Spontaneous Dieting Behaviour"; Eva Kemps, Marika Tiggemann, and Kelly Marshall, "Relationship between Dieting to Lose Weight and the Functioning of the Central Executive," *Appetite* 45, no. 3 (2005): 287–94; Eva Kemps and Marika Tiggemann, "Working Memory Performance and Preoccupying Thoughts in Female Dieters: Evidence for a Selective Central Executive Impairment," *British Journal of Clinical Psychology* 44, Pt. 3 (September 2005): 357–66, doi:10.1348/014466505X35272; Vreugdenburg, Bryan, and Kemps, "The Effect of Self-Initiated Weight-Loss Dieting on Working Memory."

13. Nicola Jones and Peter J. Rogers, "Preoccupation, Food, and Failure: An Investigation of Cognitive Performance Deficits in Dieters," *International Journal of Eating Disorders* 33, no. 2 (March 2003): 185–92, doi:10.1002/eat.10124.

14. Michael W. Green and Peter J. Rogers, "Impaired Cognitive Functioning during Spontaneous Dieting," *Psychological Medicine* 25, no. 05 (July 9, 1995): 1003, doi:10.1017/S0033291700037491; Kemps, Tiggemann, and Marshall, "Relationship between Dieting to Lose Weight and the Functioning of the Central Executive"; Vreugdenburg, Bryan, and Kemps, "The Effect of Self-Initiated Weight-Loss Dieting on Working Memory."

15. Vanessa Engle, quoted in Ermine Saner, "The Fat Controllers," *Guardian*, August 8, 2013.

16. Kemps, Tiggemann, and Marshall, "Relationship between Dieting to Lose Weight and the Functioning of the Central Executive"; Kemps and Tiggemann, "Working Memory Performance and Preoccupying Thoughts in Female Dieters"; Vreugdenburg, Bryan, and Kemps, "The Effect of Self-

Initiated Weight-Loss Dieting on Working Memory."

17.    Jones and Rogers, "Preoccupation, Food, and Failure."

18.    Green and Rogers, "Impaired Cognitive Functioning during Spontaneous Dieting"; Kemps and Tiggemann, "Working Memory Performance and Preoccupying Thoughts in Female Dieters"; Kemps, Tiggemann, and Marshall, "Relationship between Dieting to Lose Weight and the Functioning of the Central Executive"; Vreugdenburg, Bryan, and Kemps, "The Effect of Self-Initiated Weight-Loss Dieting on Working Memory."

19.    Green and Rogers, "Impaired Cognitive Functioning during Spontaneous Dieting."

20.    Hirsch, "Obesity: Matter over Mind."

21.    Kathleen D. Vohs and Brandon J. Schmeichel, "Self-Regulation and Extended Now: Controlling the Self Alters the Subjective Experience of Time," *Journal of Personality and Social Psychology* 85 (2003): 217–30.

22.    It's possible I am the person who said this. I've said it a lot over the years. I searched the Internet and can't find it at all.

23.    A. Janet Tomiyama et al., "Low Calorie Dieting Increases Cortisol," *Psychosomatic Medicine* 72, no. 4 (May 2010): 357–64, doi:10.1097/PSY.0b013e3181d9523c. Also see: Michael W. Green, Nicola A. Elliman, and Mary J. Kretsch, "Weight Loss Strategies, Stress, and Cognitive Function: Supervised versus Unsupervised Dieting," *Psychoneuroendocrinology* 30, no. 9 (2005): 908–18.

24.    Everything I say about stress in this paragraph and the next comes from Robert Sapolsky's brilliant book, *Why Zebras Don't Get Ulcers*, 3rd ed.

25.    A. Janet Tomiyama et al., "Does Cellular Aging Relate to Patterns of Allostasis? An Examination of Basal and Stress Reactive HPA Axis Activity and Telomere Length," *Physiology & Behavior* 106, no. 1 (April 12, 2012): 40–45, doi:10.1016/j.physbeh.2011.11.016.

26.    Amy Kiefer et al., "Dietary Restraint and Telomere Length in Pre- and Post-Menopausal Women," *Psychosomatic Medicine* 70, no. 8 (October 1, 2008): 845–49, doi:10.1097/PSY.0b013e318187d05e.

27.    David Gal and Wendy Liu, "Grapes of Wrath: The Angry Effects of Self-Control," *Journal of Consumer Research* 38, no. 3 (2011): 445–58.

28.    Keys et al., *The Biology of Human Starvation*, vols. 1 and 2, p. 907.

29.    Smith, "Battles of Belief in World War II."

30.    Thomas A. Wadden et al., "Dieting and the Development of Eating Disorders in Obese Women: Results of a Randomized Controlled Trial," *American Journal of Clinical Nutrition* 80, no. 3 (September 1, 2004): 560–68; Diann M. Ackard, Jillian K. Croll, and Ann Kearney-Cooke, "Dieting Frequency among College Females: Association with Disordered Eating, Body Image, and Related Psychological Problems," *Journal of Psychosomatic Research* 52, no. 3 (2002): 129–36; F. M. Cachelin and P. C. Regan, "Prevalence and Correlates of Chronic Dieting in a Multi-Ethnic U.S. Community Sample," *Eating and Weight Disorders* 11, no. 2 (June 1, 2006): 91–99; Scott Crow et al., "Psychosocial and Behavioral Correlates of Dieting among Overweight

and Non-Overweight Adolescents," *Journal of Adolescent Health* 38, no. 5 (2006): 569–74; Meghan M. Gillen, Charlotte N. Markey, and Patrick M. Markey, "An Examination of Dieting Behaviors among Adults: Links with Depression," *Eating Behaviors* 13, no. 2 (2012): 88–93; T. A. Wadden, A. J. Stunkard, and J. W. Smoller, "Dieting and Depression: A Methodological Study," *Journal of Consulting and Clinical Psychology* 54, no. 6 (1986): 869.

31. Reviewed in Rena R. Wing et al., "Mood Changes in Behavioral Weight Loss Programs," *Journal of Psychosomatic Research* 28, no. 3 (1984): 189–96.

32. Ibid.

33. Reviewed in Jordan W. Smoller, Thomas A. Wadden, and Albert J. Stunkard, "Dieting and Depression: A Critical Review," *Journal of Psychosomatic Research* 31, no. 4 (1987): 429–40.

34. Dacher Keltner, "Evidence for the Distinctness of Embarrassment, Shame, and Guilt: A Study of Recalled Antecedents and Facial Expressions of Emotion," *Cognition & Emotion* 10, no. 2 (March 1996): 155–72, doi:10.1080/026999396380312.

35. Ben C. Fletcher et al., "How Visual Images of Chocolate Affect the Craving and Guilt of Female Dieters," *Appetite* 48, no. 2 (2007): 211–17; Gillian A. King, C. Peter Herman, and Janet Polivy, "Food Perception in Dieters and Non-Dieters," *Appetite* 8, no. 2 (1987): 147–58.

36. B. Wansink, M. Cheney, and N. Chan, "Exploring Comfort Food Preferences Across Age and Gender," *Physiology & Behavior* 79, nos. 4–5 (September 2003): 739–47, doi:10.1016/S0031-9384(03)00203-8.

37. Michael Prager, "I Don't Consider Fatness a Problem," MichaelPrager .com/blog, 2013, http://michaelprager.com/content/i-dont-consider-fatness-problem-Deb-Burgard-Health-At-Every-Size.

38. June Price Tangney, Jeff Stuewig, and Debra J Mashek, "Moral Emotions and Moral Behavior," *Annual Review of Psychology* 58 (January 2007): 345–72, doi:10.1146/annurev.psych.56.091103.070145.

39. Tara L. Gruenewald et al., "Acute Threat to the Social Self: Shame, Social Self-Esteem, and Cortisol Activity," *Psychosomatic Medicine* 66, no. 6 (January 1, 2004): 915–24, doi:10.1097/01.psy.0000143639.61693.ef.

40. Sally S. Dickerson et al., "Immunological Effects of Induced Shame and Guilt," *Psychosomatic Medicine* 66, no. 1 (2004): 124–31.

41. Tangney, Stuewig, and Mashek, "Moral Emotions and Moral Behavior."

42. Eric Stice, "Risk and Maintenance Factors for Eating Pathology: A Meta-Analytic Review," *Psychological Bulletin* 128, no. 5 (September 2002): 825–48.

43. Ibid.

44. Eric Stice et al., "Fasting Increases Risk for Onset of Binge Eating and Bulimic Pathology: A 5-Year Prospective Study," *Journal of Abnormal Psychology* 117, no. 4 (November 1, 2008): 941–46, doi:10.1037/a0013644.

45. Wadden et al., "Dieting and the Development of Eating Disorders in Obese Women."

46. Donald A. Williamson et al., "Is Caloric Restriction Associated with

Development of Eating-Disorder Symptoms? Results from the CAL-ERIE Trial," *Health Psychology* 27, no. 1 Suppl. (January 2008): S32–42, doi:10.1037/0278-6133.27.1.S32.

47.  Stice, Burger, and Yokum, "Caloric Deprivation Increases Responsivity of Attention and Reward Brain Regions to Intake, Anticipated Intake, and Images of Palatable Foods."

48.  Gene-Jack Wang et al., "Regional Brain Metabolic Activation during Craving Elicited by Recall of Previous Drug Experiences," *Life Sciences* 64, no. 9 (1999): 775–84.

49.  A. E. Field et al., "Weight Cycling, Weight Gain, and Risk of Hypertension in Women," *American Journal of Epidemiology* 150, no. 6 (1999): 573–79.

50.  Richard L. Atkinson, "Weight Cycling," *JAMA* 272, no. 15 (October 19, 1994): 1196, doi:10.1001/jama.1994.03520150064038.

51.  Mette K. Simonsen et al., "Intentional Weight Loss and Mortality among Initially Healthy Men and Women," *Nutrition Reviews* 66, no. 7 (July 2008): 375–86, doi:10.1111/j.1753-4887.2008.00047.x; M. E. Perez Morales, A. Jimenez Cruz, and M. Bacardi Gascon, "The Effect of Weight Loss on Mortality: A Systematic Review from 2000 to 2009," *Nutrición Hospitalaria* 25, no. 5 (2010): 718–24, doi:S0212-16112010000500006 [pii].

52.  M. Harrington, S. Gibson, and R. C. Cottrell, "A Review and Meta-Analysis of the Effect of Weight Loss on All-Cause Mortality Risk," *Nutrition Research Reviews* 22, no. 1 (2009): 93–108, doi:10.1017/S0954422409990035; Victoria L Stevens et al., "Weight Cycling and Mortality in a Large Prospective US Study," *American Journal of Epidemiology* 175, no. 8 (April 15, 2012): 785–92, doi:10.1093/aje/kwr378.

53.  Kelly D. Brownell and Judith Rodin, "Medical, Metabolic, and Psychological Effects of Weight Cycling," *Archives of Internal Medicine* 154, no. 12 (1994): 1325; Reubin Andres, "Long-Term Effects of Change in Body Weight on All-Cause Mortality: A Review," *Annals of Internal Medicine* 119, no. 7, Part 2 (October 1, 1993): 737, doi:10.7326/0003-4819-119-7_Part_2-199310011-00022; Perez Morales, Jimenez Cruz, and Bacardi Gascon, "The Effect of Weight Loss on Mortality: A Systematic Review from 2000 to 2009"; Simonsen et al., "Intentional Weight Loss and Mortality among Initially Healthy Men and Women."

54.  Because only 6 percent of the population is obesity class III or heavier, most people in the sample were probably obesity class I or II. It may not be the case that having a stable weight in one of the heavier obese classes is as safe. Peter Rzehak et al., "Weight Change, Weight Cycling and Mortality in the ERFORT Male Cohort Study," *European Journal of Epidemiology* 22, no. 10 (January 2007): 665–73, doi:10.1007/s10654-007-9167-5.

55.  Elizabeth Abbess, "Cabbage Soup Diet: What You Need to Know," *Discovery Fit and Health*, 2013, http://health.howstuffworks.com/wellness/diet-fitness/diets/cabbage-soup-diet2.htm.

56.  "Xenical Orlistat: Information for Consumers," 2013, http://www.xenical.com/xenical/default.do.

## CHAPTER 5: OBESITY IS NOT A DEATH SENTENCE

1.    Danielle Dellorto, "Obesity Bigger Health Crisis Than Hunger," CNN.com, 2012, http://edition.cnn.com/2012/12/13/health/global-burden-report/.

2.    Nanci Hellmich, "Obesity on Track as No. 1 Killer," USAToday.com, March 9, 2004, http://usatoday30.usatoday.com/news/health/2004-03-09-obesity_x.htm.

3.    Nanci Hellmich, "Obesity Threatens Life Expectancy," USAToday.com, 2005, http://usatoday30.usatoday.com/news/health/2005-03-16-obesity-lifespan_x.htm.

4.    National Center for Health Statistics, *Health, United States, 2013: With Special Feature on Prescription Drugs* (Hyattsville, MD, 2014), Table 69.

5.    S. Jay Olshansky et al., "A Potential Decline in Life Expectancy in the United States in the 21st Century," *New England Journal of Medicine* 352, no. 11 (March 17, 2005): 1138–45, doi:10.1056/NEJMsr043743.

6.    N. Christenfeld, D. P. Phillips, and L. M. Glynn, "What's in a Name: Mortality and the Power of Symbols," *Journal of Psychosomatic Research* 47, no. 3 (September 1999): 241–54.

7.    Katherine M. Flegal et al., "Association of All-Cause Mortality with Overweight and Obesity Using Standard Body Mass Index Categories: A Systematic Review and Meta-Analysis," *JAMA* 309, no. 1 (January 2, 2013): 71–82, doi:10.1001/jama.2012.113905.

8.    These are technically hazard ratios.

9.    In these paragraphs, when I say the ratio equals 1, I mean the 95 percent confidence interval around the ratio includes 1. Similarly, if I say the ratio is over 1, I mean the lower end of the 95 percent confidence interval around the ratio is greater than 1. The number 140 refers to the number of results she looked at from a total of 97 papers, not the number of papers.

10.   Hazard ratio for lung cancer incidence in men who smoke a half a pack to a full pack of cigarettes per day, compared to never smokers. Neal D. Freedman et al., "Cigarette Smoking and Subsequent Risk of Lung Cancer in Men and Women: Analysis of a Prospective Cohort Study," *Lancet Oncology* 9, no. 7 (2008): 649–56.

11.   Katherine M. Flegal et al., "Prevalence of Obesity and Trends in the Distribution of Body Mass Index among US Adults, 1999–2010," *JAMA* 307, no. 5 (February 1, 2012): 491–97, doi:10.1001/jama.2012.39.

12.   K. M. Flegal et al., "Excess Deaths Associated with Underweight, Overweight, and Obesity," *JAMA* 293, no. 15 (2005): 1861–67, doi:10.1001/jama.293.15.1861.

13.   Daphne P. Guh et al., "The Incidence of Co-Morbidities Related to Obesity and Overweight: A Systematic Review and Meta-Analysis," *BMC Public Health* 9 (January 2009): 88, doi:10.1186/1471-2458-9-88.

14.   National Center for Health Statistics, *Health, United States, 2013: With Special Feature on Prescription Drugs*, Table 46.

15.   Ibid., Table 44.

16.    Carl J. Lavie, Richard V. Milani, and Hector O. Ventura, "Obesity and Cardiovascular Disease: Risk Factor, Paradox, and Impact of Weight Loss," *Journal of the American College of Cardiology* 53, no. 21 (May 26, 2009): 1925–32, doi:10.1016/j.jacc.2008.12.068.

17.    Konstantinos Vemmos et al., "Association between Obesity and Mortality after Acute First-Ever Stroke: The Obesity-Stroke Paradox," *Stroke* 42, no. 1 (January 2011): 30–6, doi:10.1161/STROKEAHA.110.593434.

18.    Mercedes R. Carnethon et al., "Association of Weight Status with Mortality in Adults with Incident Diabetes," *JAMA* 308, no. 6 (August 8, 2012): 581–90, doi:10.1001/jama.2012.9282.

19.    Kamyar Kalantar-Zadeh et al., "The Obesity Paradox and Mortality Associated With Surrogates of Body Size and Muscle Mass in Patients Receiving Hemodialysis," *Mayo Clinic Proceedings* 85, no. 11 (2010): 991–1001.

20.    Jordan A. Guenette, Dennis Jensen, and Denis E. O'Donnell, "Respiratory Function and the Obesity Paradox," *Current Opinion in Clinical Nutrition and Metabolic Care* 13, no. 6 (November 2010): 618–24, doi:10.1097/MCO.0b013e32833e3453.

21.    Agustín Escalante, Roy W. Haas, and Inmaculada del Rincón, "Paradoxical Effect of Body Mass Index on Survival in Rheumatoid Arthritis: Role of Comorbidity and Systemic Inflammation," *Archives of Internal Medicine* 165, no. 14 (July 25, 2005): 1624–29, doi:10.1001/archinte.165.14.1624.

22.    Vicente F. Corrales-Medina et al., "The Obesity Paradox in Community-Acquired Bacterial Pneumonia," *International Journal of Infectious Diseases* 15, no. 1 (2011): e54–e57.

23.    Relin Yang et al., "Obesity and Weight Loss at Presentation of Lung Cancer Are Associated with Opposite Effects on Survival," *Journal of Surgical Research* 170, no. 1 (2011): e75–e83.

24.    Susan Halabi et al., "Inverse Correlation between Body Mass Index and Clinical Outcomes in Men with Advanced Castration-Recurrent Prostate Cancer," *Cancer* 110, no. 7 (October 1, 2007): 1478–84, doi:10.1002/cncr.22932.

25.    Henry Oliveros and Eduardo Villamor, "Obesity and Mortality in Critically Ill Adults: A Systematic Review and Meta-Analysis," *Obesity* (Silver Spring, Md.) 16, no. 3 (March 2008): 515–21, doi:10.1038/oby.2007.102; Jeptha P Curtis et al., "The Obesity Paradox: Body Mass Index and Outcomes in Patients with Heart Failure," *Archives of Internal Medicine* 165, no. 1 (January 10, 2005): 55–61, doi:10.1001/archinte.165.1.55.

26.    Oliveros and Villamor, "Obesity and Mortality in Critically Ill Adults: A Systematic Review and Meta-Analysis."

27.    The classic citation is: R. A. Fisher, *The Design of Experiments* (Oxford, England: Oliver & Boyd, 1935). A fantastic explanation of random assignment is in my former colleagues' textbook: Brett W. Pelham and Hart Blanton, *Conducting Research in Psychology: Measuring the Weight of Smoke*, 4th ed., (Belmont, CA: Cengage Learning, 2011). They say random assignment "is the closest thing to magic that researchers have ever discovered" (p. 202).

28. You may be thinking about the studies from Chapter 2 in which prisoners and other volunteers were made temporarily obese. Those are not useful for this purpose as they did not have control groups. Sims, "Experimental Obesity, Dietary-Induced Thermogenesis, and Their Clinical Implications."

29. Mann et al., "Medicare's Search for Effective Obesity Treatments: Diets Are Not the Answer."

30. Mann, Tomiyama, and Ahlstrom, "Long-Term Effects of Dieting."

31. Look AHEAD Research Group, "Cardiovascular Effects of Intensive Lifestyle Intervention in Type 2 Diabetes," *New England Journal of Medicine* 369, no. 2 (June 24, 2013): 145–54, doi:10.1056/NEJMoa1212914.

32. Definition appears here: National Institute of Diabetes and Digestive and Kidney Diseases, "Data & Safety Monitoring Plans," *Research and Funding for Scientists*, 2013, http://www.niddk.nih.gov/research-funding/process/human-subjects-research/data-safety-monitoring-plans/Pages/data-and-safety-monitoring-plans.aspx. Statement that Look AHEAD (see previous note) was terminated for futility appears at Look AHEAD Protocol Review Committee, "Protocol: Action for Health in Diabetes: Look AHEAD Clinical Trial, 10th Revision," 2012, https://www.lookaheadtrial.org/public/LookAHEADProtocol.pdf, p. 38.

33. "Weight Loss Does Not Lower Heart Disease Risk from Type 2 Diabetes," press release, National Institutes of Health, 2012, http://www.nih.gov/news/health/oct2012/niddk-19.htm.

34. J. Bruce Redmon et al., "Effect of the Look AHEAD Study Intervention on Medication Use and Related Cost to Treat Cardiovascular Disease Risk Factors in Individuals with Type 2 Diabetes," *Diabetes Care* 33, no. 6 (June 1, 2010): 1153–58, doi:10.2337/dc09-2090.

35. This includes all of those mortality studies that Katherine Flegal reviewed.

36. If you use random assignment, you don't have to worry about any differences there might normally be between obese and non-obese people, because random assignment makes your groups pretty much equal in pretty much every way. It even makes the groups about equal on things you never thought of. This is crucial. As a professional scientist, I can say with conviction that there is an infinite number of things I have never thought of.

37. J. J. Varo et al., "Distribution and Determinants of Sedentary Lifestyles in the European Union," *International Journal of Epidemiology* 32, no. 1 (February 1, 2003): 138–46, doi:10.1093/ije/dyg116.

38. Ibid.

39. Casazza et al., "Myths, Presumptions, and Facts about Obesity."

40. Phillipa Caudwell et al., "Exercise Alone Is Not Enough: Weight Loss Also Needs a Healthy (Mediterranean) Diet?," *Public Health Nutrition* 12, no. 9A (September 1, 2009): 1663–66, doi:10.1017/S1368980009990528.

41. Scott M. Grundy et al., "Clinical Management of Metabolic Syndrome: Report of the American Heart Association/National Heart, Lung, and Blood Institute/American Diabetes Association Conference on Scientific Issues Related to Management," *Circulation* 109, no. 4 (February 3, 2004): 551–56,

doi:10.1161/01.CIR.0000112379.88385.67.

42.   D. E. Thomas, E. J. Elliott, and G. A. Naughton, "Exercise for Type 2 Diabetes Mellitus," *Evidence-Based Nursing* 10, no. 1 (2007): 11.

43.   Balraj S. Heran et al., "Exercise-Based Cardiac Rehabilitation for Coronary Heart Disease," *Cochrane Database of Systematic Reviews* no. 7 (January 2011): CD001800, doi:10.1002/14651858.CD001800.pub2.

44.   Paul D. Thompson et al., "Exercise and Physical Activity in the Prevention and Treatment of Atherosclerotic Cardiovascular Disease: A Statement from the Council on Clinical Cardiology (Subcommittee on Exercise, Rehabilitation, and Prevention) and the Council on Nutrition, Physical Activity, and Metabolism (Subcommittee on Physical Activity)," *Circulation* 107, no. 24 (June 24, 2003): 3109–16, doi:10.1161/01.CIR.0000075572.40158.77.

45.   Sean Carroll and Mike Dudfield, "What Is the Relationship between Exercise and Metabolic Abnormalities?," *Sports Medicine* 34, no. 6 (2004): 371–418, doi:10.2165/00007256-200434060-00004.

46.   Martha L. Slattery and John D. Potter, "Physical Activity and Colon Cancer: Confounding or Interaction?," *Medicine and Science in Sports and Exercise* 34, no. 6 (June 2002): 913–19.

47.   Rosalind A. Breslow et al., "Long-Term Recreational Physical Activity and Breast Cancer in the National Health and Nutrition Examination Survey I Epidemiologic Follow-up Study," *Cancer Epidemiology, Biomarkers & Prevention* 10, no. 7 (July 1, 2001): 805–8.

48.   Casazza et al., "Myths, Presumptions, and Facts about Obesity"; Breslow et al., "Long-Term Recreational Physical Activity and Breast Cancer in the National Health and Nutrition Examination Survey I Epidemiologic Follow-up Study"; Grundy et al., "Clinical Management of Metabolic Syndrome"; Thomas, Elliott, and Naughton, "Exercise for Type 2 Diabetes Mellitus"; Caudwell et al., "Exercise Alone Is Not Enough."

49.   S. N. Blair and T. S. Church, "The Fitness, Obesity, and Health Equation: Is Physical Activity the Common Denominator?," *JAMA* 292, no. 10 (2004): 1232–34, doi:10.1001/jama.292.10.1232; S. N. Blair and S. Brodney, "Effects of Physical Inactivity and Obesity on Morbidity and Mortality: Current Evidence and Research Issues," *Medicine & Science in Sports & Exercise* 31, no. 11 Suppl. (1999): S646–62; M. Fogelholm, "Physical Activity, Fitness and Fatness: Relations to Mortality, Morbidity and Disease Risk Factors: A Systematic Review," *Obesity Reviews* 11, no. 3 (2010): 202–21, doi:10.1111/j.1467-789X.2009.00653.x; M. Wei et al., "Relationship between Low Cardiorespiratory Fitness and Mortality in Normal-Weight, Overweight, and Obese Men," *JAMA* 282, no. 16 (1999): 1547–53.

50.   Paul McAuley et al., "Fitness and Fatness as Mortality Predictors in Healthy Older Men: The Veterans Exercise Testing Study," *Journals of Gerontology: Series A, Biological Sciences and Medical Sciences* 64, no. 6 (June 1, 2009): 695–99, doi:10.1093/gerona/gln039.

51.   Caitlin Mason et al., "History of Weight Cycling Does Not Impede Future Weight Loss or Metabolic Improvements in Postmenopausal Women,"

*Metabolism: Clinical and Experimental* 62, no. 1 (January 1, 2013): 127–36, doi:10.1016/j.metabol.2012.06.012.

52.  Nancy E. Adler and Joan M. Ostrove, "Socioeconomic Status and Health: What We Know and What We Don't," *Annals of the New York Academy of Sciences* 896, no. 1 (December 6, 1999): 3–15, doi:10.1111/j.1749-6632.1999. tb08101.x.

53.  M. G. Marmot, M. J. Shipley, and G. Rose, "Inequalities in Death—Specific Explanations of a General Pattern?," *Lancet* 1, no. 8384 (May 5, 1984): 1003–1006.

54.  Adler and Ostrove, "Socioeconomic Status and Health."

55.  U.S. Department of Health and Human Services, Office of Disease Prevention and Health Promotion, *Healthy People 2020* (Washington, DC, 2010).

56.  For an outstanding review, see Karen A. Matthews and Linda C. Gallo, "Psychological Perspectives on Pathways Linking Socioeconomic Status and Physical Health," *Annual Review of Psychology* 62 (January 2011): 501–30, doi:10.1146/annurev.psych.031809.130711.

57.  Bruce S. McEwen and Teresa Seeman, "Protective and Damaging Effects of Mediators of Stress: Elaborating and Testing the Concepts of Allostasis and Allostatic Load," *Annals of the New York Academy of Sciences* 896, no. 1 (December 6, 1999): 30–47, doi:10.1111/j.1749-6632.1999.tb08103.x.

58.  K. E. Pickett and M. Pearl, "Multilevel Analyses of Neighbourhood Socioeconomic Context and Health Outcomes: A Critical Review," *Journal of Epidemiology and Community Health* 55, no. 2 (February 2001): 111–22.

59.  Youfa Wang and May A. Beydoun, "The Obesity Epidemic in the United States—Gender, Age, Socioeconomic, Racial/Ethnic, and Geographic Characteristics: A Systematic Review and Meta-Regression Analysis," *Epidemiologic Reviews* 29, no. 1 (January 1, 2007): 6–28, doi:10.1093/epirev/mxm007; J. Sobal and A. J. Stunkard, "Socioeconomic Status and Obesity: A Review of the Literature," *Psychological Bulletin* 105, no. 2 (1989): 260–75.

60.  Jacob J. Feldman et al., "National Trends in Educational Differentials in Mortality," *American Journal of Epidemiology* 129, no. 5 (May 1, 1989): 919–33; M. G. Marmot et al., "Health Inequalities among British Civil Servants: The Whitehall II Study," *Lancet* 337, no. 8754 (June 8, 1991): 1387–93; Marmot, Shipley, and Rose, "Inequalities in Death—Specific Explanations of a General Pattern?"; H. Bosma et al., "Low Control Beliefs, Classical Coronary Risk Factors, and Socio-Economic Differences in Heart Disease in Older Persons," *Social Science & Medicine* 60, no. 4 (2005): 737–45.

61.  National Institutes of Health, U.S. Department of Health and Human Services, "What Is Metabolic Syndrome?," *Health Information for the Public*, accessed November 5, 2013, http://www.nhlbi.nih.gov/health/health-topics/topics/ms/.

62.  Thais Coutinho et al., "Combining Body Mass Index with Measures of Central Obesity in the Assessment of Mortality in Subjects with Coronary Disease: Role of 'Normal Weight Central Obesity,'" *Journal of the American*

*College of Cardiology* 61, no. 5 (February 5, 2013): 553–60, doi:10.1016/j. jacc.2012.10.035; Thais Coutinho et al., "Central Obesity and Survival in Subjects with Coronary Artery Disease: A Systematic Review of the Literature and Collaborative Analysis with Individual Subject Data," *Journal of the American College of Cardiology* 57, no. 19 (May 10, 2011): 1877–86, doi:10.1016/j.jacc.2010.11.058; Halfdan Petursson et al., "Body Configuration as a Predictor of Mortality: Comparison of Five Anthropometric Measures in a 12 Year Follow-up of the Norwegian HUNT 2 Study," ed. Stefan Kiechl, *PloS One* 6, no. 10 (January 2011): e26621, doi:10.1371/journal. pone.0026621.

63.   Coutinho et al., "Central Obesity and Survival in Subjects with Coronary Artery Disease."

64.   Elizabeth A. Pascoe and Laura Smart Richman, "Perceived Discrimination and Health: A Meta-Analytic Review," *Psychological Bulletin* 135, no. 4 (2009): 531–54.

65.   R. M. Puhl and C. A. Heuer, "The Stigma of Obesity: A Review and Update," *Obesity* (Silver Spring, MD) 17, no. 5 (2009): 941–64, doi:10.1038/ oby.2008.636.

66.   Drew A. Anderson and Thomas A. Wadden, "Bariatric Surgery Patients' Views of Their Physicians' Weight-Related Attitudes and Practices," *Obesity Research* 12, no. 10 (October 2004): 1587–95, doi:10.1038/oby.2004.198.

67.   Rebecca M. Puhl and Kelly D. Brownell, "Confronting and Coping with Weight Stigma: An Investigation of Overweight and Obese Adults," *Obesity* (Silver Spring, MD) 14, no. 10 (October 2006): 1802–15, doi:10.1038/ oby.2006.208.

68.   N. K. Amy et al., "Barriers to Routine Gynecological Cancer Screening for White and African-American Obese Women," *International Journal of Obesity* 30, no. 1 (January 4, 2006): 147–55, doi:10.1038/sj.ijo.0803105.

69.   G. D. Foster et al., "Primary Care Physicians' Attitudes about Obesity and Its Treatment," *Obesity Research* 11, no. 10 (2003): 1168–77, doi:10.1038/ oby.2003.161.

70.   M. B. Schwartz et al., "Weight Bias among Health Professionals Specializing in Obesity," *Obesity Research* 11, no. 9 (2003): 1033–39.

71.   M. R. Hebl and J. Xu, "Weighing the Care: Physicians' Reactions to the Size of a Patient," *International Journal of Obesity and Related Metabolic Disorders* 25, no. 8 (August 2001): 1246–52, doi:10.1038/sj.ijo.0801681.

72.   Kimberly A. Gudzune et al., "Physicians Build Less Rapport with Obese Patients," *Obesity* (Silver Spring, MD) 21, no. 10 (March 20, 2013): 2146–52, doi:10.1002/oby.20384.

73.   David P. Miller et al., "Are Medical Students Aware of Their Anti-Obesity Bias?," *Academic Medicine* 88, no. 7 (July 2013): 978–82, doi:10.1097/ ACM.0b013e318294f817; Sean M. Phelan et al., "Implicit and Explicit Weight Bias in a National Sample of 4,732 Medical Students: The Medical Student CHANGES Study," *Obesity* (Silver Spring, MD) (2013), doi:10.1002/oby.20687.

74.  Kimberly A. Gudzune et al., "Doctor Shopping by Overweight and Obese Patients Is Associated with Increased Healthcare Utilization," *Obesity* (Silver Spring, MD) 21, no. 7 (July 2013): 1328–34, doi:10.1002/oby.20189.

75.  T. Ostbye et al., "Associations between Obesity and Receipt of Screening Mammography, Papanicolaou Tests, and Influenza Vaccination: Results from the Health and Retirement Study (HRS) and the Asset and Health Dynamics among the Oldest Old (AHEAD) Study," *American Journal of Public Health* 95, no. 9 (2005): 1623–30, doi:10.2105/AJPH.2004.047803; C. C. Wee et al., "Screening for Cervical and Breast Cancer: Is Obesity an Unrecognized Barrier to Preventive Care?," *Annals of Internal Medicine* 132, no. 9 (2000): 697–704.

76.  Ostbye et al., "Associations between Obesity and Receipt of Screening Mammography, Papanicolaou Tests, and Influenza Vaccination"; Wee et al., "Screening for Cervical and Breast Cancer."

77.  Jeanne M. Ferrante et al., "Colorectal Cancer Screening among Obese Versus Non-Obese Patients in Primary Care Practices," *Cancer Detection and Prevention* 30, no. 5 (2006): 459–65; Allison B. Rosen and Eric C. Schneider, "Colorectal Cancer Screening Disparities Related to Obesity and Gender," *Journal of General Internal Medicine* 19, no. 4 (April 2004): 332–38, doi:10.1111/j.1525-1497.2004.30339.x.

78.  Ostbye et al., "Associations between Obesity and Receipt of Screening Mammography, Papanicolaou Tests, and Influenza Vaccination."

79.  Pascoe and Richman, "Perceived Discrimination and Health."

80.  B. Major, D. Eliezer, and H. Rieck, "The Psychological Weight of Weight Stigma," *Social Psychological and Personality Science* 3, no. 6 (January 19, 2012): 651–58, doi:10.1177/1948550611434400. Also see Janet Tomiyama et al., "Associations of Weight Stigma with Cortisol and Oxidative Stress Independent of Adiposity," *Health Psychology* 33, no. 8 (August 2014): 862–67, doi:10.1037/hea0000107. Another example appears in Natasha A. Schvey, Rebecca M. Puhl, and Kelly D. Brownell, "The Stress of Stigma: Exploring the Effect of Weight Stigma on Cortisol Reactivity," *Psychosomatic Medicine* (2014): PSY–0000000000000031.

81.  Puhl and Brownell, "Confronting and Coping with Weight Stigma."

82.  Jenny H. Ledikwe et al., "Dietary Energy Density Is Associated with Energy Intake and Weight Status in US Adults," *American Journal of Clinical Nutrition* 83, no. 6 (June 2006): 1362–68.

83.  Lawrence de Koning et al., "Sugar-Sweetened and Artificially Sweetened Beverage Consumption and Risk of Type 2 Diabetes in Men," *American Journal of Clinical Nutrition* 93, no. 6 (June 1, 2011): 1321–27, doi:10.3945/ajcn.110.007922. koning.

84.  Ankur Vyas et al., "Diet Drink Consumption and the Risk of Cardiovascular Events: A Report from the Women's Health Initiative," *Journal of the American College of Cardiology* 63, no. 12 (April 1, 2014): A1290, doi:10.1016/S0735-1097(14)61290-0. vyas.

85.  Jotham Suez et al., "Artificial Sweeteners Induce Glucose Intolerance by

Altering the Gut Microbiota," *Nature* (September 17, 2014), doi:10.1038/nature13793. suez.

86.  A. S. Levy and A. W. Heaton, "Weight Control Practices of US Adults Trying to Lose Weight," *Annals of Internal Medicine* 119, no. 7 Part 2 (1993): 661–66; Edward C. Weiss et al., "Weight-Control Practices among U.S. Adults, 2001–2002," *American Journal of Preventive Medicine* 31, no. 1 (2006): 18–24.

87.  Lisa L. Ioannides-Demos et al., "Safety of Drug Therapies Used for Weight Loss and Treatment of Obesity," *Drug Safety* 29, no. 4 (2006): 277–302, doi:10.2165/00002018-200629040-00001.

88.  M. A. Whisman, "Loneliness and the Metabolic Syndrome in a Population-Based Sample of Middle-Aged and Older Adults," *Health Psychology* 29, no. 5 (2010): 550–54, doi:10.1037/a0020760.

89.  J. Holt-Lunstad, T. B. Smith, and J. B. Layton, "Social Relationships and Mortality Risk: A Meta-Analytic Review," *PLoS Med* 7, no. 7 (2010): e1000316, doi:10.1371/journal.pmed.1000316.

90.  These came from the online supplemental materials to the article. They don't have a freestanding URL of their own, but can be reached from the main article: Flegal et al., "Association of All-Cause Mortality with Overweight and Obesity Using Standard Body Mass Index Categories."

91.  They had to do so by measuring at least two of the three components (for example, education and income) of SES, according to P. A. Braveman et al., "Socioeconomic Status in Health Research: One Size Does Not Fit All," *JAMA* 294, no. 22 (2005): 2879–88, doi:10.1001/jama.294.22.2879.

92.  I reported the number for white people who had never smoked. Eric A. Finkelstein et al., "Individual and Aggregate Years-of-Life-Lost Associated with Overweight and Obesity," *Obesity* 18, no. 2 (February 2010): 333–39, doi:10.1038/oby.2009.253.

93.  Ibid.

94.  Christenfeld, Phillips, and Glynn, "What's in a Name."

95.  P. Campos et al., "The Epidemiology of Overweight and Obesity: Public Health Crisis or Moral Panic?," *International Journal of Epidemiology* 35, no. 1 (2006): 55–60, doi:10.1093/ije/dyi254.

96.  Davidoff, "Sponsorship, Authorship, and Accountability."

97.  Olshansky et al., "A Potential Decline in Life Expectancy in the United States in the 21st Century."

98.  W. Wayt Gibbs, "Obesity: An Overblown Epidemic?," *Scientific American* 292, no. 6 (June 2005): 70–77, doi:10.1038/scientificamerican0605-70.

99.  Olshansky et al., "A Potential Decline in Life Expectancy in the United States in the 21st Century"; David Allison, "Disclosure of Financial Information," *New England Journal of Medicine*, 2005, http://www.nejm.org/doi/suppl/10.1056/NEJMsr043743/suppl_file/1138sa1.pdf.

100.  Flegal et al., "Association of All-Cause Mortality with Overweight and Obesity Using Standard Body Mass Index Categories."

## CHAPTER 6: LESSONS FROM A LEAN PIG

1.    I have changed his name at his request.

2.    Walter Mischel, "From Good Intentions to Willpower," in *The Psychology of Action: Linking Cognition and Motivation to Behavior*, ed. Peter Gollwitzer and John Bargh (New York: Guilford Press, 1996), 197–218.

3.    We cover this strategy (and many others) in our review of self-control strategies: Traci Mann, Denise de Ridder, and Kentaro Fujita, "Self-Regulation of Health Behavior: Social Psychological Approaches to Goal Setting and Goal Striving," *Health Psychology* 32, no. 5 (May 2013): 487–98, doi:10.1037/a0028533.

4.    Lisa R. Young and Marion Nestle, "The Contribution of Expanding Portion Sizes to the US Obesity Epidemic," *American Journal of Public Health* 92, no. 2 (February 1, 2002): 246–49.

5.    Ibid.

6.    Nancy Rivera, "Ice Cream Firm Turns 40: Baskin-Robbins Starts Program to Revitalize," *Los Angeles Times*, May 6, 1985.

7.    Young and Nestle, "The Contribution of Expanding Portion Sizes to the US Obesity Epidemic."

8.    Ibid.

9.    B. Wansink and C. S. Wansink, "The Largest Last Supper: Depictions of Food Portions and Plate Size Increased Over the Millennium," *International Journal of Obesity* (2005) 34, no. 5 (May 2010): 943–4, doi:10.1038/ijo.2010.37.

10.   Ibid.

11.   For a review, see Brian Wansink, "Environmental Factors That Increase the Food Intake and Consumption Volume of Unknowing Consumers," *Annual Review of Nutrition* 24 (January 2004): 455–79, doi:10.1146/annurev.nutr.24.012003.132140. Also see Carmen Piernas and Barry M. Popkin, "Increased Portion Sizes from Energy-Dense Foods Affect Total Energy Intake at Eating Occasions in US Children and Adolescents: Patterns and Trends by Age Group and Sociodemographic Characteristics, 1977–2006," *American Journal of Clinical Nutrition* 94, no. 5 (November 1, 2011): 1324–32, doi:10.3945/ajcn.110.008466; David A. Levitsky and Trisha Youn, "The More Food Young Adults Are Served, the More They Overeat," *Journal of Nutrition* 134, no. 10 (October 1, 2004): 2546–49.

12.   Brian Wansink, "Can Package Size Accelerate Usage Volume?," *Journal of Marketing* 60, no. 3 (1996): 1–14, doi:10.2307/1251838.

13.   Brian Wansink, Koert van Ittersum, and James E. Painter, "Ice Cream Illusions: Bowls, Spoons, and Self-Served Portion Sizes," *American Journal of Preventive Medicine* 31, no. 3 (2006): 240–43.

14.   Ellen van Kleef, Christos Kavvouris, and Hans C. M. van Trijp, "The Unit Size Effect of Indulgent Food: How Eating Smaller Sized Items Signals Impulsivity and Makes Consumers Eat Less," *Psychology & Health* 29, no. 9 (September 2014): 1081–1103, doi:10.1080/08870446.2014.909426.

15. Brian Wansink, James E. Painter, and Jill North, "Bottomless Bowls: Why Visual Cues of Portion Size May Influence Intake," *Obesity Research* 13, no. 1 (January 2005): 93–100, doi:10.1038/oby.2005.12.

16. Ibid.

17. B. Wansink and K. Van Ittersum, "Illusive Consumption Behavior and the DelBoeuf Illusion: Are the Eyes Really Bigger than the Stomach?," *Annual Review of Nutrition* 24 (2004): 455–79.

18. Wansink, Painter, and North, "Bottomless Bowls."

19. Piernas and Popkin, "Increased Portion Sizes from Energy-Dense Foods Affect Total Energy Intake at Eating Occasions in US Children and Adolescents."

20. Frank McIntyre, "U.S. Companies Shrink Packages as Food Prices Rise," *Daily Finance*, 2011, http://www.dailyfinance.com/2011/04/04/u-s-companies-shrink-packages-as-food-prices-rise/.

21. "Saving on Toilet Paper," OccupiedLife.com, 2011, http://occupiedlife.com/saving-on-toilet-paper/; Peggy Wang, "46 Penny-Pinching Ways to Save a Lot of Money This Year," Buzzfeed.com, 2013, http://www.buzzfeed.com/peggy/46-penny-pinching-ways-to-save-a-lot-of-money-this.

22. Keith Hawton et al., "Long Term Effect of Reduced Pack Sizes of Paracetamol on Poisoning Deaths and Liver Transplant Activity in England and Wales: Interrupted Time Series Analyses," *BMJ (Clinical Research Ed.)* 346 (January 2013): f403; K. Hawton, "Effects of Legislation Restricting Pack Sizes of Paracetamol and Salicylate on Self Poisoning in the United Kingdom: Before and After Study," *BMJ* 322, no. 7296 (May 19, 2001): 1203, doi:10.1136/bmj.322.7296.1203.

23. Josje Maas et al., "Do Distant Foods Decrease Intake? The Effect of Food Accessibility on Consumption," *Psychology & Health* 27, Suppl. 2 (October 2012): 59–73, doi:10.1080/08870446.2011.565341. Also see Gregory J. Privitera and Faris M. Zuraikat, "Proximity of Foods in a Competitive Food Environment Influences Consumption of a Low Calorie and a High Calorie Food," *Appetite* 76 (May 2014): 175–79, doi:10.1016/j.appet.2014.02.004.

24. Maas et al., "Do Distant Foods Decrease Intake?"

25. Paul Rozin et al., "Nudge to Nobesity I: Minor Changes in Accessibility Decrease Food Intake," *Judgment and Decision Making* 6, no. 4 (2011): 323–32.

26. As far as I can tell, nobody's done this study, so this is just a speculation.

27. For example, Frances Martel, "Jon Stewart Rails Against Bloomberg's 'Draconian' Soda Ban with Piles of Gross 'Legal' Food," Mediaite.com, 2012, http://www.mediaite.com/tv/jon-stewart-rails-against-bloombergs-draconian-soda-ban-with-piles-of-gross-legal-food/.

28. Cecilia Kang, "Google Crunches Data on Munching in Office," *Washington Post*, September 1, 2013. Also see B. Wansink, J. E. Painter, and Y. K. Lee, "The Office Candy Dish: Proximity's Influence on Estimated and Actual Consumption," *International Journal of Obesity* 30, no. 5 (May 17, 2006): 871–75, doi:10.1038/sj.ijo.0803217; James E. Painter, Brian Wansink, and Julie B. Hieggelke, "How Visibility and Convenience Influence

Candy Consumption," *Appetite* 38, no. 3 (June 2002): 237–38, doi:10.1006/
appe.2002.0485.

29.   Carol E. Cornell, Judith Rodin, and Harvey Weingarten, "Stimulus-Induced
Eating When Satiated," *Physiology & Behavior* 45, no. 4 (1989): 695–704.

30.   If you want to be inspired to attempt it, the chef and writer Tamar Adler has
posted a video online that shows her washing and roasting a huge amount of
vegetables at once, which she then puts in jars in her fridge to eat on their own
or use in recipes during the week. (It's a lot more exciting than it sounds.)
Tamar E. Adler, "How to Stride Ahead: Part 2," Tamareadler.com, 2011,
http://www.tamareadler.com/2011/10/10/how-to-stride-ahead-part-2/.

31.   Joe Redden, Zata Vickers, Marla Reicks, and Elton Mykerezi, along with
graduate students Stephanie Elsbernd and Nikki Miller.

32.   All of the tests appear in Joseph P. Redden et al., "The Effect of Juxtaposition
on the Intake of Healthy Foods" (n.d.).

## CHAPTER 7: HOW TO TRICK YOUR FRIENDS INTO IGNORING A COOKIE

1.   Solomon E. Asch, "Studies of Independence and Conformity: I. A Minority
of One against a Unanimous Majority, *Psychological Monographs: General and
Applied*" 70, no. 9 (1956) 1–70.

2.   This effect has been replicated over 100 times across 17 countries. For a review, see Rod Bond and Peter B. Smith, "Culture and Conformity: A Meta-
Analysis of Studies Using Asch's (1952b, 1956) Line Judgment Task," *Psychological Bulletin* 119, no. 1 (1996): 111–37.

3.   M. Sherif, *The Psychology of Social Norms* (Oxford, England: Harper, 1936).

4.   Paul Rozin, "The Integration of Biological, Social, Cultural and Psychological Influences on Food Choice," in *The Psychology of Food Choice*, ed. Richard
Shepherd and Monique Raats (Oxfordshire, England: CABI, 2006), 19–40.

5.   John M. de Castro and E. Marie Brewer, "The Amount Eaten in Meals by
Humans Is a Power Function of the Number of People Present," *Physiology &
Behavior* 51, no. 1 (1992): 121–25.

6.   Ibid.; A. Ward and T. Mann, "Don't Mind If I Do: Disinhibited Eating
Under Cognitive Load," *Journal of Personality and Social Psychology* 78, no. 4
(April 2000): 753–63.

7.   Vanessa I. Clendenen, C. Peter Herman, and Janet Polivy, "Social Facilita-
tion of Eating among Friends and Strangers," *Appetite* 23, no. 1 (1994): 1–13;
Sarah-Jeanne Salvy et al., "Effects of Social Influence on Eating in Couples,
Friends and Strangers," *Appetite* 49, no. 1 (July 2007): 92–99, doi:10.1016/j.
appet.2006.12.004.

8.   de Castro and Brewer, "The Amount Eaten in Meals by Humans Is a Power
Function of the Number of People Present."

9.   Maryhope Howland, Jeffrey M. Hunger, and Traci Mann, "Friends Don't
Let Friends Eat Cookies: Effects of Restrictive Eating Norms on Consumption among Friends," *Appetite* 59, no. 2 (October 2012): 505–9, doi:10.1016/

j.appet.2012.06.020. The day after our paper came out an article was published saying that people don't take research findings seriously if they come from a paper with a silly title. Uh-oh.

10.     Leon Festinger, "A Theory of Social Comparison Processes," *Human Relations* 7, no. 2 (1954): 117–40.

11.     Noah J. Goldstein, Robert B. Cialdini, and Vladas Griskevicius, "A Room with a Viewpoint: Using Social Norms to Motivate Environmental Conservation in Hotels," *Journal of Consumer Research* 35, no. 3 (October 3, 2008): 472–82, doi:10.1086/586910.

12.     Other factors matter, too, including convenience and effort, but these are equated in many countries and you still see these differences. Eric J. Johnson and Daniel Goldstein, "Do Defaults Save Lives?," *Science* 302, no. 5649 (November 21, 2003): 1338–39, doi:10.1126/science.1091721.

13.     Ervin Staub, "Instigation to Goodness: The Role of Social Norms and Interpersonal Influence," *Journal of Social Issues* 28, no. 3 (July 1972): 131–50, doi:10.1111/j.1540-4560.1972.tb00036.x.

14.     Howland, Hunger, and Mann, "Friends Don't Let Friends Eat Cookies." Other studies also show the effect of implied norms on eating, for example, Eric Robinson, Helen Benwell, and Suzanne Higgs, "Food Intake Norms Increase and Decrease Snack Food Intake in a Remote Confederate Study," *Appetite* 65 (2013): 20–24. For a review, see Eric Robinson et al., "What Everyone Else Is Eating: A Systematic Review and Meta-Analysis of the Effect of Informational Eating Norms on Eating Behavior," *Journal of the Academy of Nutrition and Dietetics* 114, no. 3 (2013): 414–29.

15.     F. Marijn Stok et al., "Minority Talks: The Influence of Descriptive Social Norms on Fruit Intake," *Psychology & Health* 27, no. 8 (January 2012): 956–70, doi:10.1080/08870446.2011.635303.

16.     Clayton Neighbors, Mary E. Larimer, and Melissa A. Lewis, "Targeting Misperceptions of Descriptive Drinking Norms: Efficacy of a Computer-Delivered Personalized Normative Feedback Intervention," *Journal of Consulting and Clinical Psychology* 72, no. 3 (June 2004): 434–47, doi:10.1037/0022-006X.72.3.434.

17.     Elizabeth M. Condon, Mary Kay Crepinsek, and Mary Kay Fox, "School Meals: Types of Foods Offered to and Consumed by Children at Lunch and Breakfast," *Journal of the American Dietetic Association* 109, no. 2 (2009): S67–S78.

18.     I worked on this with my University of Minnesota colleagues Marla Reicks, Zata Vickers, Joe Redden, and Elton Mykerezi. Marla Reicks et al., "Photographs in Lunch Tray Compartments and Vegetable Consumption among Children in Elementary School Cafeterias," *JAMA* 307, no. 8 (February 22, 2012): 784–85, doi:10.1001/jama.2012.170.

19.     Ibid.

20.     A classic finding in cognitive psychology is that people cannot remember which elements go where on a penny. Raymond S. Nickerson and Marilyn Jager Adams, "Long-Term Memory for a Common Object," *Cognitive*

*Psychology* 11, no. 3 (1979): 287–307.

21.    Heather Barry Kappes and Patrick E. Shrout, "When Goal Sharing Produces Support That Is Not Caring," *Personality & Social Psychology Bulletin* 37, no. 5 (May 1, 2011): 662–73, doi:10.1177/0146167211399926.

22.    Mary Ann Parris Stephens et al., "Spouses' Attempts to Regulate Day-to-Day Dietary Adherence among Patients with Type 2 Diabetes," *Health Psychology* 32, no. 10 (October 2013): 1029–37, doi:10.1037/a0030018; J. S. Tucker and J. S. Mueller, "Spouses' Social Control of Health Behaviors: Use and Effectiveness of Specific Strategies," *Personality and Social Psychology Bulletin* 26, no. 9 (November 1, 2000): 1120–30, doi:10.1177/01461672002611008.

23.    Ibid.

24.    Maryhope Howland and Jeffry A. Simpson, "Getting in Under the Radar. A Dyadic View of Invisible Support," *Psychological Science* 21, no. 12 (December 1, 2010): 1878–85, doi:10.1177/0956797610388817.

25.    Marci E. J. Gleason et al., "Daily Supportive Equity in Close Relationships," *Personality & Social Psychology Bulletin* 29, no. 8 (August 1, 2003): 1036–45, doi:10.1177/0146167203253473.

## CHAPTER 8: DON'T CALL THAT APPLE HEALTHY

1.     The classic work on this in social psychology is in Lee Ross and Richard E. Nisbett, *The Person and the Situation* (New York: McGraw-Hill, 1991). Cognitive-behavioral therapy has a similar conceptual backbone, and is summarized nicely in David D. Burns, *Feeling Good: The New Mood Therapy*, rev. ed. (New York: William Morrow Paperbacks, 1999).

2.     Brian Wansink, Koert van Ittersum, and James E. Painter, "How Descriptive Food Names Bias Sensory Perceptions in Restaurants," *Food Quality and Preference* 16, no. 5 (2005): 393–400.

3.     Alia J. Crum et al., "Mind Over Milkshakes: Mindsets, Not Just Nutrients, Determine Ghrelin Response," *Health Psychology* 30, no. 4 (2011): 424–29.

4.     Ibid.

5.     Calorie information is per slice, six slices per pie. "Bakers Square Restaurant and Bakery Nutritional Information," Bakerssquare.com, accessed February 7, 2014, http://www.bakerssquare.com/files/nutrition.pdf.

6.     H.R. 3590, 111th Congress: Patient Protection and Affordable Care Act. Public Law No. 111-148, www.GovTrack.us, 2010.

7.     Kamila M Kiszko et al., "The Influence of Calorie Labeling on Food Orders and Consumption: A Review of the Literature," *Journal of Community Health* (April 24, 2014), doi:10.1007/s10900-014-9876-0. Also see Table 2 in: J. Krieger and B. E. Saelens, *Impact of Menu Labeling on Consumer Behavior: A 2008–2012 Update* (Minneapolis, MN, 2013).

8.     Brian Elbel et al., "Calorie Labeling, Fast Food Purchasing and Restaurant Visits," *Obesity* (Silver Spring, MD) (October 17, 2013), doi:10.1002/oby.20550.

9.    Sarah Campos, Juliana Doxey, and David Hammond, "Nutrition Labels on Pre-Packaged Foods: A Systematic Review," *Public Health Nutrition* 14, no. 8 (2011): 1496; Klaus G. Grunert and Josephine M. Wills, "A Review of European Research on Consumer Response to Nutrition Information on Food Labels," *Journal of Public Health* 15, no. 5 (April 14, 2007): 385–99, doi:10.1007/s10389-007-0101-9; Gill Cowburn and Lynn Stockley, "Consumer Understanding and Use of Nutrition Labelling: A Systematic Review," *Public Health Nutrition* 8, no. 1 (February 2005): 21–28.

10.   Grunert and Wills, "A Review of European Research on Consumer Response to Nutrition Information on Food Labels"; Cowburn and Stockley, "Consumer Understanding and Use of Nutrition Labelling."

11.   E. A. Wartella et al., *Front-of-Package Nutrition Rating Systems and Symbols: Promoting Healthier Choices: Phase II Report* (Washington, DC: National Academies Press, Institute of Medicine, 2011).

12.   American Heart Association, "Heart Check Food Certification Program," 2014, http://www.heart.org/HEARTORG/GettingHealthy/NutritionCenter/HeartSmartShopping/Heart-Check-Program_UCM_300133_Article.jsp.

13.   Christina A. Roberto et al., "Facts Up Front Versus Traffic Light Food Labels: A Randomized Controlled Trial," *American Journal of Preventive Medicine* 43, no. 2 (August 1, 2012): 134–41, doi:10.1016/j.amepre.2012.04.022.

14.   We call it a check mark. "Heart Foundation Tick," Heart Foundation New Zealand, 2014, http://www.heartfoundation.org.nz/healthy-living/healthy-eating/heart-foundation-tick.

15.   Ellis L. Vyth et al., "A Front-of-Pack Nutrition Logo: A Quantitative and Qualitative Process Evaluation in the Netherlands," *Journal of Health Communication* 14, no. 7 (January 2009): 631–45, doi:10.1080/10810730903204247; Gray Nathan, "Healthy Logo: Netherlands 'Choices' Logo Confirmed as First Government-Backed Scheme in EU," FoodNavigator.com, 2016, http://www.foodnavigator.com/Legislation/Healthy-logo-Netherlands-Choices-logo-confirmed-as-first-government-backed-scheme-in-EU.

16.   Wartella et al., *Front-of-Package Nutrition Rating Systems and Symbols*; Roberto et al., "Facts Up Front Versus Traffic Light Food Labels."

17.   Kelly D. Brownell and Jeffrey P. Koplan, "Front-of-Package Nutrition Labeling—An Abuse of Trust by the Food Industry?," *New England Journal of Medicine* 364, no. 25 (June 22, 2011): 2373–75, doi:10.1056/NEJMp1101033.

18.   It was originally called Nutrition Keys. "GMA and FMI Select Agency Partners to Support $50 Million Nutrition Keys Consumer Education Campaign," FactsUpFront.org, 2011, http://www.factsupfront.org/Newsroom/5.

19.   Brownell and Koplan, "Front-of-Package Nutrition Labeling."

20.   Roberto et al., "Facts Up Front Versus Traffic Light Food Labels."

21.   At least in the United States. Rajagopal Raghunathan, Rebecca Walker Naylor, and Wayne D. Hoyer, "The Unhealthy=Tasty Intuition and Its Effects on Taste Inferences, Enjoyment, and Choice of Food Products," *Journal of Marketing* 70 (2006): 170–84. But this may not be true in France.

Carolina O. C. Werle, Olivier Trendel, and Gauthier Ardito, "Unhealthy Food Is Not Tastier for Everybody: The 'Healthy=Tasty' French Intuition," *Food Quality and Preference* 28, no. 1 (April 2013): 116–21, doi:10.1016/j.foodqual.2012.07.007.

22. Stacey R. Finkelstein and Ayelet Fishbach, "When Healthy Food Makes You Hungry," *Journal of Consumer Research* 37, no. 3 (October 2010): 357–67, doi:10.1086/652248.

23. My colleagues were not aware that my lab was collecting data on these foods at the conference. They are in no way complicit in my deception.

24. American Heart Association, "Heart Check Food Certification Program."

25. Richard E. Nisbett and Timothy D. Wilson, "Telling More Than We Can Know: Verbal Reports on Mental Processes," *Psychological Review* 84, no. 3 (1977): 231–59.

26. Heather Scherschel Wagner, Maryhope Howland, and Traci Mann, "Effects of Subtle and Explicit Health Messages on Food Choice," *Health Psychology*, 2014, doi:10.1037/hea0000045.

27. Sharon S. Brehm and Jack Williams Brehm, *Psychological Reactance: A Theory of Freedom and Control* (New York: Academic Press, 1981).

28. Including future honors student Hallie Espel and future lab manager Britt Ahlstrom.

29. Maryhope Howland and my lab manager Toni Gabrieli.

30. Theresa Marteau and her lab at the University of Cambridge have also shown that the word "healthy" does not lead more people to take apples, although "healthy and succulent" does. Suzanna E. Forwood et al., "Choosing between an Apple and a Chocolate Bar: The Impact of Health and Taste Labels," ed. Sidney Arthur Simon, *PloS One* 8, no. 10 (January 2013): e77500, doi:10.1371/journal.pone.0077500.

31. Finkelstein and Fishbach, "When Healthy Food Makes You Hungry."

32. This study is a little tricky. Both sandwiches are unhealthy, but participants believe the Big Mac is unhealthy and the Subway sandwich is healthy. P. Chandon and Brian Wansink, "The Biasing Health Halos of Fast Food Restaurant Health Claims: Lower Calorie Estimates and Higher Side Dish Consumption Intentions," *Journal of Consumer Research* 34, no. October (2007): 301–14.

33. It's a brilliant and hugely influential study. I've never taught a course on eating, health psychology, or research methods without discussing it. Herman and Mack, "Restrained and Unrestrained Eating."

34. Janet Polivy and C. Peter Herman, "Dieting and Binging: A Causal Analysis," *American Psychologist* 40, no. 2 (1985): 193–201.

35. Janet Tomiyama and Ashley Moskovich.

36. Janet Tomiyama et al., "Consumption after a Diet Violation: Disinhibition or Compensation?," *Psychological Science* 20, no. 10 (October 2009): 1275–81, doi:10.1111/j.1467-9280.2009.02436.x.

37. Ravi Dhar and Itamar Simonson, "Making Complementary Choices in Consumption Episodes: Highlighting Versus Balancing," *Journal of Marketing Research* (1999): 29–44.

38.    Kentaro Fujita et al., "Construal Levels and Self-Control," *Journal of Person-
       ality and Social Psychology* 90, no. 3 (March 2006): 351–67, doi:10.1037/002
       2-3514.90.3.351.

39.    Tinuke Oluyomi Daniel, Christina M Stanton, and Leonard H. Epstein,
       "The Future Is Now: Reducing Impulsivity and Energy Intake Using Epi-
       sodic Future Thinking," *Psychological Science* 24, no. 11 (November 1, 2013):
       2339–42, doi:10.1177/0956797613488780.

40.    K. Fujita and J. J. Carnevale, "Transcending Temptation Through Ab-
       straction: The Role of Construal Level in Self-Control," *Current Di-
       rections in Psychological Science* 21, no. 4 (July 25, 2012): 248–52,
       doi:10.1177/0963721412449169.

41.    Wansink, van Ittersum, and Painter, "How Descriptive Food Names Bias
       Sensory Perceptions in Restaurants."

42.    Walter Mischel and Nancy Baker, "Cognitive Appraisals and Transforma-
       tions in Delay Behavior," *Journal of Personality and Social Psychology* 31, no. 2
       (1975): 254.

43.    Remember when I said only one out of three hundred social psychologists at
       the conference figured out we were doing an experiment on them (with the
       apples)? That would be Ken Fujita. You can't get anything past him.

44.    Kentaro Fujita and H. Anna Han, "Moving Beyond Deliberative Control of
       Impulses: The Effect of Construal Levels on Evaluative Associations in Self-
       Control Conflicts," *Psychological Science* 20, no. 7 (July 1, 2009): 799–804,
       doi:10.1111/j.1467-9280.2009.02372.x; Kentaro Fujita, "Seeing the Forest
       Beyond the Trees: A Construal-Level Approach to Self-Control," *Social and
       Personality Psychology Compass* 2, no. 3 (May 2008): 1475–96, doi:10.1111/
       j.1751-9004.2008.00118.x.

45.    Fujita and Han, "Moving Beyond Deliberative Control of Impulses."

## CHAPTER 9: KNOW WHEN TO TURN OFF YOUR BRAIN

1.     Jon Henley, "Merde Most Foul," *Guardian*, April 12, 2002, http://www
       .theguardian.com/world/2002/apr/12/worlddispatch.jonhenley.

2.     Suzanne Daley, "Budget Cuts May Foul Sidewalks of Paris," *New York Times*,
       November 6, 2001, http://www.nytimes.com/2001/11/06/world/budget-
       cuts-may-foul-sidewalks-of-paris.html.

3.     D. Neal, W Wood, and J. Quinn, "Habits—A Repeat Performance," *Current
       Directions in Psychological Science* 15, no. 4 (2006): 198–202; Judith A. Ouel-
       lette and Wendy Wood, "Habit and Intention in Everyday Life: The Mul-
       tiple Processes by Which Past Behavior Predicts Future Behavior," *Psycho-
       logical Bulletin* 124, no. 1 (1998): 54–74, doi:10.1037//0033-2909.124.1.54;
       Wendy Wood and David T. Neal, "A New Look at Habits and the Habit-
       Goal Interface," *Psychological Review* 114, no. 4 (October 2007): 843–63,
       doi:10.1037/0033-295X.114.4.843.

4.     I am oversimplifying a giant research literature on automatic versus con-
       trolled processing. For an interesting overview, see: J. A. Bargh and M. J.

Ferguson, "Beyond Behaviorism: On the Automaticity of Higher Mental Processes," *Psychological Bulletin* 126, no. 6 (November 2000): 925–45.

5.    Joanna Robertson, "The Pampered Pooches of Paris," BBC, 2011, http://www.bbc.co.uk/news/magazine-16268890.

6.    The dozens of studies showing that our intentions do not predict our behavior very well are documented in a thorough quantitative review: Thomas L. Webb and Paschal Sheeran, "Does Changing Behavioral Intentions Engender Behavior Change? A Meta-Analysis of the Experimental Evidence," *Psychological Bulletin* 132, no. 2 (March 2006): 249–68, doi:10.1037/0033-2909.132.2.249.

7.    Phillippa Lally et al., "How Are Habits Formed: Modelling Habit Formation in the Real World," *European Journal of Social Psychology* 40, no. 6 (October 16, 2010): 998–1009, doi:10.1002/ejsp.674.

8.    Heather Barry Kappes and Gabriele Oettingen, "Positive Fantasies about Idealized Futures Sap Energy," *Journal of Experimental Social Psychology* 47, no. 4 (July 2011): 719–29, doi:10.1016/j.jesp.2011.02.003.

9.    Compared to people who had visualized having already succeeded. Shelley E. Taylor et al., "Harnessing the Imagination: Mental Simulation, Self-Regulation, and Coping," *American Psychologist* 53, no. 4 (1998): 429–39.

10.    Evidence that the performance of one habitual behavior can cue the performance of another: Stef P. J. Kremers, Klazine van der Horst, and Johannes Brug, "Adolescent Screen-Viewing Behaviour Is Associated with Consumption of Sugar-Sweetened Beverages: The Role of Habit Strength and Perceived Parental Norms," *Appetite* 48, no. 3 (May 2007): 345–50, doi:10.1016/j.appet.2006.10.002; Judith A Ouellette and Wendy Wood, "Habit and Intention in Everyday Life: The Multiple Processes by Which Past Behavior Predicts Future Behavior," *Psychological Bulletin* 124, no. 1 (1998): 54–74; Glenn J. Wagner and Gery W. Ryan, "Relationship between Routinization of Daily Behaviors and Medication Adherence in HIV-Positive Drug Users," *AIDS Patient Care and STDs* 18, no. 7 (July 2004): 385–93, doi:10.1089/1087291041518238.

11.    M. Ji and W. Wood, "Purchase and Consumption Habits: Not Necessarily What You Intend," *Journal of Consumer Psychology* 17, no. 4 (October 2007): 261–76, doi:10.1016/S1057-7408(07)70037-2.

12.    This has been shown with exercise, in Wendy Wood, Leona Tam, and Melissa Guerrero Witt, "Changing Circumstances, Disrupting Habits," *Journal of Personality and Social Psychology* 88, no. 6 (2005): 918–33. It's also been shown with making environmentally friendly transportation choices, in Bas Verplanken et al., "Context Change and Travel Mode Choice: Combining the Habit Discontinuity and Self-Activation Hypotheses," *Journal of Environmental Psychology* 28, no. 2 (June 2008): 121–27, doi:10.1016/j.jenvp.2007.10.005. It has not yet been carefully tested with eating, according to Johannes Brug et al., "Environmental Determinants of Healthy Eating: In Need of Theory and Evidence," *Proceedings of the Nutrition Society* 67, no. 3 (August 1, 2008): 307–16, doi:10.1017/S0029665108008616.

13.    Jayne Hurley and Bonnie Liebman, "Big: Movie Theaters Fill Buckets . . . and Bellies," *Nutrition Action Health Letter*, December 2009.

14.    David T. Neal et al., "The Pull of the Past: When Do Habits Persist Despite Conflict with Motives?," *Personality & Social Psychology Bulletin* 37, no. 11 (November 1, 2011): 1428–37, doi:10.1177/0146167211419863.

15.    Don't say I told you to, because movie theaters do not like that.

16.    Bas Verplanken and Wendy Wood, "Interventions to Break and Create Consumer Habits," *Journal of Public Policy & Marketing* 25, no. 1 (2006): 90–103.

17.    Wood, Tam, and Witt, "Changing Circumstances, Disrupting Habits."

18.    Nor do I necessarily recommend eating healthily on vacations. Or perhaps this is a handy rationalization as I happen to be in Paris as I write this and I am eating more than my share of pastries.

19.    Peter M. Gollwitzer, "Implementation Intentions: Strong Effects of Simple Plans," *American Psychologist* 54, no. 7 (1999): 493–503.

20.    For a review of the evidence, see Peter M. Gollwitzer and Paschal Sheeran, "Implementation Intentions and Goal Achievement: A Meta-Analysis of Effects and Processes" *Advances in Experimental Social Psychology* 38 (2006): 69–119, doi:10.1016/S0065-2601(06)38002-1. A good example can be found in Peter M Gollwitzer and Veronika Brandstätter, "Implementation Intentions and Effective Goal Pursuit," *Journal of Personality and Social Psychology* 73, no. 1 (1997): 186–99.

21.    Marieke A. Adriaanse et al., "Do Implementation Intentions Help to Eat a Healthy Diet? A Systematic Review and Meta-Analysis of the Empirical Evidence," *Appetite* 56, no. 1 (February 2011): 183–93, doi:10.1016/j.appet.2010.10.012.

22.    Bas Verplanken and Suzanne Faes, "Good Intentions, Bad Habits, and Effects of Forming Implementation Intentions on Healthy Eating," *European Journal of Social Psychology* 29, no. 5–6 (August 1999): 591–604, doi:10.1002/(SICI)1099-0992(199908/09)29:5/6<591::AID-EJSP948>3.0.CO;2-H.

23.    Paraphrased from Gollwitzer, "Implementation Intentions." For evidence that implementation intentions help prevent getting derailed by distractions, see Gollwitzer and Sheeran, "Implementation Intentions and Goal Achievement." For evidence that implementation intentions work automatically, see Ute C. Bayer et al., "Responding to Subliminal Cues: Do If-Then Plans Facilitate Action Preparation and Initiation Without Conscious Intent?," *Social Cognition* 27, no. 2 (April 21, 2009): 183–201, doi:10.1521/soco.2009.27.2.183.

24.    For evidence that implementation intentions help with the problem of failing to notice or act on an opportunity to fulfill a goal, see Gollwitzer and Sheeran, "Implementation Intentions and Goal Achievement."

25.    Janine Chapman, Christopher J. Armitage, and Paul Norman, "Comparing Implementation Intention Interventions in Relation to Young Adults' Intake of Fruit and Vegetables," *Psychology & Health* 24, no. 3 (March 2009): 317–32, doi:10.1080/08870440701864538.

26. Marieke A. Adriaanse et al., "Planning What Not to Eat: Ironic Effects of Implementation Intentions Negating Unhealthy Habits," *Personality & Social Psychology Bulletin* 37, no. 1 (January 1, 2011): 69–81, doi:10.1177/0146167210390523.

27. Adriaanse et al., "Do Implementation Intentions Help to Eat a Healthy Diet?"

28. This study comes from Charlotte Vinkers's dissertation, which I had the pleasure of watching her defend in Utrecht. In Dutch. Charlotte Vinkers, "Future-Oriented Self-Regulation in Eating Behavior" (diss., University of Utrecht, 2013).

29. This example was mentioned in Molly J. Crockett et al., "Restricting Temptations: Neural Mechanisms of Precommitment," *Neuron* 79, no. 2 (2013): 391–401.

30. D. Ariely and K. Wertenbroch, "Procrastination, Deadlines, and Performance: Self-Control by Precommitment," *Psychological Science* 13, no. 3 (May 1, 2002): 219–24, doi:10.1111/1467-9280.00441.

31. Yaacov Trope and Ayelet Fishbach, "Counteractive Self-Control in Overcoming Temptation," *Journal of Personality and Social Psychology* 79, no. 4 (2000): 493–506. Also see the excellently titled article by Xavier Giné, Dean Karlan, and Jonathan Zinman, "Put Your Money Where Your Butt Is: A Commitment Contract for Smoking Cessation," *American Economic Journal: Applied Economics* 2, no. 4 (2010): 213–35.

32. Janet Schwartz et al., "Healthier by Precommitment," *Psychological Science* 25 (January 3, 2014): 538–46, doi:10.1177/0956797613510950.

33. George Loewenstein, "Out of Control: Visceral Influences on Behavior," *Organizational Behavior and Human Decision Processes* 65, no. 3 (March 1996): 272–92, doi:10.1006/obhd.1996.0028; Loran F. Nordgren, Frenk van Harreveld, and Joop van der Pligt, "The Restraint Bias: How the Illusion of Self-Restraint Promotes Impulsive Behavior," *Psychological Science* 20, no. 12 (December 1, 2009): 1523–28, doi:10.1111/j.1467-9280.2009.02468.x.

## CHAPTER 10: HOW TO COMFORT AN ASTRONAUT

1. NASA publishes its evidence in Michele Perchonok and Grace Douglas, "Risk Factor of Inadequate Food System," in *Human Health Performance Risks of Space Exploration Missions: Evidence Reviewed by the NASA Human Research Program*, ed. Jancy C. McPhee and John B. Charles (Houston: NASA, 2009), 295–316.

2. Charles T. Bourland and Gregory L. Vogt, *The Astronaut's Cookbook: Tales, Recipes, and More* (New York: Springer International, 2009).

3. B. J. Caldwell et al., "Fluid Shift to the Upper Body Reduces Nasal Cavity Dimension and Airflow in Head-Down Bed Rest Subjects," in *NASA Human Research Program Investigators' Workshop* (Houston, 2012).

4. Barb Stuckey, *Taste: Surprising Stories and Science About why Food Tastes Good* (New York: Simon & Schuster, 2012).

5.    Perchonok and Douglas, "Risk Factor of Inadequate Food System."

6.    See, for example: D. J. Wallis and M. M. Hetherington, "Emotions and Eating. Self-Reported and Experimentally Induced Changes in Food Intake under Stress," *Appetite* 52, no. 2 (April 2009): 355–62, doi:10.1016/j .appet.2008.11.007. For a review, see: C. Greeno and R Wing, "Stress-Induced Eating," *Psychological Bulletin* 115 (1994): 444.

7.    J. McPhee and J. Charles, eds., *Human Health Performance Risks of Space Exploration Missions: Evidence Reviewed by the NASA Human Research Program* (Houston: NASA, 2009).

8.    Joe Redden and Zata Vickers, along with our graduate students Heather Wagner, Rachel Burns, and Katie Osdoba, and lab manager Britt Ahlstrom.

9.    Well, nobody had ever tested it the way we thought it should be done—by giving people their own idiosyncratic comfort food, though there is one rigorous test of chocolate on moods: Michael Macht and Jochen Mueller, "Immediate Effects of Chocolate on Experimentally Induced Mood States," *Appetite* 49, no. 3 (November 2007): 667–74, doi:10.1016/j.appet.2007.05.004.

10.   This shows just how strongly we believed in the ability of comfort food to improve mood.

11.   Britt Ahlstrom, my lab manager at the time, deserves all the credit for finding the foods.

12.   The four comfort food studies described in this chapter are published in Heather Wagner et al., "The Myth of Comfort Food," *Health Psychology* (2014).

13.   The research methodologists among you might be wondering if we had simply improved their moods as far as it was possible to improve them, leaving no "room" for comfort food to outperform the other food, called a ceiling effect. This was not the case, as we show most clearly in the fourth study in the article.

14.   There may be chemical properties of chocolate that cause it to make you feel good over a longer amount of time, but not immediately, the way we all expect comfort food to work. For a review, see Andrew Scholey and Lauren Owen, "Effects of Chocolate on Cognitive Function and Mood: A Systematic Review," *Nutrition Reviews* 71, no. 10 (October 2013): 665–81, doi:10.1111/ nure.12065.

15.   Wagner et al., "The Myth of Comfort Food."

16.   This is a popular comfort food among astronauts.

17.   There are people who are particularly likely to seek out comfort food or to eat when they feel bad. They are called emotional eaters. There is no evidence that comfort food helps them more than it does any other eaters. A measure of this appears in Tatjana van Strien et al., "The Dutch Eating Behavior Questionnaire (DEBQ) for Assessment of Restrained, Emotional, and External Eating Behavior," *International Journal of Eating Disorders* 5, no. 2 (February 1986): 295–315, doi:10.1002/1098-108X(198602)5:2<295::AID-EAT2260050209>3.0.CO;2-T.

18.   Meryl P. Gardner et al., "Better Moods for Better Eating? How Mood Influences Food Choice," *Journal of Consumer Psychology* (January 2014),

doi:10.1016/j.jcps.2014.01.002.

19. Yann Cornil and Pierre Chandon, "From Fan to Fat? Vicarious Losing Increases Unhealthy Eating, but Self-Affirmation Is an Effective Remedy," *Psychological Science* 24, no. 10 (October 1, 2013): 1936–46, doi:10.1177/0956797613481232.

20. Michael Macht, Jessica Meininger, and Jochen Roth, "The Pleasures of Eating: A Qualitative Analysis," *Journal of Happiness Studies* 6, no. 2 (June 2005): 137–60, doi:10.1007/s10902-005-0287-x; Jordi Quoidbach et al., "Positive Emotion Regulation and Well-Being: Comparing the Impact of Eight Savoring and Dampening Strategies," *Personality and Individual Differences* 49, no. 5 (October 2010): 368–73, doi:10.1016/j.paid.2010.03.048.

21. E. K. Papies, L. W. Barsalou, and R. Custers, "Mindful Attention Prevents Mindless Impulses," *Social Psychological and Personality Science* 3, no. 3 (August 29, 2011): 291–99, doi:10.1177/1948550611419031. Also see P. Rozin et al., "The Ecology of Eating: Smaller Portion Sizes in France Than in the United States Help Explain the French Paradox," *Psychological Science* 14, no. 5 (September 1, 2003): 450–54, doi:10.1111/1467-9280.02452.

22. This is true for dieters or people trying not to eat, as Andrew Ward and I found in our early eating studies. Ward and Mann, "Don't Mind If I Do: Disinhibited Eating Under Cognitive Load," April 1, 2000; Traci Mann and Andrew Ward, "To Eat or Not to Eat: Implications of the Attentional Myopia Model for Restrained Eaters," *Journal of Abnormal Psychology* 113, no. 1 (2004): 90–98.

23. Reine C. van der Wal and Lotte F. van Dillen, "Leaving a Flat Taste in Your Mouth: Task Load Reduces Taste Perception," *Psychological Science* 24, no. 7 (July 1, 2013): 1277–84, doi:10.1177/0956797612471953.

24. There is a slight difference. Intuitive eaters specifically reject following diet rules or plans and only eat what their body "tells" them it wants. Mindful eaters might follow an eating plan, so long as they are attentive to their eating and hunger. For specific measures of each, see Tracy L. Tylka, "Development and Psychometric Evaluation of a Measure of Intuitive Eating," *Journal of Counseling Psychology* 53, no. 2 (2006): 226–40; Celia Framson et al., "Development and Validation of the Mindful Eating Questionnaire," *Journal of the American Dietetic Association* 109, no. 8 (August 2009): 1439–44, doi:10.1016/j.jada.2009.05.006.

25. For an example, see Gayle M. Timmerman and Adama Brown, "The Effect of a Mindful Restaurant Eating Intervention on Weight Management in Women," *Journal of Nutrition Education and Behavior* 44, no. 1 (January 2012): 22–28, doi:10.1016/j.jneb.2011.03.143. For a review, see G. A. O'Reilly et al., "Mindfulness-Based Interventions for Obesity-Related Eating Behaviours: A Literature Review," *Obesity Reviews* (March 18, 2014), doi:10.1111/obr.12156.

26. Linda Bacon et al., "Size Acceptance and Intuitive Eating Improve Health for Obese, Female Chronic Dieters," *Journal of the American Dietetic Association* 105, no. 6 (June 2005): 929–36, doi:10.1016/j.jada.2005.03.011.

27. This was found in two of the three studies reviewed in O'Reilly et al., "Mindfulness-Based Interventions for Obesity-Related Eating Behaviours."

28. Megan Spanjers, "A Nutritious Diet Without Calorie Counting and Restrictive Rules? An Analysis of Nutrition Trends among Intuitive Eaters," (University of Minnesota, 2013).

29. This is shown in 11 out of 12 studies in O'Reilly et al., "Mindfulness-Based Interventions for Obesity-Related Eating Behaviours." For an example, see Jean Kristeller, Ruth Q. Wolever, and Virgil Sheets, "Mindfulness-Based Eating Awareness Training (MB-EAT) for Binge Eating: A Randomized Clinical Trial," *Mindfulness* (February 1, 2013), doi:10.1007/s12671-012-0179-1.

30. P. Rozin et al., "Attitudes to Food and the Role of Food in Life in the U.S.A., Japan, Flemish Belgium and France: Possible Implications for the Diet-Health Debate," *Appetite* 33, no. 2 (October 1999): 163–80, doi:10.1006/appe.1999.0244.

31. My kids call this behavior "the commercial chew."

32. Rozin et al., "The Ecology of Eating."

33. Rozin et al., "Attitudes to Food and the Role of Food in Life in the U.S.A., Japan, Flemish Belgium and France."

34. Ibid.

35. Jordi Quoidbach et al., "Money Giveth, Money Taketh Away: The Dual Effect of Wealth on Happiness," *Psychological Science* 21, no. 6 (June 1, 2010): 759–63, doi:10.1177/0956797610371963.

36. Ibid.

37. Richard Kirshenbaum, "Let Them Eat Kale: Extreme Dieters Ruining Dinner Parties for Everyone Else. Two Almonds Is Now Considered a Meal?," *New York Observer*, January 21, 2014.

## CHAPTER 11: WHY TO STOP OBSESSING AND BE OKAY WITH YOUR BODY

1. Art Caplan, "New Zealand's Solution for Rising Health Costs? Deport Fat People," NBC News, 2013, http://www.nbcnews.com/health/diet-fitness/new-zealands-solution-rising-health-costs-deport-fat-people-f6C10861122.

2. Helen Carter, "Too Fat to Adopt—the Married, Teetotal Couple Rejected by Council Because of Man's Weight," *Guardian*, January 16, 2009.

3. Mark V. Roehling et al., "The Effects of Weight Bias on Job-Related Outcomes: A Meta-Analysis of Experimental Studies," in Academy of Management Annual Meeting, Anaheim, CA, 2008.

4. M. V. Roehling, P. V. Roehling, and L. M. Odland, "Investigating the Validity of Stereotypes about Overweight Employees: The Relationship between Body Weight and Normal Personality Traits," *Group & Organization Management* 33, no. 4 (May 28, 2008): 392–424, doi:10.1177/1059601108321518.

5. Brian A. Nosek et al., "Pervasiveness and Correlates of Implicit Attitudes and Stereotypes," *European Review of Social Psychology* 18, no. 1 (January 2007):

36–88, doi:10.1080/10463280701489053. Sixty-nine percent of participants implicitly preferred thin people over obese people.

6.   Ibid.

7.   R. T. Azevedo et al., "Weighing the Stigma of Weight: An fMRI Study of Neural Reactivity to the Pain of Obese Individuals," *NeuroImage* 91 (May 1, 2014): 109–19, doi:10.1016/j.neuroimage.2013.11.041.

8.   R. M. Puhl, T. Andreyeva, and K. D. Brownell, "Perceptions of Weight Discrimination: Prevalence and Comparison to Race and Gender Discrimination in America," *International Journal of Obesity* 32, no. 6 (2008): 992–1000, doi:10.1038/ijo.2008.22.

9.   Puhl and Heuer, "The Stigma of Obesity: A Review and Update," 2009.

10.  Examples of the above, for college admissions, see Jane Wardle, Jo Waller, and Martin J. Jarvis, "Sex Differences in the Association of Socioeconomic Status with Obesity," *American Journal of Public Health* 92, no. 8 (August 10, 2002): 1299–1304, doi:10.2105/AJPH.92.8.1299. For health insurance, see Walter Hamilton, "Report: CVS Caremark Demands Workers Disclose Weight, Health Info," *Los Angeles Times*, March 20, 2013.

11.  Legal remedies are reviewed, and new laws suggested, in Young Suh et al., "Support for Laws to Prohibit Weight Discrimination in the United States: Public Attitudes from 2011 to 2013," *Obesity* (Silver Spring, MD) 22, no.8 (April 8, 2014):1872–9, doi:10.1002/oby.20750.

12.  For boys, see Nina Karnehed et al., "Obesity and Attained Education: Cohort Study of More than 700,000 Swedish Men," *Obesity* (Silver Spring, MD) 14, no. 8 (August 2006): 1421–28, doi:10.1038/oby.2006.161. For girls but not boys: R. Crosnoe, "Gender, Obesity, and Education," *Sociology of Education* 80, no. 3 (July 1, 2007): 241–60, doi:10.1177/003804070708000303. For girls and boys, but these researchers did not control for intelligence: Wardle, Waller, and Jarvis, "Sex Differences in the Association of Socioeconomic Status with Obesity."

13.  Jacob M Burmeister et al., "Weight Bias in Graduate School Admissions," *Obesity* (Silver Spring, MD) 21, no. 5 (May 2013): 918–20, doi:10.1002/oby.20171.

14.  For a review, see R. Puhl and C. Heuer, "The Stigma of Obesity: A Review and Update," *Obesity* 17, no. 5 (2009): 941–64.

15.  Scott Klarenbach et al., "Population-Based Analysis of Obesity and Workforce Participation," *Obesity* (Silver Spring, MD) 14, no. 5 (May 2006): 920–27, doi:10.1038/oby.2006.106.

16.  Roehling et al., "The Effects of Weight Bias on Job-Related Outcomes."

17.  K. S. O'Brien et al., "Obesity Discrimination: The Role of Physical Appearance, Personal Ideology, and Anti-Fat Prejudice," *International Journal of Obesity* 37, no. 3 (March 2013): 455–60, doi:10.1038/ijo.2012.52.

18.  Klarenbach et al., "Population-Based Analysis of Obesity and Workforce Participation."

19.  They rescinded the policy after getting unfavorable media attention. James Zervios, "Texas-Based Hospital 'Citizens Medical Center' Suspends Body

Mass Index Employment Requirement," *Obesity Action Coalition*, 2012, http://www.obesityaction.org/newsroom/news-releases/2012-news-releases/texas-based-hospital-citizens-medical-center-suspends-body-mass-index-employment-requirement.

20. Roehling et al., "The Effects of Weight Bias on Job-Related Outcomes."

21. For a thorough discussion, see Chapter 6 of Terry Poulton, *No Fat Chicks: How Big Business Profits by Making Women Hate Their Bodies—And How to Fight Back* (New York: Birch Lane Press, 1997).

22. Ibid.

23. Charles L. Baum and William F. Ford, "The Wage Effects of Obesity: A Longitudinal Study," *Health Economics* 13, no. 9 (September 2004): 885–99, doi:10.1002/hec.881. For similar data from Europe, see Giorgio Brunello and Béatrice D'Hombres, "Does Body Weight Affect Wages? Evidence from Europe," *Economics and Human Biology* 5, no. 1 (March 2007): 1–19, doi:10.1016/j.ehb.2006.11.002.

24. Timothy A. Judge and Daniel M. Cable, "When It Comes to Pay, Do the Thin Win? The Effect of Weight on Pay for Men and Women," *Journal of Applied Psychology* 96, no. 1 (January 1, 2011): 95–112, doi:10.1037/a0020860.

25. Baum and Ford, "The Wage Effects of Obesity."

26. Patricia V. Roehling et al., "Weight Discrimination and the Glass Ceiling Effect among Top US CEOs," *Equal Opportunities International* 28, no. 2 (February 13, 2009): 179–96, doi:10.1108/02610150910937916.

27. Patricia V. Roehling et al., "Weight Bias in US Candidate Selection and Election," *Equality, Diversity and Inclusion* 33, no. 4 (May 13, 2014): 334–46, doi:10.1108/EDI-10-2013-0081.

28. N. A. Schvey et al., "The Influence of a Defendant's Body Weight on Perceptions of Guilt," *International Journal of Obesity (2005)* 37, no. 9 (September 2013): 1275–81, doi:10.1038/ijo.2012.211.

29. Jason D. Seacat, Sarah C. Dougal, and Dooti Roy, "A Daily Diary Assessment of Female Weight Stigmatization," *Journal of Health Psychology* (March 18, 2014): 1359105314525067–, doi:10.1177/1359105314525067.

30. See also Puhl and Brownell, "Confronting and Coping with Weight Stigma."

31. Michael Scherer, "The Elephant in the Room: How Chris Christie Can Win Over the GOP," *Time*, November 18, 2013.

32. Puhl and Brownell, "Confronting and Coping with Weight Stigma."

33. See Chapter 4 of Poulton, *No Fat Chicks*. Also see Lesley, "What's Wrong with Fat-Shaming?," XOJane.com, 2012, http://www.xojane.com/issues/whats-wrong-fat-shaming. This beautifully written and heartbreaking column is worth reading in full.

34. Poulton, *No Fat Chicks*; Lesley, "What's Wrong With Fat-Shaming?"

35. For example, see Rod Liddle, "If We Don't Stigmatise Fat People, There'll Be Lots More of Them," *Spectator*, October 19, 2013.

36. Daniel Callahan, "Obesity: Chasing an Elusive Epidemic," *Hastings Center Report* 43, no. 1 (2013): 34–40, doi:10.1002/hast.114. He also argues that stigmatizing smokers was partly responsible for reductions in smoking in the

last few decades. It's not clear if that is true, but even if it is, that doesn't mean it would work for obesity (and the evidence in this part of the chapter shows it does not).

37.   Liddle, "If We Don't Stigmatise Fat People, There'll Be Lots More of Them."

38.   Brenda Major et al., "The Ironic Effects of Weight Stigma," *Journal of Experimental Social Psychology* 51 (March 2014): 74–80, doi:10.1016/j.jesp.2013.11.009.

39.   Other studies show this as well. See Elizabeth A. Pascoe and Laura Smart Richman, "Effect of Discrimination on Food Decisions," *Self and Identity* 10, no. 3 (July 2011): 396–406, doi:10.1080/15298868.2010.526384; Natasha A. Schvey, Rebecca M. Puhl, and Kelly D. Brownell, "The Impact of Weight Stigma on Caloric Consumption," *Obesity* (Silver Spring, MD) 19, no. 10 (October 2011): 1957–62, doi:10.1038/oby.2011.204; Rebecca Puhl, Joerg Luedicke, and Jamie Lee Peterson, "Public Reactions to Obesity-Related Health Campaigns: A Randomized Controlled Trial," *American Journal of Preventive Medicine* 45, no. 1 (July 1, 2013): 36–48, doi:10.1016/j.amepre.2013.02.010.

40.   Lenny R. Vartanian and Sarah A. Novak, "Internalized Societal Attitudes Moderate the Impact of Weight Stigma on Avoidance of Exercise," *Obesity* (Silver Spring, MD) 19, no. 4 (April 2011): 757–62, doi:10.1038/oby.2010.234; Lenny R. Vartanian and Jacqueline G. Shaprow, "Effects of Weight Stigma on Exercise Motivation and Behavior: A Preliminary Investigation among College-Aged Females," *Journal of Health Psychology* 13, no. 1 (January 1, 2008): 131–38, doi:10.1177/1359105307084318.

41.   Jason D. Seacat and Kristin D. Mickelson, "Stereotype Threat and the Exercise/Dietary Health Intentions of Overweight Women," *Journal of Health Psychology* 14, no. 4 (May 1, 2009): 556–67, doi:10.1177/1359105309103575.

42.   Vartanian and Shaprow, "Effects of Weight Stigma on Exercise Motivation and Behavior"; Vartanian and Novak, "Internalized Societal Attitudes Moderate the Impact of Weight Stigma on Avoidance of Exercise."

43.   Technically, it prevented an expected decrease in cortisol: Schvey, Puhl, and Brownell, "The Stress of Stigma." Also see Tomiyama et al., "Associations of Weight Stigma with Cortisol and Oxidative Stress Independent of Adiposity."

44.   Only 5 percent of lead characters on television shows are played by obese people, and in movies, obese actors and actresses aren't even necessarily hired to play obese characters. Bradley S. Greenberg et al., "Portrayals of Overweight and Obese Individuals on Commercial Television," *American Journal of Public Health* 93, no. 8 (August 10, 2003): 1342–48, doi:10.2105/AJPH.93.8.1342.

45.   Jeffrey M. Hunger and A. Janet Tomiyama, "Weight Labeling and Obesity," *JAMA Pediatrics* (April 28, 2014), doi:10.1001/jamapediatrics.2014.122. For similar findings with adults, see Angelina R. Sutin and Antonio Terracciano, "Perceived Weight Discrimination and Obesity," ed. Robert L. Newton, *PloS One* 8, no. 7 (January 2013): e70048, doi:10.1371/journal.pone.0070048.

46.  Flegal et al., "Prevalence of Obesity and Trends in the Distribution of Body Mass Index among US Adults, 1999–2010."

47.  Tatiana Andreyeva, Rebecca M. Puhl, and Kelly D. Brownell, "Changes in Perceived Weight Discrimination among Americans, 1995–1996 through 2004–2006," *Obesity* (Silver Spring, MD) 16, no. 5 (May 2008): 1129–34, doi:10.1038/oby.2008.35.

48.  Gordon W. Allport, *The Nature of Prejudice* (Reading, MA: Addison-Wesley, 1954). For the specific example of homophobia, see Sebastian E. Barto, Israel Berger, and Peter Hegarty, "Interventions to Reduce Sexual Prejudice: A Study-Space Analysis and Meta-Analytic Review," *Journal of Sex Research* 51, no. 4 (January 2014): 363–82, doi:10.1080/00224499.2013.871625.

49.  S. S. Wang, K. D. Brownell, and T. A. Wadden, "The Influence of the Stigma of Obesity on Overweight Individuals," *International Journal of Obesity and Related Metabolic Disorders* 28, no. 10 (October 1, 2004): 1333–7, doi:10.1038/sj.ijo.0802730.

50.  Tracy Moore, "I Don't Love (or Hate) My Body—and So Can You!," Jezebel.com, 2014, http://jezebel.com/i-dont-love-or-hate-my-body-and-so-can-you-1557099034.

51.  Joan Jacobs Brumberg, *The Body Project: An Intimate History of American Girls* (New York: Vintage Books, 1998).

52.  Ibid.

53.  "Gym, Health & Fitness Clubs in the US: Market Research Report," IBISWorld.com, 2014, http://www.ibisworld.com/industry/default.aspx?indid=1655.

54.  Se-Jin Lee, "Regulation of Muscle Mass by Myostatin," *Annual Review of Cell and Developmental Biology* 20 (January 8, 2004): 61–86, doi:10.1146/annurev.cellbio.20.012103.135836.

55.  Frank Bruni, "These Wretched Vessels," *New York Times*, December 24, 2012.

## CHAPTER 12: THE REAL REASONS TO EXERCISE AND STRATEGIES FOR STICKING WITH IT

1.  A strong case is made by Amy Luke and Richard S Cooper, "Physical Activity Does Not Influence Obesity Risk: Time to Clarify the Public Health Message," *International Journal of Epidemiology* 42, no. 6 (December 1, 2013): 1831–36, doi:10.1093/ije/dyt159. Also see the following for a rebuttal: James O Hill and John C. Peters, "Commentary: Physical Activity and Weight Control," *International Journal of Epidemiology* 42, no. 6 (December 1, 2013): 1840–42, doi:10.1093/ije/dyt161.

2.  This point is presented as one of nine facts about obesity in Casazza et al., "Myths, Presumptions, and Facts about Obesity."

3.  Petra Stiegler and Adam Cunliffe, "The Role of Diet and Exercise for the Maintenance of Fat-Free Mass and Resting Metabolic Rate during Weight Loss," *Sports Medicine* (Auckland, NZ) 36, no. 3 (January 2006): 239–62.

4.    N. A. King et al., "The Interaction between Exercise, Appetite, and Food
      Intake: Implications for Weight Control," *American Journal of Lifestyle Med-
      icine* 7, no. 4 (February 6, 2013): 265–73, doi:10.1177/1559827613475584;
      Catia Martins et al., "Effects of Exercise on Gut Peptides, Energy Intake
      and Appetite," *Journal of Endocrinology* 193, no. 2 (May 1, 2007): 251–58,
      doi:10.1677/JOE-06-0030.
5.    Carolina O. C. Werle, Brian Wansink, and Collin R. Payne, "Just Think-
      ing about Exercise Makes Me Serve More Food: Physical Activity and Cal-
      orie Compensation," *Appetite* 56, no. 2 (April 2011): 332–35, doi:10.1016/j
      .appet.2010.12.016.
6.    The government recommends 150 minutes of moderate exercise (or 75 of in-
      tense exercise) per week for health, but 300 minutes of moderate exercise per
      week (or 150 minutes of intense exercise) for weight loss. U.S. Department of
      Health and Human Services, "2008 Physical Activity Guidelines for Ameri-
      cans," http://www.health.gov/paguidelines/.
7.    This comes from a review of eighty studies that included over a million par-
      ticipants. About half of the studies made a point of controlling for weight.
      Guenther Samitz, Matthias Egger, and Marcel Zwahlen, "Domains of Physi-
      cal Activity and All-Cause Mortality: Systematic Review and Dose-Response
      Meta-Analysis of Cohort Studies," *International Journal of Epidemiology* 40,
      no. 5 (October 1, 2011): 1382–400, doi:10.1093/ije/dyr112.
8.    These patients were followed for over eight years. Edward W Gregg et al.,
      "Relationship of Walking to Mortality among US Adults with Diabetes," *Ar-
      chives of Internal Medicine* 163, no. 12 (June 23, 2003): 1440–7, doi:10.1001/
      archinte.163.12.1440.
9.    Samitz, Egger, and Zwahlen, "Domains of Physical Activity and All-Cause
      Mortality."
10.   Huseyin Naci and John P. A. Ioannidis, "Comparative Effectiveness of Ex-
      ercise and Drug Interventions on Mortality Outcomes: Metaepidemiological
      Study," *BMJ* (Clinical Research Ed.) 347 (January 2013): f5577.
11.   Ibid.
12.   Mark Hamer, Kim L. Lavoie, and Simon L. Bacon, "Taking Up Physical
      Activity in Later Life and Healthy Ageing: The English Longitudinal Study
      of Ageing," *British Journal of Sports Medicine* 48, no. 3 (February 1, 2014):
      239–43, doi:10.1136/bjsports-2013-092993.
13.   Francesco Sofi et al., "Physical Activity during Leisure Time and Primary
      Prevention of Coronary Heart Disease: An Updated Meta-Analysis of Co-
      hort Studies," *European Journal of Cardiovascular Prevention and Rehabilita-
      tion* 15, no. 3 (June 1, 2008): 247–57, doi:10.1097/HJR.0b013e3282f232ac.
14.   Chong Do Lee, Aaron R. Folsom, and Steven N. Blair, "Physical Activity
      and Stroke Risk: A Meta-Analysis," *Stroke* 34, no. 10 (October 1, 2003):
      2475–81, doi:10.1161/01.STR.0000091843.02517.9D.
15.   Frank B. Hu et al., "Walking Compared with Vigorous Physical Activity
      and Risk of Type 2 Diabetes in Women," *JAMA* 282, no. 15 (October 20,
      1999): 1433, doi:10.1001/jama.282.15.1433; S. P. Helmrich et al., "Physical

Activity and Reduced Occurrence of Non-Insulin-Dependent Diabetes Mellitus," *New England Journal of Medicine* 325, no. 3 (July 18, 1991): 147–52, doi:10.1056/NEJM199107183250302; Bridget M. Kuehn, "Physical Activity May Stave Off Diabetes for Women at Risk," *JAMA{dec63}* 311, no. 22 (June 11, 2014): 2263, doi:10.1001/jama.2014.6862.

16.    Inger Thune and Anne-Sofie Furberg, "Physical Activity and Cancer Risk: Dose-Response and Cancer, All Sites and Site-Specific," *Medicine and Science in Sports and Exercise* 33, Suppl. (June 1, 2001): S530–S550, doi:10.1097/00005768-200106001-00025.

17.    This was true regardless of whether they lost weight. Sean Carroll and Mike Dudfield, "What Is the Relationship between Exercise and Metabolic Abnormalities?," *Sports Medicine* 34, no. 6 (2004): 371–418, doi:10.2165/00007256-200434060-00004.

18.    Kelly M. Naugle, Roger B. Fillingim, and Joseph L. Riley, "A Meta-Analytic Review of the Hypoalgesic Effects of Exercise," *Journal of Pain* 13, no. 12 (December 2012): 1139–50, doi:10.1016/j.jpain.2012.09.006.

19.    Liisa Byberg et al., "Total Mortality After Changes in Leisure Time Physical Activity in 50 Year Old Men: 35 Year Follow-up of Population Based Cohort," *BMJ* (Clinical Research Ed.) 338, no. mar05_2 (January 5, 2009): b688, doi:10.1136/bmj.b688.

20.    Caudwell et al., "Exercise Alone Is Not Enough."

21.    Ibid.

22.    This is presented as one of nine facts about obesity in Casazza et al., "Myths, Presumptions, and Facts about Obesity."

23.    Petri Wiklund et al., "Metabolic Response to 6-Week Aerobic Exercise Training and Dieting in Previously Sedentary Overweight and Obese Pre-Menopausal Women: A Randomized Trial," *Journal of Sport and Health Science* (June 2014), doi:10.1016/j.jshs.2014.03.013.

24.    Organisation for Economic Co-operation and Development Better Life Index, 2014, Center for Economic and Policy Research, http://www.cepr.net/index.php/publications/reports/no-vacation-nation-2013.

25.    Rebecca Ray, Milla Sanes, and John Schmitt, *No-Vacation Nation Revisited* (Washington, DC: Center for Economic and Policy Research, 2013).

26.    The overall evidence for the effects of stress on health is summarized in the thorough and readable book by Robert Sapolsky, *Why Zebras Don't Get Ulcers*, 3rd ed. (New York: Holt Paperbacks, 2004). The classic scholarly review is McEwen and Seeman, "Protective and Damaging Effects of Mediators of Stress."

27.    This is nicely demonstrated in studies of parachute jumps, for example, Manfred Schedlowski et al., "Changes of Natural Killer Cells during Acute Psychological Stress," *Journal of Clinical Immunology* 13, no. 2 (March 1993): 119–26, doi:10.1007/BF00919268.

28.    S. Cohen, D. Janicki-Deverts, and G. E. Miller, "Psychological Stress and Disease," *JAMA* 298, no. 14 (2007): 1685–87, doi:10.1001/jama.298.14.1685.

29.    Sapolsky, *Why Zebras Don't Get Ulcers*.

30.    Ibid.

31.  Ibid.

32.  Sally S. Dickerson and Margaret E. Kemeny, "Acute Stressors and Cortisol
     Responses: A Theoretical Integration and Synthesis of Laboratory Research,"
     *Psychological Bulletin* 130, no. 3 (May 1, 2004): 355–91, doi:10.1037/003
     3-2909.130.3.355; Gregory E. Miller, Edith Chen, and Eric S. Zhou, "If
     It Goes Up, Must It Come Down? Chronic Stress and the Hypothalamic-
     Pituitary-Adrenocortical Axis in Humans," *Psychological Bulletin* 133, no. 1
     (2007): 25–45.

33.  P. Bjorntorp, "Do Stress Reactions Cause Abdominal Obesity and Comor-
     bidities?," *Obesity Reviews* 2, no. 2 (May 2001): 73–86, doi:10.1046/j.1467
     789x.2001.00027.x; E. S Epel et al., "Stress and Body Shape: Stress-Induced
     Cortisol Secretion Is Consistently Greater among Women with Central Fat,"
     *Psychosomatic Medicine* 62, no. 5 (2000): 623–32.

34.  Suzanne C. Segerstrom and Gregory E. Miller, "Psychological Stress and
     the Human Immune System: A Meta-Analytic Study of 30 Years of In-
     quiry," *Psychological Bulletin* 130, no. 4 (July 1, 2004): 601–30, doi:10.1037
     /0033-2909.130.4.601; Theodore F. Robles, Ronald Glaser, and Janice K.
     Kiecolt-Glaser, "Out of Balance. A New Look at Chronic Stress, Depression,
     and Immunity," *Current Directions in Psychological Science* 14, no. 2 (April
     2005): 111–15, doi:10.1111/j.0963-7214.2005.00345.x; Schedlowski et al.,
     "Changes of Natural Killer Cells during Acute Psychological Stress."

35.  Sheldon Cohen, David A. Tyrrell, and Andrew P. Smith, "Psychological
     Stress and Susceptibility to the Common Cold," *New England Journal of
     Medicine* 325, no. 9 (1991): 606–12.

36.  Jessica Walburn et al., "Psychological Stress and Wound Healing in Humans:
     A Systematic Review and Meta-Analysis," *Journal of Psychosomatic Research*
     67, no. 3 (September 2009): 253–71, doi:10.1016/j.jpsychores.2009.04.002.

37.  Elissa S. Epel et al., "Accelerated Telomere Shortening in Response to
     Life Stress," *Proceedings of the National Academy of Sciences of the United
     States of America* 101, no. 49 (December 7, 2004): 17312–15, doi:10.1073/
     pnas.0407162101.

38.  Kimberly A. Brownley et al., "Sympathoadrenergic Mechanisms in Re-
     duced Hemodynamic Stress Responses After Exercise," *Medicine and Sci-
     ence in Sports and Exercise* 35, no. 6 (June 2003): 978–86, doi:10.1249/01.
     MSS.0000069335.12756.1B.

39.  Peter Salmon, "Effects of Physical Exercise on Anxiety, Depression, and
     Sensitivity to Stress," *Clinical Psychology Review* 21, no. 1 (February 2001):
     33–61, doi:10.1016/S0272-7358(99)00032-X.

40.  Cheryl J. Hansen, Larry C. Stevens, and J. Richard Coast, "Exercise Dura-
     tion and Mood State: How Much Is Enough to Feel Better?," *Health Psychol-
     ogy* 20, no. 4 (July 1, 2001): 267–75, doi:10.1037/0278-6133.20.4.267.

41.  J. C. Coulson, J. McKenna, and M. Field, "Exercising at Work and
     Self-Reported Work Performance," *International Journal of Work-
     place Health Management* 1, no. 3 (September 26, 2008): 176–97,
     doi:10.1108/17538350810926534; Robert R. Yeung, "The Acute Effects of

Exercise on Mood State," *Journal of Psychosomatic Research* 40, no. 2 (February 1996): 123–41, doi:10.1016/0022-3999(95)00554-4.

42.  Salmon, "Effects of Physical Exercise on Anxiety, Depression, and Sensitivity to Stress."

43.  Steven J. Petruzzello et al., "A Meta-Analysis on the Anxiety-Reducing Effects of Acute and Chronic Exercise," *Sports Medicine* 11, no. 3 (March 1991): 143–82, doi:10.2165/00007256-199111030-00002.

44.  Peter J. Carek, Sarah E. Laibstain, and Stephen M. Carek, "Exercise for the Treatment of Depression and Anxiety," *International Journal of Psychiatry in Medicine* 41, no. 1 (January 1, 2011): 15–28, doi:10.2190/PM.41.1.c; Andreas Broocks et al., "Comparison of Aerobic Exercise, Clomipramine, and Placebo in the Treatment of Panic Disorder," *American Journal of Psychiatry* 155, no. 5 (May 1, 1998): 603–9.

45.  Carek, Laibstain, and Carek, "Exercise for the Treatment of Depression and Anxiety"; Gillian E. Mead et al., "Exercise for Depression," *Cochrane Database of Systematic Reviews* no. 4 (January 2008): CD004366, doi:10.1002/14651858.CD004366.pub3.

46.  Hamer, Lavoie, and Bacon, "Taking Up Physical Activity in Later Life and Healthy Ageing."

47.  Daniel Y. T. Fong et al., "Physical Activity for Cancer Survivors: Meta-Analysis of Randomised Controlled Trials," *BMJ* (Clinical Research Ed.) 344, no. jan30_5 (January 31, 2012): e70, doi:10.1136/bmj.e70.

48.  M E. Hopkins et al., "Differential Effects of Acute and Regular Physical Exercise on Cognition and Affect," *Neuroscience* 215 (July 26, 2012): 59–68, doi:10.1016/j.neuroscience.2012.04.056; Hamer, Lavoie, and Bacon, "Taking Up Physical Activity in Later Life and Healthy Ageing"; Maria A. I. Aberg et al., "Cardiovascular Fitness Is Associated with Cognition in Young Adulthood," *Proceedings of the National Academy of Sciences of the United States of America* 106, no. 49 (December 8, 2009): 20906–11, doi:10.1073/pnas.0905307106; Arthur F. Kramer, Kirk I. Erickson, and Stanley J. Colcombe, "Exercise, Cognition, and the Aging Brain," *Journal of Applied Physiology* 101, no. 4 (October 1, 2006): 1237–42, doi:10.1152/japplphysiol.00500.2006.

49.  Kate Lambourne and Phillip Tomporowski, "The Effect of Exercise-Induced Arousal on Cognitive Task Performance: A Meta-Regression Analysis," *Brain Research* 1341 (June 23, 2010): 12–24, doi:10.1016/j.brainres.2010.03.091.

50.  Marily Oppezzo and Daniel L. Schwartz, "Give Your Ideas Some Legs: The Positive Effect of Walking on Creative Thinking," *Journal of Experimental Psychology* (2014).

51.  Shelley S. Tworoger et al., "Effects of a Yearlong Moderate-Intensity Exercise and a Stretching Intervention on Sleep Quality in Postmenopausal Women," *Sleep* 26, no. 7 (2003): 830–38.

52.  Abby C. King et al., "Moderate-Intensity Exercise and Self-Rated Quality of Sleep in Older Adults," *JAMA* 277, no. 1 (January 1, 1997): 32–37, doi:10.1001/jama.1997.03540250040029.

53. This study did not control for weight or weight loss. Hamer, Lavoie, and Bacon, "Taking Up Physical Activity in Later Life and Healthy Ageing."

54. B. L. Tracy et al., "Muscle Quality. II. Effects of Strength Training in 65- to 75-Yr-Old Men and Women," *Journal of Applied Physiology* 86, no. 1 (January 1, 1999): 195–201.

55. Kramer, Erickson, and Colcombe, "Exercise, Cognition, and the Aging Brain."

56. U.S. Department of Health and Human Services, "2008 Physical Activity Guidelines for Americans."

57. Your maximum heart rate can be calculated here: http://www.ntnu.edu/cerg/hrmax.

58. Karissa L. Canning et al., "Individuals Underestimate Moderate and Vigorous Intensity Physical Activity," ed. Conrad P. Earnest, *PloS One* 9, no. 5 (January 2014): e97927, doi:10.1371/journal.pone.0097927.

59. U.S. Department of Health and Human Services, "2008 Physical Activity Guidelines for Americans."

60. Ross C. Brownson, Tegan K. Boehmer, and Douglas A. Luke, "Declining Rates of Physical Activity in the United States: What Are the Contributors?," *Annual Review of Public Health* 26 (October 7, 2005): 421–43.

61. Ibid.

62. Ibid.

63. Uri Ladabaum et al., "Obesity, Abdominal Obesity, Physical Activity, and Caloric Intake in US Adults: 1988 to 2010," *American Journal of Medicine* 127, no. 8 (August 2014): 717–727.e12, doi:10.1016/j.amjmed.2014.02.026.

64. The Exercise Is Medicine campaign is dedicated to making exercise a standard part of disease prevention and to include questions about physical activity in all patient visits. It is endorsed by hundreds of health-related organizations. The list can be found at http://www.exerciseismedicine.org/supporters.htm.

65. Susan A Carlson et al., "Trend and Prevalence Estimates Based on the 2008 Physical Activity Guidelines for Americans," *American Journal of Preventive Medicine* 39, no. 4 (October 2010): 305–13, doi:10.1016/j.amepre.2010.06.006.

66. Jared M. Tucker, Gregory J. Welk, and Nicholas K. Beyler, "Physical Activity in U.S.: Adults Compliance with the Physical Activity Guidelines for Americans," *American Journal of Preventive Medicine* 40, no. 4 (April 2011): 454–61, doi:10.1016/j.amepre.2010.12.016.

67. Ibid.

68. Ibid. Accelerometers aren't perfect, and they are more likely to underestimate exercise than to overestimate it.

69. Ryan E. Rhodes and Gert-Jan de Bruijn, "How Big Is the Physical Activity Intention-Behaviour Gap? A Meta-Analysis Using the Action Control Framework," *British Journal of Health Psychology* 18, no. 2 (May 2013): 296–309, doi:10.1111/bjhp.12032.

70. Geoff Williams, "The Heavy Price of Losing Weight," *U.S. News & World Report*, January 2, 2013, http://money.usnews.com/money/personal-

finance/articles/2013/01/02/the-heavy-price-of-losing-weight.     Williams cites: "Gym Membership Statistics," StatisticsBrain.com, 2012, http://www .statisticbrain.com/gym-membership-statistics/.

71.     Thirty billion dollars per year are spent on fitness clothes in the United States, according to sportsbusinessdaily.com, cited in: Amber Goodfellow, "The Athletic Apparel Industry: Fitness or Fashion?," *Digital Universe*, 2013, http://universe.byu.edu/2013/07/30/the-athletic-apparel-industry-fitness-or-fashion/.

72.     Entire books and thousands of articles have been written on this point alone. This book is a nice summary: Mark Conner et al., *Predicting Health Behaviour* (Maidenhead, England: McGraw-Hill International, 2005). This article is also helpful: Ralf Schwarzer, "Modeling Health Behavior Change: How to Predict and Modify the Adoption and Maintenance of Health Behaviors," *Applied Psychology* 57, no. 1 (January 2008): 1–29, doi:10.1111/ j.1464-0597.2007.00325.x.

73.     Conner et al., *Predicting Health Behaviour*.

74.     Marcel den Hoed et al., "Heritability of Objectively Assessed Daily Physical Activity and Sedentary Behavior," *American Journal of Clinical Nutrition* 98, no. 5 (November 18, 2013): 1317–25, doi:10.3945/ajcn.113.069849.

75.     Justin S. Rhodes, Theodore Garland, and Stephen C. Gammie, "Patterns of Brain Activity Associated with Variation in Voluntary Wheel-Running Behavior," *Behavioral Neuroscience* 117, no. 6 (December 1, 2003): 1243–56, doi:10.1037/0735-7044.117.6.1243.

76.     Ibid.

77.     Rachel J. Burns et al., "A Theoretically Grounded Systematic Review of Material Incentives for Weight Loss: Implications for Interventions," *Annals of Behavioral Medicine* 44, no. 3 (December 2012): 375–88, doi:10.1007/ s12160-012-9403-4.

78.     The student was Rachel Burns.

79.     Rachel J. Burns, "Can We Pay People to Act Healthily? Testing the Relative Effectiveness of Incentive Dimensions and Underlying Psychological Mediators," (University of Minnesota, 2014).

80.     I'm not alone in this experience. Benjamin Lorr describes something similar in his book (though he takes things a bit far). Benjamin Lorr, *Hell-Bent: Obsession, Pain, and the Search for Something Like Transcendence in Competitive Yoga* (New York: St. Martin's Press, 2012).

81.     The following makes the point that reinforcers need to be immediate: C. B. Ferster and B. F. Skinner, *Schedules of Reinforcement* (East Norwalk, CT: Appleton-Century-Crofts, 1957). I have not seen specific research evidence for the effectiveness of fitness feedback over weight feedback on long-term exercise maintenance. I am conducting research on this now.

82.     Carolina O. C. Werle, Brian Wansink, and Collin R. Payne, "Is It Fun or Exercise? The Framing of Physical Activity Biases Subsequent Snacking," *Marketing Letters* (May 15, 2014), doi:10.1007/s11002-014-9301-6.

83.     Staub, "Instigation to Goodness"; Howland, Hunger, and Mann, "Friends

Don't Let Friends Eat Cookies."

84.  Staub, "Instigation to Goodness"; Howland, Hunger, and Mann, "Friends
     Don't Let Friends Eat Cookies."
85.  Gollwitzer and Sheeran, "Implementation Intentions and Goal Achieve-
     ment."
86.  Sarah Milne, Sheina Orbell, and Paschal Sheeran, "Combining Motivational
     and Volitional Interventions to Promote Exercise Participation: Protection
     Motivation Theory and Implementation Intentions," *British Journal of Health
     Psychology* 7, no. Pt 2 (May 2002): 163–84, doi:10.1348/135910702169420.
87.  Ibid.
88.  Gollwitzer and Sheeran, "Implementation Intentions and Goal Achieve-
     ment."
89.  Williams, "The Heavy Price of Losing Weight."
90.  Schwartz et al., "Healthier by Precommitment."
91.  E. Kahn et al., "The Effectiveness of Interventions to Increase Physical Ac-
     tivity: A Systematic Review," *American Journal of Preventive Medicine* 22,
     no. 4 (May 2002): 73–107, doi:10.1016/S0749-3797(02)00434-8; G. Neil
     Thomas et al., "Health Promotion in Older Chinese: A 12-Month Clus-
     ter Randomized Controlled Trial of Pedometry and 'Peer Support,'" *Med-
     icine and Science in Sports and Exercise* 44, no. 6 (June 2012): 1157–66,
     doi:10.1249/MSS.0b013e318244314a.

## FINAL WORDS: DIET SCHMIET

1.   Tomiyama et al., "Low Calorie Dieting Increases Cortisol."
2.   Glennon Doyle Melton, "Your Body Is Not Your Masterpiece," Momas-
     tery blog, July 6, 2014, http://momastery.com/blog/2014/07/06/body-
     masterpiece/.

# INDEX

# ABOUT THE AUTHOR

Traci Mann is professor of social and health psychology at the University of Minnesota. She received her Ph.D. in psychology from Stanford University and was a tenured professor at UCLA before moving to the University of Minnesota in 2007, where she founded the Health and Eating Lab. Her research has been funded by the National Institutes of Health, the United States Department of Agriculture, and the National Aeronautics and Space Association (NASA). She lives with her husband, University of Minnesota professor of psychology Stephen Engel, and their two sons in Edina, Minnesota.

# The Lupus Book
## A Guide for Patients and Their Families

## Sixth Edition

DANIEL J. WALLACE, MD, FACP, MACR

Professor of Medicine

Associate Director, Rheumatology Fellowship Program

Cedars-Sinai Medical Center

David Geffen School of Medicine at UCLA

Los Angeles, California

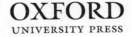

OXFORD
UNIVERSITY PRESS

# OXFORD
UNIVERSITY PRESS

Oxford University Press is a department of the University of Oxford. It furthers the University's objective of excellence in research, scholarship, and education by publishing worldwide. Oxford is a registered trade mark of Oxford University Press in the UK and certain other countries.

Published in the United States of America by Oxford University Press
198 Madison Avenue, New York, NY 10016, United States of America.

© Oxford University Press 2019

First Edition published in 1995
Second Edition published in 2000
Third Edition published in 2005
Fourth Edition published in 2009
Fifth Edition published in 2012

Library of Congress Cataloging-in-Publication Data
Names: Wallace, Daniel J. (Daniel Jeffrey), 1949- author.
Title: The lupus book : a guide for patients and
their families / Daniel J. Wallace, MD.
Description: Sixth edition. | New York, NY : Oxford University Press, [2019] |
Includes bibliographical references and index.
Identifiers: LCCN 2018036152 | ISBN 9780190876203
Subjects: LCSH: Systemic lupus erythematosus—Popular works.
Classification: LCC RC924.5.L85 W35 2019 | DDC 616.7/72—dc23
LC record available at https://lccn.loc.gov/2018036152

5 7 9 8 6

Printed by Sheridan Books, Inc., United States of America

# Contents

# Preface to the Sixth Edition

I am amazed at the number of lupus patients referred to me who have received only a cursory explanation of their disease and a brief discussion of its management. They have no idea what to expect and therefore usually have many questions, some of which I cannot yet answer. I have written this book for them, their caregivers, and their physicians.

*The Lupus Book* has sold nearly 200,000 copies since it was first published in 1995. The sixth edition adds numerous tables, extensively revises basic science and research sections, and adds sections on new emerging areas such as the microbiome, lupus clinical trials, and developing therapies. Over 500 changes have been made in the text since the previous edition. For those interested in additional resources, a "Further Reading" listing has been added for each chapter.

I hope you find this work informative and enjoyable to read. If you are reading this book, you may have been diagnosed with lupus or suspect that you have it. It is my hope that this book will help you work with your physician. In some instances, to flesh out the details, I have used composite cases based on real people I treat. Of course—as I learned early in my practice—no two patients have exactly the same experience with the disease. But some of the patients' personal stories may ring true and help you cope with your own symptoms.

This book is not intended to be a substitute for advice given by your family physician or the specialist you have been referred to. These doctors know your medical history and related problems far better than I ever will and can provide you with a perspective that is not possible for me to impart.

*The Lupus Book* is not meant to be read from front to back. It is intended to be a resource for patients and caregivers who are interested in how various aspects are approached in particular. Chapters 5 through 9 may be very technical. The reader should not get discouraged; understanding immunology is a daunting task, even for physicians.

As a physician who specializes in rheumatology and has a special interest in lupus, I have tried to anticipate your questions with the most up-to-date information we now have on causes, prevention, cure, exercise, diet, and many other important topics. This book is a distillation of my experience in treating over several thousand lupus patients. It is aimed at patients and allied health professionals (e.g., physical therapists, nurses, occupational therapists, social workers, psychologists, and others) who may be involved in the care of lupus patients.

I am indebted to my wife and our three children (Phil, Sarah, and Naomi) and amazing grandchildren for my imposition on their time in preparing this book, as well as my research and administrative staff (especially Jody Stanley and Jennifer Nelson) for their patience and support.

# Part I

# INTRODUCTION AND DEFINITIONS

Where should we start? The most logical place is with a definition of lupus. We look at how it is classified as a disease and place it in its proper historical perspective. This is followed by an overview of how lupus is distributed in the population—in other words, who gets the disease, which parts of the world have the highest prevalence of lupus, how many people have lupus in the United States and at what age, and which sex is most affected.

# 1

# *Why Write a Book on Lupus?*

The first time someone hears the words "lupus erythematosus," he or she usually says, "What?" When I first started my practice, patients identified the term with Peter Lupus, one of the characters on *Mission Impossible*, a popular television series (antedating the movies) in the late 1960s. Sometimes it looks as though finding a cure for lupus is an impossible mission, but there is much we do know, and the aim of this book is to share that knowledge.

Lupus is the common name for the disorder known technically as lupus erythematosus. This formal name includes systemic lupus erythematosus—where *systemic* means affecting the entire body or internal system—or SLE for short. Although underrecognized, lupus is an extremely important disease for many reasons:

- *In the United States, nearly 1 million people suffer from lupus* related disorders (put in italics). It is more common than better-known disorders such as leukemia, multiple sclerosis, cystic fibrosis, and muscular dystrophy combined. Those who develop SLE do so in the prime of life. Ninety percent of these sufferers are women, 90 percent of whom are in their childbearing years. Moreover, the effects of the disease disrupt family life and account for billions of dollars in lost work productivity.
- *Understanding the immunology of lupus will help us better understand HIV, infections in general, allergies, and cancer.* Medical students are often told, "Know lupus and you know medicine," and lupus is the paradigm of autoimmunity. This is because SLE can affect every part of the body. The basic immunopathology of lupus, or the factors that cause the disease, get to the core of how the human immune system functions. Nearly every major advance in understanding lupus immunology has had a spillover effect—it has helped not only SLE patients but also those with immune-related disorders such as HIV, other infectious processes, allergies, and cancer.
- *Lupus can be a very difficult disease to diagnose.* Many lupus patients look perfectly healthy, but surveys have shown that newly diagnosed patients have had symptoms or signs for an average of 3 years. A young woman who

complains of fatigue, achiness, stiffness, and low-grade fevers or swollen glands is often told she is experiencing stress, has picked up a virus that is going around, or—worse—that she is exaggerating her symptoms. By the time she is diagnosed with SLE, permanent damage to vital organs such as the lungs or kidneys may have occurred. (Advanced lupus is usually easy to diagnose.) This book attempts to increase public awareness of the disease, which could lead to earlier diagnosis.

- *There is a shortage of doctors capable of diagnosing and treating SLE, a disease studied and managed by rheumatologists.* Rheumatology is one of the recognized subspecialties of internal medicine, along with cardiology, gastroenterology, and pulmonary medicine, a field in which only 1 percent of physicians in the United States are certified to practice. The American College of Rheumatology (ACR) has estimated that the United States will be short nearly 3,000 rheumatologists by 2030. Only 4,000 rheumatologists are in active private full-time practice as of this writing.

- *Many patients who are told they have SLE do not.* Some 10 million Americans have a positive lupus blood screen (called antinuclear antibody, or ANA), but only about 1 million of these actually have SLE or lupus-related disorders. Since normal patients and healthy relatives of those with autoimmune disease can have positive tests for lupus, some physicians take the test results at face value and inform their patients (especially young women) that they do indeed have the disease or may succumb to it in the future. Such patients may suffer ill effects, especially if unnecessary treatments are prescribed. Also, many disorders mimic SLE. A positive blood test for lupus may be found during a viral illness, and unsuspecting physicians may draw the wrong conclusions. Disorders closely related to SLE such as scleroderma or polymyositis (see the glossary for definitions of technical terms) may exhibit similar test results but are treated quite differently. In discerning among these conditions, a complex diagnostic workup is often necessary, and few physicians are equipped to interpret the necessary battery of tests. In these instances, most physicians will consult a board-certified rheumatologist or recommend that their patients visit such a specialist.

Now let's get started. We'll begin by discussing what lupus really is.

## FURTHER READING

1. FitzGerald JD, Battistone M, Brown CR Jr, et al. American College of Rheumatology Committee on Rheumatology Training and Workforce Issues. Regional distribution of adult rheumatologists. *Arthritis Rheum.* 2013;65(12):3017–3025.
2. Al Daabil M, Massarotti EM, Fine A, et al. Development of SLE among "potential SLE" patients seen in consultation: long-term follow-up. *Int J Clin Pract.* 2014;68(12):1508–1513.

# 2
## *What Is Lupus?*

In simple terms, lupus erythematosus develops when the body becomes allergic to itself. Immunologically speaking, it is the opposite of what takes place in cancer or HIV. In lupus, the body overreacts to an unknown stimulus and makes too many antibodies, or proteins directed against body tissue. Thus, lupus is called an *autoimmune disease* (*auto* meaning *self*).

### IS THERE AN "OFFICIAL" DEFINITION OF LUPUS?

The American College of Rheumatology (ACR), a professional association to which nearly all rheumatologists in the United States belong, devised criteria for clinical trials and population studies rather than for diagnostic purposes in 1971. These criteria were revised in 1982 and 1997, and they are shown in Table 2.1. The presence of 4 of the 11 criteria confirms the diagnosis. These criteria apply only to systemic lupus erythematosus (SLE) and not to drug-induced or discoid (cutaneous) lupus. (These various forms of lupus are discussed in the section What Types of Lupus Are There?)

The first four criteria concern the skin: sun sensitivity, mouth sores, butterfly rashes, and discoid lesions (sores resembling a disk).

The second four criteria are associated with specific organ areas: the lining of the heart or lung, the kidneys, the central nervous system, and the joints.

The remaining three criteria specify relevant laboratory abnormalities: altered blood counts (low red blood cells, white blood cells, or platelets), positive antinuclear antibody (ANA) testing, and other blood antibody abnormalities of the disease. The ANA test is used as the primary diagnostic tool to determine whether a person has lupus, but there are limits to its reliability, which we discuss in Chapter 6. A patient can have SLE without fulfilling ACR criteria. For example, a patient with a positive kidney biopsy for lupus may meet only two criteria if the ANA is also positive. Though they are over 90 percent sensitive and specific for the diagnosis of SLE, the ACR criteria are primarily used for research purposes as entry criteria for a study.

**Table 2.1.** *American College of Rheumatology (1997) Revised Criteria for the Classification of Systemic Lupus Erythematosus (SLE)*

A person is said to have SLE if 4 of the following 11 criteria are present at any time:

*Skin criteria*

1. Butterfly rash (lupus rash over the cheeks and nose)
2. Discoid rash (a thick, disk-like rash that scars, usually on sun-exposed areas)
3. Sun sensitivity (rash after being exposed to ultraviolet A and B light)
4. Oral ulcerations (recurrent sores in the mouth or nose)

*Systemic criteria*

5. Arthritis (inflammation of two peripheral joints with tenderness, swelling, or fluid)
6. Serositis (inflammation of the lining of the pleura [lung] or the pericardium [heart])
7. Kidney disorder (protein in urine samples or abnormal sediment in urine seen under the microscope)
8. Neurologic disorder (seizures or psychosis with no other explanation)

*Laboratory criteria*

9. Blood abnormalities (hemolytic anemia, low white blood cell counts, low platelet counts)
10. Immunologic disorder (blood testing indicating either antiphospholipid antibodies, lupus anti-coagulant, anti-DNA, false-positive syphilis test, or a positive anti-Smith antibody [anti-Sm])
11. Positive antinuclear antibody blood test

Many other manifestations of SLE are not included in the ACR criteria. They are excluded because they are not *statistically* important in differentiating SLE from other rheumatic diseases. For example, a condition known as Raynaud's phenomenon (when one's fingers turn white and then blue in cold weather) is present in one third of lupus patients. But it is not included in the criteria because 95 percent of those suffering from scleroderma also have Raynaud's. In other words, Raynaud's is not specific to SLE and therefore does not provide enough proof to classify someone as having SLE. In 2012, the Systemic Lupus International Collaborative Clinics (SLICC) proposed a classification for SLE that takes into account recent advances. It is as sensitive and specific as the ACR criteria, but it allows patients to be diagnosed with SLE who have a positive biopsy, additional laboratory tests, and neurologic findings. See Table 2.2. A committee of the ACR and the European League Against Rheumatism (EULAR) is currently working on an international criteria set based on an updated means of ascertainment known as the Delphi method that has proven successful for other rheumatic diseases. The preliminary criteria are shown in Table 2.3.

These particular manifestations of SLE will be covered in detail in later chapters.

## WHAT TYPES OF LUPUS ARE THERE?

Sometimes the autoimmune reaction of lupus can be limited just to the skin and may result in a negative ANA blood test. This condition is called *cutaneous* or *discoid lupus erythematosus* (DLE). Though DLE is not an entirely accurate term

**Table 2.2.** *Systemic Lupus Erythematosus International Collaborative Clinics (SLICC)*
*Classification for Systemic Lupus Erythematosus*

I. Biopsy documented nephritis excluding other causes *or*
II. One clinical and one immunologic criterion from the following:
   A. Clinical criteria in the absence of other causes
      1. Acute cutaneous rash (malar, sun sensitive, maculopapular, toxic epidermal necrolysis variant)
      2. Chronic cutaneous lupus (discoid, hypertrophic, profundus, tumidus, chilblains, mucosal, lichenoid)
      3. Oral ulcers (buccal, tongue, or nasal)
      4. Nonscarring alopecia
      5. Nonerosive inflammatory arthritis
      6. Serositis (pleural, pericardial)
      7. >0.5 G/day equivalent proteinuria or red blood cell urinary casts
      8. Neurologic (seizures, psychosis, mononeuritis multiplex, myelitis, peripheral/cranial neuropathy, acute confusional state)
      9. Hemolytic anemia
     10. Leukopenia (<4 K) or lymphopenia (<1 K)
     11. Thrombocytopenia (<100 K)
   B. Immunologic criteria
      1. Antinuclear antibody present above reference range
      2. Anti-double-stranded DNA >2 times reference range
      3. Antiphospholipid antibody (lupus anticoagulant, false-positive syphilis serology, anticardiolipin antibody greater than twice normal range, or anti-beta-2 glycoprotein)
      4. Anti-Sm
      5. Low C3, C4, or CH50 (total hemolytic complement)
      6. Positive direct Coombs without hemolytic anemia

From Petri M, Orbai AM, Alarcón GS, et al. Derivation and validation of the Systemic Lupus International Collaborating Clinics classification criteria for systemic lupus erythematous. *Arthritis Rheum.* 2012;64(8):2677–2686.

(see Chapter 12), it helps distinguish these patients from those suffering with systemic lupus. About 40% of lupus patients exhibit this condition. When internal features are also present and fulfil criteria, we describe the condition as SLE.

SLE patients who have symptoms of achiness, fatigue, pain on taking a deep breath, fever, swollen glands, and signs of swollen joints or rashes but whose internal organs are not involved (e.g., the heart, lungs, kidneys, or liver) are said to have *non-organ-threatening disease*. Statistics vary, but on the basis of my own clinical experience, I estimate that about 25 percent of all lupus patients fall into this category. Patients with non-organ-threatening disease have a normal life expectancy, and it is uncommon for them to develop disease in the major organs after the first 5 years of having the disease.

On the other hand, involvement of the heart, lungs, or kidneys, or the presence of liver or serious blood abnormalities indicates that an *organ-threatening disease* is at work. This may become life-threatening if the patient is not treated with corticosteroids or other interventions. Another 25 percent of all lupus patients fall into this category.

**Table 2.3.** *Proposed ACR/EULAR classification criteria: ANA ≥ 1:80 and score ≥ 10 points across 22 domains*

| Clinical Domain | Criteria | Weight |
|---|---|---|
| Constitutional domain | Fever | 2 |
| Cutaneous domain | Non scarring alopecia | 2 |
| | Oral ulcers | 2 |
| | Subacute cutaneous or discoid lupus | 4 |
| | Acute cutanous lupus | 6 |
| Arthritis domain | Synovitis >=2 joints or tenderness >=2 joints and >=30 minutes of morning stiffness | 6 |
| Neurological domain | Delirium | 2 |
| | Psychosis | 3 |
| | Seizure | 5 |
| Serositis domain | Pleural of pericardial effusion | 5 |
| | Acute pericarditis | 6 |
| Hematological domain | Leukopenia | 3 |
| | Thrombocytopenia | 4 |
| | Autoimmune hemolysis | 4 |
| Renal domain | Proteinuria > 0.5g/24 hours | 4 |
| | Class II or V Lupus nephritis | 8 |
| | Class III or IV Lupus nephritis | 10 |
| *Immunological domain* | | |
| Antiphospholipid antibody domain | Anti-Cardiolipin IgG or Anti-Beta2 GP IgG or Lupus anticoagulant | 2 |
| Complement Protein domain | Low C3 or Low C4 | 3 |
| | Low C3 and Low C4 | 4 |
| SLE specific antibody domain | Anti-dsDNA | 6 |
| | Anti-Smith | 6 |

Aringer M et al. *Annals of the Rheumatic Diseases* 2018;77:60.

Some patients with lupus develop the disease for the first time from a prescription drug and have what is termed *drug-induced lupus erythematosus*. The drug-induced form is usually less severe than SLE and usually disappears after the patient stops taking the particular drug. Occasionally, however, short courses of lupus medication are required for these patients.

Perhaps 5 to 10 percent of the individuals who fulfill the ACR criteria for SLE may also fulfill the ACR criteria for another autoimmune disorder such as scleroderma (tight skin with arthritis), dermato-/polymyositis (inflammation of the muscles), or rheumatoid arthritis (a potentially deforming joint inflammation). These patients are said to have *mixed connective tissue disease* (MCTD) if they possess a particular autoantibody (anti-RNP). If they do not, the patients are said to have a *crossover* or *overlap syndrome*. This classification system is summarized in Table 2.4. A group of patients who have lupus-associated symptoms, signs, or laboratory abnormalities but do not fulfill ACR criteria

**Table 2.4.** *Types of Lupus Erythematosus*

| |
|---|
| Cutaneous (discoid) lupus erythematosus (40%) |
| Systemic lupus erythematosus (50%) |
|    Non-organ-threatening disease (25%) |
|    Organ-threatening disease (25%) |
| Drug-induced lupus erythematosus (<1%) |
| Crossover or overlap syndrome and/or mixed connective tissue disease (10%) |
| Neonatal lupus (<1%) |

for any rheumatic disorders have an *undifferentiated connective tissue disease* (UCTD), which is reviewed in Chapter 23.

Finally, the presence of a lupus rash at birth or congenital heart block with a positive SSA (Ro) antibody is termed *neonatal lupus*. Several hundred cases have been reported in the United States.

## WHAT'S IN STORE FOR THE READER

Don't be overwhelmed by all these facts and figures. This chapter has simply provided you with an overview of the book, and all the points mentioned will be discussed again in more detail in later chapters.

We close this first part with a brief historical background and an overview about who gets lupus (Chapters 3 and 4). In Parts II and III, the heart of the book, we look at the immune system and how it relates to SLE (Chapters 5–9). We discuss the manifestation of the disease in different areas of the body, such as the joints, the gastrointestinal system, the kidneys, and other organs (Chapters 12–20), and talk about the role of blood testing (Chapter 11). We will review the necessary clinical and diagnostic studies (X-rays, scans, etc.) that are used in assessing lupus (Chapters 12–20), as well as problems unique to specific circumstances, such as pregnancy, infection, and lupus in children and the elderly (Chapters 22, 23, 29, and 30). Next, we take up the treatment of lupus—the physical measures we can take to combat the disease, the various medications, and the emotional support a patient will need from his or her family and physician (Chapters 24–28). Finally, future directions and advances soon to take place are detailed in Chapters 32 and 33.

## FURTHER READING

1. Hochberg MC. Updating the American College of Rheumatology revised criteria for the classification of systemic lupus erythematosus. *Arthritis Rheum.* 1997;40(9):1725.
2. Tan EM, Cohen AS, Fries JF, et al. The 1982 revised criteria for the classification of systemic lupus erythematosus. *Arthritis Rheum.* 1982;25(11):1271–1217.

3. Petri M, Orbai AM, Alarcón GS, et al. Derivation and validation of the Systemic Lupus International Collaborating Clinics classification criteria for systemic lupus erythematous. *Arthritis Rheum.* 2012;64(8):2677–2686.

4. Wallace DJ. *Lupus: The Essential Clinician's Guide.* 2nd ed. New York: Oxford University Press: 5–10.

# 3
## *The History of Lupus*

*Lupus* is the Latin word for *wolf*, and it is common medical lore that the "butterfly rash" seen on the cheeks of many lupus patients is so similar to the facial markings of a wolf that our ancestors chose the name for this reason. The technical name for the disease we know of as lupus—*lupus erythematosus*—was first applied to a skin disorder by a Frenchman, Pierre Cazenave, in 1851, though descriptive articles detailing the condition date back to Hippocrates in ancient Greece (Figure 3.1).

Accurate treatises on the skin disorders associated with lupus were published in the mid-1800s by the great Viennese physicians Ferdinand von Hebra and his son-in-law Moriz Kaposi (for whom Kaposi's sarcoma is named). The first suggestions that the disease could be internal (more than skin deep and affecting the organs of the body) appeared in these writings. However, it was Sir William Osler (the founder of our first real medical internship and residency programs in the 1890s at Johns Hopkins) who wrote the earliest complete treatises on lupus erythematosus between 1895 and 1903. In addition to describing such symptoms as fevers and aching, he clearly showed that the central nervous, musculoskeletal, pulmonary, and cardiac systems could be part of the disease.

The golden age of pathology in the 1920s and 1930s led to the first detailed pathologic descriptions of lupus and showed how it affected kidney, heart, and lung tissues. Early discussions of abnormal blood findings such as anemia (low red blood cell count or low hemoglobin) and low platelet count (cells that clot blood) appeared during this time. We had to wait until 1941 for the next breakthrough, which took place at Mount Sinai Hospital in New York City. There, Dr. Paul Klemperer and his colleagues coined the term "collagen disease" on the basis of their clinical research. Although this term is a misnomer (collagen tissues are not necessarily involved in lupus), the evolution of this line of thinking led to our contemporary classification of lupus as an "autoimmune disorder," based on the presence of antinuclear antibody (ANA) and other autoantibodies.

The first arthritis unit with a special interest in lupus was started by Marian Ropes at the Massachusetts General Hospital in Boston in 1922. In those days, no blood test to diagnose lupus was available. In fact, until 1948 there were no

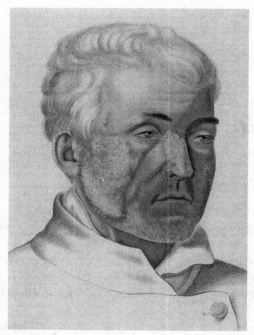

**Figure 3.1.** *A Patient with Lupus from Pierre Cazenave's Monograph, 1846*

effective treatments for lupus except for local skin salves or aspirin. Dr. Ropes observed that half of her patients got better and half of them died during the first 2 years of treatment. Indirectly, she was classifying her patients into "organ-threatening" and "non-organ-threatening" categories, but in many cases she had no way short of a tissue biopsy to determine to which subset a patient belonged.

In 1946, a Mayo Clinic pathologist named Malcolm Hargraves performed a bone marrow examination on a patient and absentmindedly kept a tube from the procedure in his pocket for several days. In a bone marrow examination, the physician removes a tissue sample from bone (usually from the sternum or pelvis, where blood components are made). After finally retrieving the tube, Hargraves observed a unique cell on his microscope slides, which became known as the LE cell. Published in 1948, his description of the LE, or lupus erythematosus, cell was one of the landmark developments in the history of rheumatology. This cell was representative of the systemic inflammatory process; its identification allowed doctors for the first time to diagnose the disease faster and more reliably. Dr. Hargraves and others were quick to show how LE cells could be looked for in peripheral blood samples and found that 70 to 80 percent of patients with active systematic lupus erythematosus (SLE) possessed these cells. At long last, patients with the disease could be readily identified. Researchers were on a roll: in the following year, 1949, another landmark event took place. Dr. Phillip Hench, another

Mayo Clinic physician and one of two rheumatologists ever to win the Nobel Prize in Medicine, demonstrated that a newly discovered hormone known as cortisone could treat rheumatoid arthritis. This hormone was administered to SLE patients throughout the country, and immediately dramatic life-saving took place.

The final chapter of our story evolved during the 1950s, when the concept of autoimmune disease was formalized and the LE cell was shown to be part of an ANA reaction. This led to the development of other tests for autoantibodies, which enabled researchers to characterize the disease in a more detailed and definitive manner. My mentor, Dr. Edmund Dubois, amassed an incredible 1,000 patients with lupus at the Los Angeles County/University of Southern California School of Medicine and in his private practice based at Cedars-Sinai Medical Center and was among the first researchers to explore the natural course of the disease and advise how best to treat it. Also during this time, cancer chemotherapy agents such as nitrogen mustard were shown to be effective in the management of serious organ-threatening complications of SLE when used together with corticosteroids. In 2011, the first new drug approved for lupus by the Food and Drug Administration, belimumab, came on the market. This occasion marked the advent of "targeted" or "biologic therapies" and ushered in a new age of lupus management.

With this historical context in mind, we now turn our attention to the present and a discussion of who gets lupus and why.

## FURTHER READING

1. Wallace DJ, Lyon I. Pierre Cazenave and the first detailed modern description of lupus erythematosus. *Semin Arthritis Rheum.* 1999;28(5):305–313.
2. Benedek, T. The history of lupus. In Wallace DJ, Hahn BH, eds. *Dubois' Lupus Erythematosus.* 9th ed. Philadelphia: Elsevier, 2018.

# 4

## Who Gets Lupus?

If we include thyroiditis, 3 to 5 percent of Americans develop an autoimmune disease in their lifetime. How many lupus patients are there in the United States? It is not as easy to answer this question as it might seem. In the 1990s, the National Arthritis Data Workshop estimated that there were 239,000 Americans with systemic lupus erythematosus (SLE). These numbers, however, do not include those patients who have discoid lupus or drug-induced lupus. However, based on patients being told that they had lupus by at least one doctor, a Lupus Foundation of America survey suggested that the prevalence of SLE could be as high as 2 million in the United States. This has led to misleading assumptions about the true number of people with SLE in the United States. The *incidence* of a disease is defined as the number of new cases per time period (e.g., year), whereas *prevalence* denotes the number of sufferers in the population.

In 2004, the Centers for Disease Control (CDC) funded the creation of national lupus registries in parts of Georgia, Michigan, Manhattan, and northern California. They utilized a methodology that collected reports of lupus from hospitals and discharge diagnoses, integrated health care systems, the US Renal Data System, pharmacy records, and commercial laboratories. The diagnosis of lupus was validated by a consensus panel of rheumatologists to assure they fulfilled either the ACR criteria or had a positive renal biopsy. The findings were published between 2014 and 2017 in multiple publications. In all, a population of 6.4 million was surveyed. The CDC found that the incidence and prevalence were remarkably similar in all regions: 64/100,000 individuals had lupus, or roughly 1 case per 1,500 people. Women had a nine- to tenfold increased risk compared to men, and blacks and Native Americans had a three- to fourfold risk for developing the disease. Hispanics and Asians had greater risk and were between the black and white population. Hence, there are approximately 250,000 people in the United States fulfilling the accepted criteria not counting those who clearly have the disease but do not meet the criteria, which are only 90 percent accurate. See Table 4.1.

Chronic cutaneous (mostly discoid) is three times more common in women than men with a prevalence of 30 per 100,000 individuals. The actual number

**Table 4.1.** *Who Gets Lupus?*

1. There are probably 300,000 cases of true SLE in the United States.
2. The risk for developing SLE is threefold in African Americans and Native Americans, ninefold in females versus males, and probably doubled in US Asians and Hispanics.
3. One in 1,500 people in the United States have SLE, including 1 in 250 African American women and 1 in 10,000 white males.
4. There are probably 1,000 children born each year with neonatal lupus in the United States.
5. 17,000 of the 300,000 with SLE were diagnosed lupus before the age of 18.
6. There are probably 300,000 cases of cutaneous lupus (without SLE) in the United States.
7. 10,000 cases of drug induced lupus are diagnosed annually in the United States. It resolves within months in 95%.
8. The prevalence of lupus throughout the world is greatest in South America and Asia and the least in Europe.

approaches the same number as SLE since these patients often do not often seek medical attention (other than dermatology) and are rarely hospitalized. The prevalence of children under the age of 18 developing lupus is 6 per 100,000 people, or 1 case per 17,000. There are probably seven cases of undifferentiated connective tissue disease for every patient with lupus.

International surveys have come to similar conclusions. The prevalence of lupus in the Caribbean is 48/100,000, Mexico 60/100,000, South America 98/100,000, Asia 59/100,000, and Europe 20/100,000 in work published since 2000.

## AGE OF ONSET

Lupus has been recorded in individuals at birth (*neonatal lupus*) and has been diagnosed in some people as old as 89. Nevertheless, 80 percent of those afflicted with SLE develop it between the ages of 15 and 45. Neonatal lupus is limited to children of mothers who carry a specific autoantibody (an antibody that reacts against the body's own tissues) called the anti-Ro (or SSA) antibody, which will be discussed in Chapter 30. This is one of the autoantibodies that crosses the placenta. For example, the skin rash of neonatal lupus is a self-limited process that disappears during the first year of life because the mother's antibody gets "used up" and the baby cannot make more of it. Children may develop SLE between the age of 3 years and the onset of puberty. This form of lupus is usually a severe, organ-threatening disease but fortunately accounts for less than 5 percent of all lupus cases. The onset of lupus after age 45 or after menopause is uncommon, and a diagnosis of lupus past the age of 70 is extremely unusual. Late-onset lupus infrequently threatens organ systems, and it can be mistaken for rheumatoid arthritis, Sjögren's syndrome, or polymyalgia rheumatica (see Chapters 22 and 23 for a discussion of these conditions).

**Table 4.2.** *Sex Ratios of Onset or at First Diagnosis of Systemic Lupus Erythematosus*

| Age (Years) | Female-to-Male Ratio |
|---|---|
| 0–4 | 1.4:1 |
| 5–9 | 2.3:1 |
| 10–14 | 5.8:1 |
| 15–19 | 5.4:1 |
| 20–29 | 7.5:1 |
| 30–39 | 8.1:1 |
| 40–49 | 5.2:1 |
| 50–59 | 3.9:1 |
| 60–69 | 2.2:1 |

## SEX OF SLE PATIENTS AND TRENDS

In children and in adults over the age of 50, the incidence of lupus demonstrates only a slight female predominance; however, between the ages of 15 and 45, close to 90 percent of diagnosed patients are women. The reasons for this are discussed in Chapter 17. Overall, 80 to 92 percent of all Americans with SLE are women. The percentages are less for discoid lupus, where 70 to 80 percent are women, and for drug-induced lupus, which occurs equally in males and females. In light of these statistics, lupus has been called a "women's disease." To view the prevalence of lupus in men and women by ages, see Table 4.2, which summarizes some of the studies relating to sex and incidence.

The prevalence of lupus may be moderately increasing. Whether this represents a true trend or simply that our methods of ascertainment and availability of additional autoantibodies lead to diagnosing more difficult cases has not been resolved.

## WHY DO PEOPLE GET LUPUS?

Lupus results when a specific predisposing set of genes is exposed to the right combination of environmental elements, infectious agents, lupus-inducing drugs, excessive ultraviolet light, physical trauma, emotional stress, or other factors. The next few chapters detail the circumstances that make certain populations more susceptible to the disorder than others.

## FURTHER READING

1. Izmirly PM, Wan I, Sahl S, et al. The incidence and prevalence of systemic lupus erythematosus in New York County (Manhattan) New York: the Manhattan Lupus Surveillance Program. *Arthritis Rheumatol.* 2017;69(10):2006–2017.

2. Dall'Era M, Cisternas MG, Snipes K, Herrinton LJ, Gordon C, Helmick CG. The incidence and prevalence of systemic lupus erythematosus in San Francisco County, California: the California Lupus Surveillance Project. *Arthritis Rheumatol.* 2017;69(10):1996–2005.
3. van Vollenhoven RF. Editorial: who gets lupus? Clues to a tantalizing syndrome, *Arthritis Rheumatol.* 2017;69(3):483–486.
4. Lim SS, Drenkard C. Epidemiology of lupus: an update. *Curr Opin Rheumatol.* 2015;27(5):427–432.

# Part II
# INFLAMMATION AND IMMUNITY

Part I defined and classified lupus, explored the historical context of this disease, and reviewed the populations afflicted by lupus. The next two parts look at how lupus damages body tissue and why it occurs. Scientifically speaking, this is the most difficult part of the book because we tackle complex immunologic concepts and discuss how inflammation takes place. Tables and summaries are provided throughout to assist the reader. Feel free to skip this section or skim it. First, we turn to the workings of the normal immune and inflammatory response so that the abnormal responses observed in lupus will be better understood.

# 5

# *The Body's Protection Plan*

Inflammatory and immune responses account for many of the symptoms observed in systemic lupus. This chapter reviews concepts of immunity and inflammation; the following chapters discuss how these concepts apply to rheumatic diseases.

## WHAT ARE THE COMPONENTS OF THE NORMAL INFLAMMATORY AND IMMUNE SYSTEM?

The body is always on the lookout for foreign substances that may pose a threat to its intricate workings. Its monitoring system consists of blood and tissue components, including certain proteins and blood cells that travel back and forth between blood and tissues.

### Blood Components

A 150-pound (70-kilogram) person has about 6 liters of blood, which contains several components. These include *red blood cells*, called *erythrocytes*, which are responsible for carrying and exchanging oxygen. If a person has a low count of red blood cells, she is suffering from anemia. *White blood cells*, called *leukocytes*, constitute the body's main defense system. Other blood components are *platelets*, which clot blood, and *plasma*, which includes serum. Plasma makes up most of our blood volume. It contains many proteins and other substances being carried to different parts of the body, including clotting factors that are not present in serum.

White blood cells play a central role in inflammation. Five types of white blood cells have been identified by scientists; all are relevant to lupus. These include the following.

#### Polymorphonuclear Cells

These cells are also called *neutrophils* or *granulocytes* and, like all other blood components, they are made in our bone marrow (blood-making parts of our bone in the pelvis and sternum). After being produced, they circulate in the blood for a few days and then pass into tissues. Some 50 to 70 percent of our circulating white cells are neutrophils.

### Eosinophils

These white blood cells make up 0 to 5 percent of all our white blood cells. Their life cycle is similar to that of granulocytes. Eosinophils are involved in allergic responses.

### Basophils

These cells do not have a clearly defined function and constitute less than 1 percent of our white blood cells. Tissue-based basophils are termed *mast cells*. These specialized cells combat parasitic or fungal invasion. They also play a role in allergy.

### Lymphocytes

These make up 20 to 45 percent of our white blood cells and are the gatekeepers of our immune responses. Produced in the bone marrow, they migrate constantly between blood and tissue and can survive as long as 20 years. Lymphocytes can be T (thymus-derived) or B (derived from the mythical "Bursa of Fabricius") cells.

### Monocytes

These cells represent about 5 percent of our circulating blood cells. They are the circulating blood component of what is called the "monocyte–macrophage" network because these cells are responsible for processing foreign materials (*antigens*) and destroying cells and tissue debris that are by-products of inflammation. In circulating blood, these cells are called monocytes; macrophages can also be present in blood, but they are mostly in tissues (see Table 5.1 and Figures 5.1 and 5.3).

## Lymphoid Tissue and the Thymus

Lymphoid tissue is a key part of the immune system and represents up to 3 percent of a person's body weight. It includes our *lymph nodes* (or lymph glands), the *circulating lymphocytes*, and fixed *lymphoid tissue* (i.e., spleen). A 150-pound person has $10^{12}$, or 100 billion, lymphocytes. They are widely distributed throughout the body and consist of long- and short-lived populations.

Bone marrow is the source of primitive ancestors of the *T* and *B lymphocytes*. These precursors migrate to the thymus, a gland just below the neck, which processes them into immunologically competent and knowledgeable *T cells*. These T cells provide cellular immunity and are the body's memory cells. About 70 percent of the lymphocytes are T cells. They remember what is foreign, go on to alert the body when a person re-encounters a foreign substance, and formulate a response that protects the body.

Blood is carried to tissues by the arteries and returns to the heart through the veins. Blood components, cellular waste and debris, and other materials can also return by another system—a chain of lymph nodes that starts in our toes and fingers and ends up in the chest area. (See Figure 5.1.)

Lymphoid tissue contains T cells, *B cells*, and *natural killer cells*. B cells, which make up 10 to 15 percent of the lymphocytes, produce antibodies that eliminate what is foreign. Natural killer cells destroy targeted cells without having been sensitized to them in the past.

There are various types of T cells, which are identified by their surface markings and appearance. These types are labeled by the cumbersome term *cluster-determined*, or *CD*. Nearly all T cells have markers associated with *CD3*. *CD4* cells are those that "help" or promote immune responses, whereas *CD8* cells usually "suppress" or block the immune response. Approximately 50 percent of T cells have the CD4 marker, and 20 percent have the CD8 marker. Other markers are also present.

### Our Antibody Response: The Gamma Globulins

When you were growing up, there may have been an occasion when your pediatrician gave you gamma globulin shots to minimize certain infections that were going around. A type of gamma globulin, *immunoglobulin*, is responsible for our antibody response. In response to an antigen our bodies produce antibodies. With appropriate signaling by T cells, B cells transform themselves into *plasma cells*. Plasma cells make immunoglobulins. These gamma globulins circulate in the plasma and protect the body from infection and other foreign material. There are five types of immunoglobulins:

*IgG* (immunoglobulin G) is the major antibody of plasma and the most important part of our antibody response. Most autoimmune diseases are characterized by IgG autoantibodies. IgG is made up of four subclasses known as Ig1, IgG2, IgG3, and IgG4. Deficiencies in these proteins or subclasses can lead to recurrent infections. Known as *common variable immunodeficiency, or CVID,* patients are often treated with different forms of intramuscular, subcutaneous, or intravenous gamma globulin.

*IgM* (immunoglobulin M) is initially produced to fight antigens but soon decreases and allows IgG to take over. It plays an important but secondary role in autoimmunity.

*IgA* is the major antibody of external secretions (tears, gastrointestinal tract secretions, and respiratory tract secretions). It is important in *Sjögren's syndrome* (a combination of dry eyes, dry mouth, and arthritis seen in many lupus patients) and autoimmune diseases of the bowel (ulcerative colitis and Crohn's).

*IgD* is poorly understood but has a role in helping B cells recognize antigens.

*IgE* binds to mast cells and mediates allergic reactions.

This categorization is summarized in Table 5.1 and Figure 5.1.

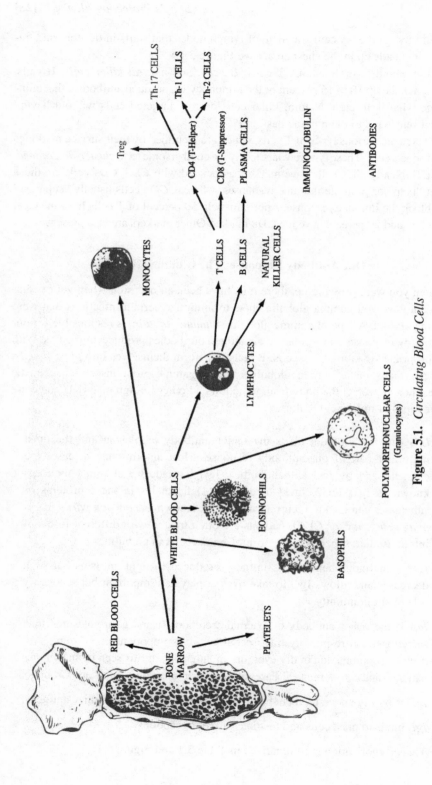

**Figure 5.1.** *Circulating Blood Cells*

**Table 5.1.** *Circulating Components of Whole Blood Important to the Immune System*

Red blood cells
Platelets
White blood cells (leukocytes)
   Basophils (called mast cells in tissue)
   Eosinophils
   Polymorphonuclear cells (granulocytes, neutrophils)
   Monocytes (called macrophages in tissues)
   Lymphocytes
      T cells
         CD4 cells (usually helpers)
         CD8 cells (usually suppressors)
      Natural killer cells
      B cells
Plasma (includes serum)
   Albumin
   Globulin
      Alpha globulins
      Beta globulins (includes complement)
      Gamma globulins (includes immunoglobulins, listed below)
         IgG (subclasses IgG1, IgG2, IgG3, IgG4)
         IgA
         IgM
         IgD
         IgE

## Cytokines and Complement

*Cytokines* are hormonelike substances that promote various activities in the body, but in lupus their functions are altered. Cytokines play a role in the growth and development of cells and include various interleukins (mostly produced by T helper cells), chemokines (mediate chemoattraction between cells), lymphokines (make by lymphocytes), tumor necrosis factors, colony-stimulating factors (promote cell growth), and interferons. For example, interleukin-1 has many actions. Secreted during the course of an immune response, it exerts effects by binding to receptors on the cell surface. Interleukin-1 can stimulate T cells to make interleukin-2, trigger the liver to make chemicals that perpetuate inflammation, allow certain cells to proliferate, and promote the production of growth factors that, in turn, make more white blood cells and other growth factors, thus amplifying or "gearing up" the immune system. *Interferons* were originally described as proteins that interfered with the growth of viruses. Their levels are increased in the sera of lupus patients as well as in genes expressed, and they are important in the inflammatory process.

Cytokines are made by a variety of cells, especially lymphocytes and macrophages. CD4 helper cells elaborate cytokines that promote inflammation. They are called *Th-1*, or *T helper-one cells*, and go by several names: interferon, interleukin-2, and tumor necrosis factor. Other CD4 helper cells can promote the

| | |
|---|---|
| TNF-alpha | Promotes rheumatoid-like inflammation; blocked by several available rheumatoid arthritis drugs: etanercept, adalimumab, infliximab |
| IL-1 | Pro-inflammatory, stimulated by TNF-alpha, blocked by anakinra |
| IL-2 | T-cell growth factor |
| IL-4 | Anti-inflammatory |
| IL-6 | Tocilizumab is used to treat lupus, rheumatoid arthritis, vasculitis, Still's disease |
| IL-8 | Promotes chemotaxis (a chemokine) and inflammation, increased with autonomic nervous dysfunction |
| IL-10 | Anti-inflammatory and pro-inflammatory |
| IL-12, 15, 17, 18,23 | Pro-inflammatory; drugs that block it (ustekinumab an anti IL-12/23 is approved for psoriasis and inflammatory bowel disease |
| Interferon-alpha | Increased expression in SLE, which promotes inflammation |
| Interferon-beta | Made by fibroblasts; used to treat multiple sclerosis |
| Interferon-gamma | Antiviral made by T helper cells, dysregulated in lupus |
| TGF-beta | Partly responsible for tight skin in scleroderma |

IL, interleukin; SLE, systemic lupus erythematosus; TGF, transforming growth factor; TNF, tumor necrosis factor.

formation of antibodies, such as interleukins-4, -6, -10, and -13; these are known as *Th-2*, or *T helper-two cells* and fight inflammation. *Treg* cells are CD4+ cells that downregulate the immune response, whereas *Th-17* cells upregulate it and promote inflammation. Table 5.2 lists some of the more important cytokines.

*Complement* refers to a group of 28 plasma proteins whose interactions clear away immune complexes (antigens mixed with antibodies) and kill bacteria. They are consumed (serum levels decrease) during inflammation, and low complement levels are an important indicator of lupus activity. Blood testing may indicate activation of complement products, which is also associated with inflammation. (See Chapter 11.)

## THE INFLAMMATORY PROCESS

We have described the key fighters in the body's defensive army against immunologic and inflammatory attack. We can imagine them as a highly disciplined force, each member of which carries out a specialized task in the course of battling against foreign invaders. Neutrophils, lymphocytes, and macrophage-monocytes are all involved in the body's inflammatory and immune process in critical but distinct ways.

### Neutrophils, Inflammation, and NETs

In healthy people, neutrophils have only one known function: they kill foreign invaders such as bacteria. If the level of neutrophils in the blood is low, we know this decreases our ability to fight infection and increases our risk of contracting it.

In rheumatic diseases such as gout, neutrophils can ingest, or swallow, immune complexes and crystalline material. Neutrophils are part of the acute (early, initial) inflammatory process, whereas lymphocytes are part of a chronic (later, ongoing) inflammatory process.

The process by which neutrophils kill foreign material occurs in several stages, which can be visualized in Figure 5.2. First, imagine neutrophils, or antibodies, as guns and cytokines, or complement, as bullets, which cause tissue destruction. By adhering to the surface of veins and emigrating through them, neutrophils turn on a system of attractants that includes activated complement, adhesion molecules, chemokines, histamine, leukotrienes, prostaglandins, nitric oxide, reactive oxygen intermediates, and cytokines, which are important for cell destruction and inflammation. These mediators generate chemicals that can be suppressed by lupus medicines such as steroids and nonsteroidal anti-inflammatories (e.g., Advil, Naprosyn). The end result is the coating of bacteria with IgG and activated complement, which then adheres to the neutrophil. Finally, the neutrophil discharges its granules, thus completing the killing process.

*Neutrophil extracellular traps*, or *NETs*, are networks of extracellular fibers, primarily composed of DNA from neutrophils, which bind pathogens. In addition, engulfing microbes and secreting antimicrobials, neutrophils also kill extracellular pathogens while minimizing damage to host cells. In lupus, exposed extracellular histone complexes in NETs can promote inflammation, or have the opposite of their intended effect.

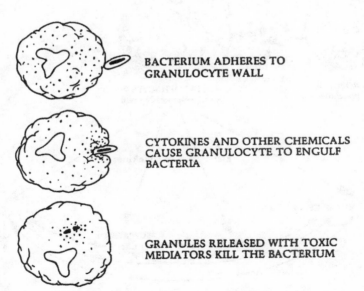

BACTERIUM ADHERES TO
GRANULOCYTE WALL

CYTOKINES AND OTHER CHEMICALS
CAUSE GRANULOCYTE TO ENGULF
BACTERIA

GRANULES RELEASED WITH TOXIC
MEDIATORS KILL THE BACTERIUM

**Figure 5.2.** *How Granulocytes Kill Bacteria*

### Adaptive Immunity: The Monocyte-Macrophage and Antigen-Presenting System

The monocyte–macrophage network is an important member of the immune surveillance force; it is central because regulation of this network is what goes awry in autoimmune disease. It includes our lymph nodes and dendritic cells. In what is termed the *adaptive immune response,* the monocyte–macrophage network has several functions: it destroys microorganisms and tissue debris that result from inflammation; it clears dead and dying red cells, denatured plasma proteins, and micro-organisms from the blood; it plays a role in the recognition of foreign substances; and it promotes the secretion of cytokines.

Antigens do not generally activate T cells directly. They are usually presented to the T cells by macrophages. Antigens are present on the macrophage surface, but to respond to their presence, the T cell must recognize a code on the surface of the macrophage, called the HLA class II (or D) determinant. The HLA (or human leukocyte antigen) system is responsible for recognizing antigens. See Chapter 7 for a review of this system. This system acts in combination with a T-cell surface marker, which can then activate T cells. Class II determinants recognize surface antigens for CD4, or helper cells; class I (HLA-A, -B, or -C) determinants recognize markers for CD8 or suppressor cells. Figures 5.3 and 5.4 illustrate these complex interactions.

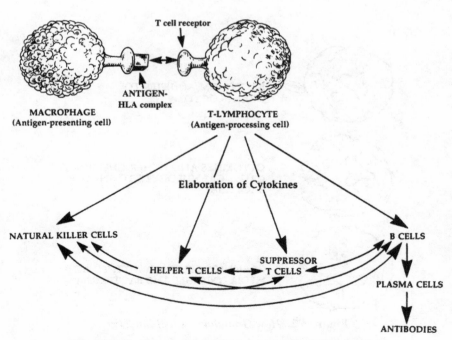

**Figure 5.3.** *How Antigens Stimulate Antibody Production*

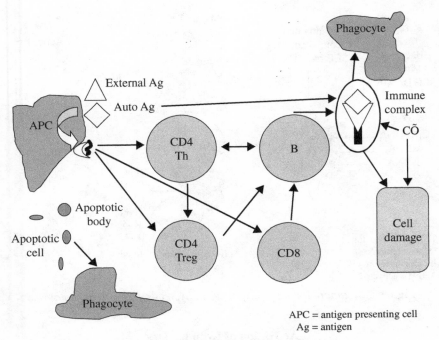

**Figure 5.4.**  *The Adaptive Immune System*

Let's summarize what happens when something foreign (e.g., a virus) enters the body. It is recognized as something that must be eliminated. The foreign body (known as the antigen) is recognized by macrophages, which roam the bloodstream keeping watch for antigens. A macrophage engulfs the antigens, and that may be the end of the story. However, in some instances, the antigens are broken into small pieces known as "antigenic peptides." If additional help is needed to destroy it, the antigenic peptide unites with an HLA molecule inside the macrophage. The HLA molecule then moves to the outside of the macrophage bound to the peptide, forming a "complex." T cells and their receptors interact with the antigen–peptide complex. T cells send chemical signals called cytokines, which bring in more T cells and alert B cells to produce antibody. Ultimately, phagocytes remove the antigen from the body.

### The Innate Immune System

Since prehistoric times, complexes of DNA and RNA as well as bacteria and viruses existed. When mammals evolved, their immune system included a "pattern recognition system" whereby foreign materials were identified for destruction. Cell receptors, known as *toll-like receptors* (TLRs), activated the macrophage–monocyte system (represented here as dendritic cells) that protected the body. This became the innate immune system. TLR7 and TLR9 expression is increased in lupus. This is shown in Figure 5.5 and in the introduction to Part III.

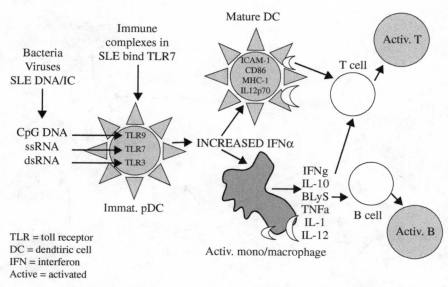

**Figure 5.5.** *Innate Immune Responses in Systemic Lupus Erythematosus*

### Activation of Lymphocytes

The T lymphocytes are made in the bone marrow and processed in the thymus. When they leave the thymus, they are able to respond selectively to environmental stimulation. Upon exposure to a foreign body or antigen and after a series of steps, T cells transform: they become larger in appearance and start to divide. This occurs in part as a result of the production of the cytokine interleukin-2 (also called *T-cell growth factor*). T cells then differentiate into helper cells, suppressor cells, effector cells (which make cytokines), and cytotoxic or killer cells, and they promote the production of B cells. Some B cells become plasma cells and make immunoglobulin, or antibody. A small number of T cells live for many years and act as memory cells for the immune system. They are capable of initiating effective and rapid immunologic responses if the body is re-exposed to the antigen.

### SUMMING UP

Whole blood consists of red blood cells, white blood cells, platelets, and plasma. There are five types of white blood cells. These include the neutrophils, which are important in acute inflammation; lymphocytes, which help regulate chronic inflammatory processes; and monocytes, which are responsible for helping the body recognize foreign material. All these cells are derived from the bone marrow. In a normal adaptive and innate immune response, these elements all work together. Lymphocytes migrate to the thymus, where they are ultimately recognized as T cells or B cells. The T cells read antigenic signals present in monocytes or macrophages and are thus able to promote or turn off inflammation and the killing of specific cells. Some B cells transform themselves into plasma cells that make immunoglobulin, which then circulates in the plasma. Immunoglobulins G, A, M, D, and E also help to destroy foreign materials. All these processes are promoted and amplified by cytokines, complement, and other mediators that constitute our normal immune surveillance network.

## FURTHER READING

1. Delves PJ Martin SJ, Burton DR, Roitt IM. *Roitt's Essential Immunology.* 13th ed. Hoboken, NJ: Wiley Blackwell, 2017.
2. Peakman M, Vergani D. *Basic and Clinical Immunology.* 2nd ed. Edinburgh, UK: Churchill Livingstone, 2009.

# 6

# *The Enemy Is Our Cells*

Chapter 5 reviewed the normal inflammatory and immune response network. Several features unique to lupus and other autoimmune processes alter this system to produce tissue injury that is not observed by the body's normal immunological surveillance system. These features will be summarized briefly here to help us understand the many antibodies that play an important role in lupus.

Lupus results when genetically susceptible individuals are exposed to certain environmental factors, and in my opinion, only 10 percent of those who carry lupus genes will ever develop the disease. These environmental factors create a setting in which things happen that normally shouldn't. *Neutrophils* (the white blood cells responsible for mediating acute inflammation) can increase inflammation in the body of lupus sufferers because of the way their blood plasma interacts with cytokines, complement, and adhesion molecules (the chemicals that draw cells closer to the site of inflammation). *Lymphocytes*, the white blood cells responsible for chronic inflammation, also have their function altered in lupus. The T helper cells become more active, and the body becomes less responsive to T suppressor cells. Natural killer lymphocytes promote inflammation and are not able to suppress or contain it. As a result, the body's system of tolerance is disrupted so much that B cells are signaled to make antibodies to the patient's own tissues, which are called *autoantibodies*. In other words, the normal immune surveillance system is altered in lupus, resulting in accelerated inflammatory responses and autoantibody formation; the autoantibodies, in turn, attack the body's own cells and tissues. It is as if the body's police force found itself unable to tolerate healthy, law-abiding cells and schemed to undermine them.

## AUTOANTIBODIES GALORE!

Autoantibodies are the hallmark of lupus. They represent antibodies to the body's own tissue—to parts of the cells or the cells themselves. In addition to having a positive result on an antinuclear antibody (ANA) test, the typical systemic lupus erythematosus (SLE) patient has at least one or two other autoantibodies. These antibodies distinguish lupus patients from others without the disease, because few healthy people have significant levels of them.

Sixteen important autoantibodies in lupus are described and defined in this chapter. In Chapter 11, the clinical importance of some of these autoantibodies is discussed in more detail; there, we will look at the blood tests a doctor will order so that the disease can be diagnosed and treated. In other words, this section defines and categorizes autoantibodies.

## WHERE DO AUTOANTIBODIES COME FROM?

Autoantibodies are triggered by antigens in the environment (e.g., foods, dyes, tobacco smoke), autoantigens (self-driven), and regions of immunoglobulin that are recognized as being foreign, or antigenic.

Even though immunologists know that B cells are critical in the formation of autoantibodies, several important issues regarding autoantibodies remain unresolved. Namely, which B cells can make autoantibodies? And what is the defect in immune response that permits the expression of pathologic or injurious autoantibodies?

In nature, autoantibodies are often produced that do not have any clinical or pathologic significance (mostly IgM antibodies). In lupus, IgG autoantibodies often correlate with disease activity. Autoantibody responses can be general or, on occasion, quite specific. Both phenomena are observed in lupus.

## WHAT KINDS OF AUTOANTIBODIES ARE THERE?

The autoantibodies important in lupus can be broken down into four categories. These include *antibodies that form against materials in the nucleus, or center, of the cell*, such as antinuclear antibody, anti-DNA, anti-Sm, anti-RNP, and antihistone antibody; *antibodies that form against cytoplasm or cell surface components*, such as anti-Ro (SSA), anti-La (SSB), antiphospholipid, and antiribosomal P antibodies; *antibodies to different types of cells*, such as red blood cells, white blood cells, platelets, or nerve cells; and *antibodies that form against circulating antigens*, such as rheumatoid factors and circulating immune complexes.

If you are a lupus patient, your doctor is likely at some time to test your blood for many if not most of these antibodies. Therefore, the following paragraphs endeavor to explain what they are. Doctors have been accused of creating their own vocabulary o make themselves indispensable. Consider this chapter a foreign language class. The next time Dr. Jones excitedly tells you that your anti-Ro (SSA) antibody is highly positive, ask him or her if it was measured using immunodiffusion or by ELISA!

## ANTIBODIES TO NUCLEAR CELLULAR COMPONENTS

Since its description in 1957, the *antinuclear antibody*, or ANA (antibody to the cell nucleus), has become the most widely known autoantibody in SLE. It is hard to imagine having lupus without it, although a person can have a positive ANA test without having systemic lupus. For many years, the test for ANA was conducted using animal cells. Human serum was placed over kidney or liver cells of the mouse, rat, or hamster, and if ANA was present, human antibody would attach to the animal cell's nucleus. Fluorescent staining of the antibody bound to animal cell nuclei was used to document these findings. Now, however, testing involves human cells in place of animal cells; as a result, the test more accurately predicts the presence of lupus. As recently as the late 1980s, 10 percent of lupus patients had false-negative results (in other words, people with lupus had a negative ANA test) and might have been told they did not have the disease. The rate of negatives at present is as low as 2 percent; however, more people now have positive ANAs without evidence of lupus.

ANA tests are analyzed according to the amount of antibody present and the pattern seen in cells recognized by antibodies in the sample. Although this is a crude measure, the amount of antibody can suggest the degree of seriousness of the disease. The patterns of antibody are classified as follows:

1. The *homogenous* pattern is seen primarily in SLE but also in other illnesses as well as in older adults. This pattern indicates the presence of antibodies to chromatin (part of the chromosomes), histone, and/or deoxy-nucleoprotein.
2. The *peripheral* or *rimmed* patterns are seen primarily in SLE and represent antibodies to DNA. Often, the concurrence of a homogenous pattern makes the peripheral pattern undetectable, because a stain that covers the entire nucleus may include its rim or margin.
3. The *speckled* pattern is seen in SLE, numerous other autoimmune diseases, and in some healthy individuals who show low amounts of antibody. "Speckled" suggests a spotty uptake of the fluorescent stain.
4. *Nucleolar* (a part of the nucleus) patterns are not often seen in SLE and suggest scleroderma.
5. *Centromere* patterns detect the central part of the chromosome. They are rarely seen in lupus, and their presence suggests a form of scleroderma called the CREST syndrome.

A large survey showed that 13.7 percent of Americans may receive a positive ANA test result, but many fewer have SLE. Positive ANAs (even in large amounts) can be found in healthy relatives of SLE patients, patients with other autoimmune diseases, and in people with normal health, especially those over the age of 60. In addition, infections with certain viruses and bacteria can stimulate the production of ANA.

*Deoxyribonucleic acid*, or *DNA*, is a molecule located in the control center of each of our cells and is responsible for the production of all the body's proteins. Antibodies to single-stranded DNA are found in many normal individuals. However, the presence of antibodies to double-stranded DNA may suggest a serious form of SLE; these antibodies, if positively charged, may damage tissue directly. Throughout, I will refer to these antibodies as *anti-DNA*. Approximately one half of SLE patients possess anti-DNA. By tracking their specific levels, I can assess my patient's response to therapy. More than 90 percent of patients with anti-DNA have SLE, especially those with serious organ-threatening (e.g., kidney) disease.

*Anti-Sm* stands for a Mrs. Smith, in whom it was first described. Antibodies to the Sm antigen are very specific for lupus (present in 20 to 30 percent of those with SLE) and are rarely observed in any other disease. These antibodies interfere with the ability to transcribe RNA (ribonucleic acid) from DNA.

The antibody directed against ribonuclear protein, *anti-RNP*, is essential for the diagnosis of mixed connective tissue disease, a lupus look-alike. However, it is not specific to this disease, since 20 to 30 percent of lupus patients and a small number with scleroderma or rheumatoid arthritis also have the antibody. Anti-RNP interferes with the ability of RNA to bind in the cytoplasm of cells.

*Histones* are structural proteins in the cell nucleus. They can be autoantigens and are observed in SLE, rheumatoid arthritis, certain cancers, and liver diseases. Histones are thought to be responsible for the LE cell phenomenon, the first immune abnormality reported in lupus. Histone deacetylation is an important feature of epigenetic modulation of SLE (see Chapter 8). Antihistone antibodies are of particular interest because they are present in 95 percent of patients with drug-induced lupus.

## ANTIBODIES TO CYTOPLASMIC COMPONENTS

Four autoantibodies to *cytoplasm* (if a cell looks like an egg, it is the egg white) are important in SLE and are discussed here. The true prevalence of many of these antibodies, however, is not known, because the levels vary according to the methods of detection employed. Although the technology is not relevant to this discussion, it is important to know that older, less sensitive methods such as immunodiffusion detect fewer positive patients than the newer ELISA and immunoblotting tests. But whereas the older tests rarely if ever gave false-positive readings, newer methods of evaluation occasionally produce misleading results. These methods nevertheless detect 30 to 50 percent more patients with the autoantibody than traditional testing. The percentages listed below for anti-Sm, anti-RNP, anti-Ro, and anti-La were derived from older methods.

*Antiphospholipid antibodies* react against *phospholipids*, which are components of the cell membrane. There are several antiphospholipid antibodies, the most important of which is anticardiolipin. These antibodies are frequently seen with the lupus anticoagulant and are discussed in detail in Chapter 21. Antiphospholipid antibodies are present in about one third of patients with SLE and are less frequently found in other autoimmune diseases.

*Anti-Ro* (SSA) is present in most patients with Sjögren's syndrome (dry eyes, dry mouth, and arthritis) and 20 to 30 percent of those with SLE. As one of the few autoantibodies that crosses the placenta, it may induce neonatal lupus and congenital heart block. Anti-Ro can impart increased sun sensitivity to its carriers and is seen in nearly all patients with a skin disorder called subacute cutaneous lupus erythematosus. It is associated immunogenetically with HLA-DR2 and HLA-DR3. Anti-Ro may interfere with the cell's ability to process RNA.

*Anti-La* (SSB) is almost always seen with anti-Ro. Rarely present by itself, it coexists with anti-Ro 40 percent of the time and may make anti-Ro less *pathogenic*, or dangerous. This statement especially applies to kidney disease. La may function as a way station on the road to where RNA transcripts are carried from the nucleus to the cytoplasm.

*Antiribosomal P* antibodies are observed in 20 percent of known patients with SLE. Found only in the cytoplasm, antiribosomal P may correlate with psychotic behavior, depression, and liver disease in lupus and its levels may decrease with response to therapy.

## ANTIBODIES TO CELLS

Lupus patients can have antibodies to red blood cells, white blood cells, platelets, and nerve cells.

*Antierythrocyte antibodies* are directed against the surface of red blood cells. One lupus patient in 10 develops *autoimmune hemolytic anemia*, or the destruction of red blood cells due to antierythrocyte antibodies. The true prevalence of these antibodies is not known, but there are probably two to three lupus patients with this antibody for every one who becomes seriously anemic.

*Antineutrophil antibodies* are occasionally observed. Antibodies that act against the cytoplasmic component of neutrophils, called *ANCA (antineutrophil cytoplasmic antibodies)*, indicate the presence of one of two types of non-lupus vasculitis (inflammation of the blood vessels) called granulomatosis with polyangiitis (formerly known as Wegener's granulomatosis), which is characterized by the c-ANCA subset and microscopic polyangiitis. The p-ANCA subset, which characterizes microscopic polyangiitis, is also positive in 20 percent of those with SLE. Antibodies to certain peptides and proteins are known as *anticyclic citrullinated peptide* (anti-CCP) antibody. A fairly specific marker for rheumatoid arthritis, but anti-CCP is found in 5 percent with SLE, many of whom have overlapping features of both disorders.

Another white blood cell antibody called *antilymphocyte antibody* is present in most lupus patients. It is a natural autoantibody; large amounts indicate greater severity of the disease, and it is responsible for the low white blood cell counts seen in many lupus patients. Most antilymphocyte antibodies are IgM antibodies that coat the surface of lymphocytes and result in the depletion of T cells.

*Antiplatelet antibodies* are present in approximately 15 percent of lupus patients and account for most *thrombocytopenia* (a condition in which platelet counts drop below 100,000 per cubic millimeter) seen in lupus patients. Although there are many other reasons for thrombocytopenia (they are discussed in detail in Chapter 20), the majority of patients have platelets coated with IgG, which assures their premature destruction. Unfortunately, the methods for detecting antiplatelet antibodies are technically difficult and not always reproducible. Antiplatelet antibodies are often seen in association with antiphospholipid antibodies.

*Antineuronal antibodies* react to nerve cell membranes, or coverings. Nerve cells, or *neurons*, look like a series of electrical wires and are responsible for storing and transmitting nerve responses throughout the body. Autoantibody reactivity to nerve cell components is not observed in healthy people, but, if tested correctly, it can be detected in 5 percent of patients with rheumatoid arthritis, in 5 to 20 percent of all lupus patients, and in up to 90 percent of patients with active central nervous system inflammation from lupus or autoimmune nervous disorders. Although blood levels may indicate the presence of central nervous system lupus, spinal fluid is a more reliable source than serum for measuring neuronal antibodies.

## ANTIBODIES THAT FORM AGAINST CIRCULATING ANTIGENS

Remember that antigens are foreign materials to which cells react. Sometimes the body makes antibodies to antigens expressed by its own cells.

In rheumatoid arthritis, it is probable that antigenic material to the *synovium* (the lining of the joint) induces an antibody response. The body then makes an antibody to this antigen–antibody complex, which is called *rheumatoid factor*. Rheumatoid factor, in turn, may release a chain of biochemical events that contributes to joint and cartilage destruction. As many as one third of lupus patients may have rheumatoid factor. Rheumatoid factor in lupus can exacerbate the inflammation of joints but may be protective of other tissues such as the kidneys. Five to 10% with SLE also have antibodies to CCP, or cyclic citrullinated peptide. About half with rheumatoid arthritis also have this antibody.

*Circulating immune complexes* are the combination of antibody and antigen circulating in the bloodstream. These complexes contain everything from rheumatoid factor to complement mixed with antigen and immunoglobulins. The true incidence of circulating immune complexes in lupus is unknown, because the methods capable of assessing them detect only certain types of complexes. Circulating immune complexes can activate complement, which, in turn, can promote inflammation. In lupus, some complexes cannot be cleared from the body by the monocyte–macrophage system, and when they settle in tissues, either directly or indirectly, they induce inflammation.

**Table 6.1.** *Important Autoantibodies and Antibodies in Lupus*

| Autoantibody | Antibody to | Percentage in Lupus | Percentage in Normals | Lupus Specificity |
|---|---|---|---|---|
| Antinuclear | Nucleus | 98 | 5–10 | Fair |
| Anti-DNA | Nucleus | 50 | <1 | Excellent |
| Antihistone | Nucleus | 50 | 1–3 | Fair |
| Anti-Sm | Nucleus | 25 | <1 | Excellent |
| Anti-RNP | Nucleus | 25 | <1 | Fair |
| Antiphospholipid | Membrane | 33 | 5 | Fair |
| Anti-Ro (SSA) | Cytoplasm | 30 | <1 | Fair |
| Anti-La (SSB) | Cytoplasm | 15 | <1 | Fair |
| Antiribosomal P | Cytoplasm | 20 | <1 | Good |
| Antierythrocyte | Red cells | 15–30 | <1 | Fair |
| ANCA | White cells | 20 | <1 | Poor |
| Antilymphocyte | White cells | Most | 20 | Poor |
| Antiplatelet | Platelets | 15–30 | <5 | Poor |
| Antineuronal | Nerve cells | 20 | <1 | Good |
| Rheumatoid factors | Ag-AB | 30 | 5–10 | Poor |
| Anti-CCP | Ag-Ab | 5–10% | 1–3% | Poor |
| Immune complexes | Ag-Ab | Most | Varies | Poor |

ANCA, antineutrophil cytoplasmic antibodies; Anti-citric citrullinated peptide. Ag-AB is an abbreviation for antigen–antibody complexes. These immune complexes are elevated with many common bacterial and viral infections, not just with lupus.

Table 6.1 summarizes these antibodies and compares their presence in normal individuals and lupus patients.

## LESSONS LEARNED FROM ANIMALS

What is fascinating about animal research is that science has found similarities between the immune systems of animals and those of humans. Much of the information presented here was derived from animal research. In addition to afflicting nearly a million Americans, lupus is also found in many animals. It has been reported to occur spontaneously in dogs (including a presidential one—George H. W. Bush's Millie), cats, rabbits, rats, mice, guinea pigs, pigs, monkeys, goats, hamsters, and Aleutian minks. One of the best described is canine lupus, which is very similar to human lupus in its presentation and management. In the 1950s and 1960s, occasional research studies utilized guinea pigs and rabbits, but these approaches have been abandoned. One laboratory has extensive experience inducing lupus in cats with an antithyroid preparation, but this has not been adopted as a research tool by other investigators. More than 95 percent of animal lupus research studies involve mice with lupus.

## WHY SHOULD WE STUDY ANIMAL MODELS OF LUPUS?

Many of the advances in lupus over the last 50 years would not have been possible without animal studies, and thousands of human lives have been saved as a result of this work. The immune system of a mouse is remarkably similar to that of a human. As hard as we try, no satisfactory computer simulation of the mouse's or human's immune system exists, in large part because there's a lot we don't know about it.

The breakthroughs resulting from mouse work in SLE include proof that genetic factors are important determinants of autoimmune disease and have led to the identification of genes important in lupus. Animal research has also proved that lupus can be influenced by environmental and hormonal factors. Therapy has pushed forward because trials of multiple therapeutic interventions that never would have worked in humans have saved years of research and lots of misery for patients. Furthermore, many of the drugs we use to treat lupus (e.g., cyclophosphamide) were first shown to be effective in mice. Three types of mice are used by researchers: breeds that spontaneously develop lupus, those in whom it can be induced, or mice missing a specific gene. There have even been strong suggestions from mouse work that "gene therapies" may become useful in the treatment of lupus, as scientists have been able to develop breeds of "knockout" mice missing a specific gene or chemical.

As long as investigators stick to well-established guidelines that mandate humane and ethical environments for animal research, these efforts can save billions of dollars and a lot of unnecessary trial and error in humans while accelerating the pace for establishing the efficacy of new treatments. For example, because mice with lupus live 1 to 2 years and humans with lupus can live up to 100 years, the influence of different therapeutic or environmental interventions can be seen more easily in animals with lupus.

## FURTHER READING

1. Satoh M, Chan EK, Ho LA, et al. Prevalence and sociodemographic correlates of antinuclear antibodies in the United States. *Arthritis Rheum.* 2012;64(7):2319–2327.
2. Summond J, Diamond B. Autoantibodies in systemic autoimmune diseases: specificity and pathogenicity. *J Clin Invest.* 2015;125(6):2194–2202.

# Part III
# WHAT CAUSES LUPUS?

In the development of systemic lupus erythematosus (SLE), several factors play a role, and these are enumerated in Chapters 7 to 9. In essence, a long period of predisposition to autoimmunity is conferred by genetic susceptibility, hormones, and environmental exposures. A small proportion of those individuals predisposed develop autoantibodies, which usually precede clinical symptoms by months to years. A proportion of those who develop autoantibodies develop clinical and laboratory abnormalities ultimately classified as SLE. These individuals undergo a course associated with disease flares and improvements, but they compile organ damage and comorbidities. This is related to genetic predisposition, chronic inflammation, activation of pathways that damage organs or induce fibrosis (scarring), and aging. The reader is not expected to readily understand the concepts discussed: *this is the most technically complicated section of the book.* Most of the topics covered here are reviewed in more detail elsewhere in the book.

1. *Genetics.* The risk for SLE is increased tenfold in monozygotic (identical) twins compared to dizygotic ones and eight- to twentyfold in siblings of SLE patients compared to the healthy population. Patients with certain HLA markers (e.g., DR3, DR2, DR4, DR8, especially in the presence of anti-SSA or anti-SSB) have a 1.5-fold greater-than-expected risk for developing lupus. Over 40 lupus associated genes have been identified, but most have odds ratios (relative risks) of less than 2.5 (1 would indicate no predisposition), and they are only of minimal clinical value. A handful of non-HLA genes (e.g., Clq deficiency, DNAsel, Trexl mutations) have an odds ratio of 2.5 or greater, but they are infrequently seen. There is some evidence that a polymorphism of TLR5 (a toll-like receptor) confers protection from SLE.
2. *Epigenetics.* Epigenetics refers to inherited or acquired modification of DNA without any changes in the DNA base sequence. These alterations occur via three mechanisms: DNA methylation, histone deacetylation, and microRNA (miRNA). SLE is associated with hypomethylation, which leads

to upregulated expression of surface molecules and T cell autoreactivity. Lupus-inducing drugs, ultraviolet light, and miRNA can promote hypomethylation. Alterations in histones conformationally influence DNA transcription and repair. Deacetylation promotes autoimmunity and alters DNA signaling. Agents that interfere with this pathway are in clinical trials for a variety of autoimmune disorders. miRNA are noncoding small RNA (19–25 nucleotides in length) "gene-silencing" sequences that regulate gene expression at posttranscriptional levels. Over 1,000 have been described in humans. Recent work has suggested that TLR2, TLR4, and TLR5 are upregulated by certain miRNAs, which promotes increased interferon-alpha activity.

3. *Gender.* Gender studies demonstrate several possible roles in SLE. In lupus mice, estradiol prolongs the life of autoreactive B and T cells, while in male mice with lupus, androgens are immune protective. After a pregnancy, a mechanism known as microchimerism (where the Y chromosome is found in cells and tissues) can produce a chronic "graft versus host," or low-grade tissue rejection that is associated with SLE. Also, inactivated X chromosomes (women have XX) enriched with hypomethylation can be bound and activated by TLR7 and 9, which is associated with SLE.

4. *Environment.* A variety of environmental factors are important in SLE, and many other putative agents have been postulated to be lupogenic or lupus associated. Definite associations have been made with ultraviolet light (especially UVB). DNA in the dermis becomes more immunogenic in the presence of UV light leading to apoptosis of keratinocytes (skin cells) and the formation of self-antigen. There is also considerable evidence that the Epstein–Barr virus activates B cells in the presence of the Ro (SSA) antigen through a mechanism known as molecular mimicry. Other than silica dust exposure (e.g., sandblasters, uranium miners) predisposing one to SLE, no other environmental agent, vocation, or other exposures have been demonstrated to induce lupus but some are have a slight statistical association.

5. *Autoantibodies and Immune Complexes.* Data from armed forces recruits show that the development of autoantibodies precedes the first symptoms of SLE by 2 to 9 years. Antinuclear antibody first forms, followed by anti-DNA, antiphospholipid antibodies, and finally antibodies to Sm and RNP. Immunoregulation of potentially pathogenic antibodies can occur for a sustained period, and in individuals whose regulation becomes "exhausted," disease appears. These autoantibodies are self-perpetuating where amino acid sequences are T cell determinants and peptides activate helper T cells and ultimately antibodies are formed. Antigen–antibody combinations (immune complexes) that are bound by complement receptors and FcR receptors on immunoglobulins and fail to be cleared become fixed in tissue where inflammation ensues.

6. *Stimulation of Innate and Adaptive Immune Responses by Autoantigens.* The innate immune system dates from primordial times and uses pattern recognition receptors to identify foreign substances (e.g., viruses, DNA, RNA, chemicals) and prevent them from inducing damage. Adaptive immune responses developed in each individual as a response to environmental insults. Normal cells die via a mechanism known as *apoptosis*. Sometimes, debris from these dying cells becomes antigenic itself (e.g., nucleosomes, Ro in surface blebs, phosphatidyl serine in the outer cell membranes), which, under the influence of oxidation, microorganisms, phosphorylation, and cleavage, are processed by antigen-presenting cells. In the innate immune system, they are activated by DNA and RNA proteins complexed with TLRs via a process known as NETosis (neutrophil extracellular traps), which traps them and activates dendritic cells, cytokines, and interferon. The consequence of this is that effector T cells activate B cells (including plasmablasts) and form autoantibodies, which deposit immunoglobulin and fix complement in tissues and promote inflammation. A similar pathway is initiated in adaptive immune responses.

7. *Regulatory Mechanisms Fail to Control Autoimmune Responses.* Immune complexes and apoptotic cells circulate in the bloodstream and need to be disposed of so they do not settle in tissues (which causes inflammation) or release chemicals (e.g., cytokines, chemokines), which also promotes inflammation. In SLE, this clearance fails due to a variety of mechanisms: defective phagocytosis, altered transport by complement receptors, defective regulation of T helper cells by regulatory T cells, inadequate production or function of regulatory cells that kill or suppress autoreactive B cells, low production of interleukin-2 by T cells, and defects in apoptosis that permit the survival of effector T and autoreactive B cells (activated B cells, memory B cells, plasma cells).

8. *Abnormalities in T and B Lymphocytes in SLE.* When activated, T and B cells produce cytokines and autoantibodies. When underactivated, cells fail to undergo apoptosis, and B and T cells become autoreactive. Both phenomena occur in lupus. Defects in immune tolerance permit prolonged survival of B and T cells, which leads to activated B cells, memory B cells, and plasma cell formation and ultimately autoreactive B cells. These are further influenced by B cell surface antigen receptors, soluble BLyS (B lymphocyte stimulation—which is what is blocked by the drug belimumab, or Benlysta), genetic polymorphisms (variations) affecting B cell receptor signaling, and the intracellular mobilization of calcium. Regulatory T cells (T reg) suppress inflammation, and their function is diminished in lupus. T-cell receptor activation is altered, and T reg mechanisms fail that allow the suppression of IL-2 and the activation of the pro-inflammatory cytokine interleukin-17. When there is a defect in T suppressor apoptosis, autoreactive B cells form. Several defects permit survival of autoreactive cell subsets

in SLE. The usual tolerance processes (apoptosis, anergy, ignorance, BCR editing, external suppression) are blunted allowing dangerous autoreactive B cells.

9. *Tissue Damage.* Tissue damage is produced by the deposition of circulating immune complexes into tissue, which, in turn, activates endothelial cells, cytokines, and chemokines. In the kidneys, this produces inflammation, followed by proliferation and ultimately fibrosis (scarring). Complement activation, overloading of the CR1 transport system, antibodies to complement components (anti-Clq), and congenital or acquired deficiency in complement components also lead to tissue inflammation and damage. Lupus is characterized by accelerated atherosclerosis. This results from circulating immune complexes and complement split products activating endothelial cells in coronary arteries, which leads to the release of chemokines, cytokines, and activated monocytes. A nidus of plaque forms that, in combination with oxidized LDL (bad cholesterol), forms "foam" cells that produce damage to coronary arteries. (See Figure III.1.)

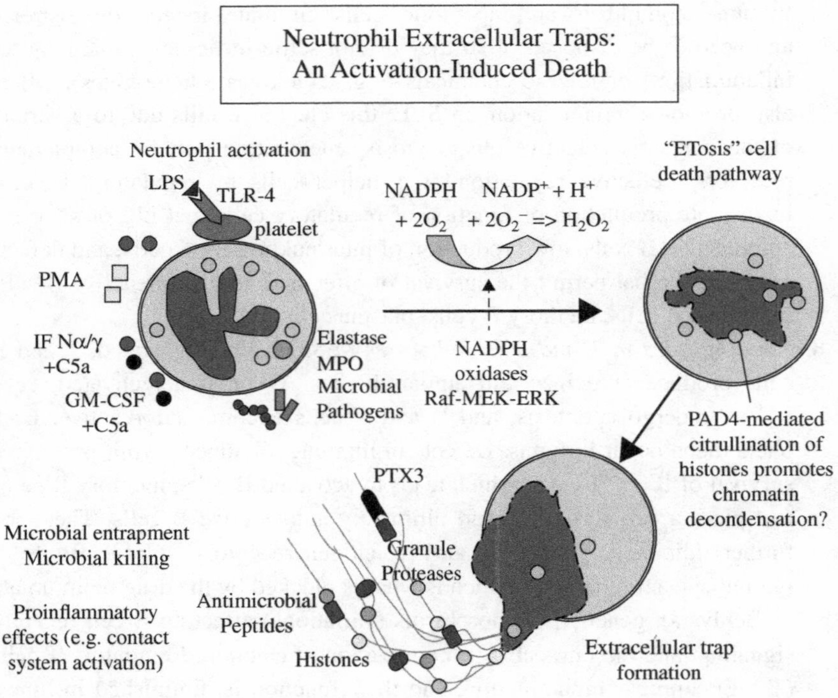

**Figure III.1.** *Factors Promoting the Development of Systemic Lupus Erythematosus*

## FURTHER READING

1. Tsokos GC, Lo MS, Costa Reis P et al. New insights into the immunopathogenesis of systemic lupus erythematosus. *Nat Rev Rheumatol.* 2016;12:716–730.
2. Mouton VR, Suarez-Fueyo A, Meidan E, et al. Pathogenesis of human systemic lupus erythematosus: a cellular perspective. *Trends Mol Med.* 2017;23:617–635.
3. Zharkova O, Celhar T, Cravens PD, et al. Pathways leadning to an immunological disease: systemic lupus erythematosus. *Rheumatology* (Oxford). 2017;56(suppl 1):i55–i66.
4. Arbuckle MR, Mc Clain MT, Rubertone MB et al. Development of autoantibodies before the clinical onset of systemic lupus erythematosus. *N Engl J Med.* 2003;349(16):1526–1533.

# 7
## *The Genetic Connection*

Is lupus a genetic disorder? Does it run in families? How can it be passed on or be inherited? These questions are commonly asked. The answer is not simple, but researchers now believe that various genes that predispose people to lupus are inherited, among them the *major histocompatibility complex*, or *MHC*, which includes the *human leukocyte antigen* (HLA) region, a specific area of the genes. Along with HLA, we also inherit T cell receptor genes and other genes relevant to systemic lupus erythematosus (SLE), such as immunoglobulin genes. Each of us inherits a unique chemical signature, just as we inherit our blood type. Over the last decade, genome-wide area studies (GWAS) followed detailed analyses have yielded substantial number of genomic loci linked to SLE susceptibility, which helps to enhance our understanding of lupus at the molecular level.

All this probably seems a little like alphabet soup, but in the next few pages we take a closer look at how the principles of genetics apply to our understanding of lupus.

## THE MAJOR HISTOCOMPATIBILITY COMPLEX: A GENE SYSTEM

Every human cell that contains a nucleus (or center) also contains 23 pairs of *chromosomes*. We inherit one member of every pair from each of our parents. These chromosomes store the genetic material responsible for determining whether you are a male or female, have red hair, are color blind, and might develop cystic fibrosis, among other characteristics. In mapping human chromosomes, geneticists have referred to the "short" and "long" arms of the chromosomes, which have been numbered for convenience. On the short arm of the sixth chromosome lie a series of specific sites, called *genetic markers*, that determine what an individual's HLA system will look like. First described in the early 1970s, the HLA region contains genes that may predispose one to a remarkable number of diseases, especially rheumatic disorders.

HLA testing is very simple. A physician needs only a few tubes of blood drawn from the arm. The HLA site consists of three well-defined and functionally distinct regions known as classes I, II, and III. Class I is expressed on all cells with a nucleus and is divided into A, B, and C subtypes. Class II is present on cells that are capable of presenting antigens (foreign material) to white blood cells and includes the D subtype. The D regions are further broken down into DP, DQ, and DR subregions, among others. Class III provides for the structural genes that produce a variety of substances important in lupus blood and tissues such as complement, tumor necrosis factor, and heat shock protein.

An HLA "marker" is given to patients based on the subtype they possess: A, B, C, or D. Numerous *alleles* ("designations" or "arrangements") can be found at the same marker or site; there are more than a hundred possible arrangements that are further subdivided. If this seems complicated, don't worry. This expanding area of knowledge often confuses the best rheumatologists.

A combination of alleles at two HLA loci is a name tag, or *haplotype*. These can differ widely among various racial and ethnic groups. For example, HLA-B27 (the marker associated with a spinal disease known as ankylosing spondylitis) is found in 8 percent of Americans of European Caucasian ancestry but is less common among African Americans.

The statistical chance that two particular haplotypes will occur together is about 2 percent (e.g., A6 with B5). However, in certain rheumatic diseases the chance that two alleles or arrangements will occur together may greatly exceed this.

Table 7.1 illustrates the classification of the HLA system. The labels themselves are not important for our purposes; what is important is that specific genes are inherited and these may predispose a person to lupus.

## WHY IS HLA IMPORTANT IN LUPUS PATIENTS?

What does all this mean for lupus? First, certain subsets of the disease are associated (in other words, they are often but not always found) with very specific HLA markers. For instance, neonatal lupus (lupus afflicting children at birth) is most often present in children who possess the A1, B8, DR3, and DQw52 haplotypes. Patients with discoid lupus tend to possess DR4 markers, and DR3 is present in those with a specific skin problem known as subacute cutaneous lupus. Sjögren's syndrome (dry eyes, dry mouth, and arthritis, which is seen in many patients with SLE) is associated with B8, DR3, and DRw52. DR2 and DR3 are more commonly observed in Caucasians of Western European descent than any other DR types. The presence of DQw1 correlates with certain autoantibodies such as anti-DNA, anti-Ro, and anti-La. "Null" or absent alleles can account for some of the deficiencies in blood complement levels that are frequently seen in SLE.

Even though medicine has yet to isolate a lupus "gene," certain genetic markers and other non-HLA genes correlate with specific lupus subsets and autoantibodies. Different sets or combinations of genes may be associated with as much as a twentyfold risk for developing SLE.

**Table 7.1.** *Monogenic Mutations with SLE and SLE-Like Diseases*

| Function | Gene | Effect | Clinical Features |
|---|---|---|---|
| **Apoptotic and IC Clearance** | | | |
| 1p36 | *C1QA, C1QB, C1QC* | Complement C1 deficiency | Early-onset severe SLE |
| 3p21 | *PRKCD* | Exonic mutation | SLE |
| 6p21 | *C4A, C4B* | Complement C4 deficiency | Early-onset severe SLE |
| 6p21 | *C2* | Complement C2 deficiency | Recurrent infections, SLE with skin involvement |
| 7q11 | *NCF1* | p47$^{phox}$ deficiency | AR-CGD, SLE |
| 12p13 | *C1R, C1S* | Complement C1 deficiency | Early-onset severe SLE |
| 19p13 | *C3* | Complement C3 deficiency | MPGN |
| 19q13 | *PEPD* | Prolidase deficiency | Cutaneous ulcers, autoantibodies |
| Xp21 | *CYBB* | gp91$^{phox}$ deficiency | X-linked CGD, SLE |
| **Nucleic Acid Sensing And IFN-I Signaling** | | | |
| 1q21 | *ADAR* | Exonic mutation | AGS |
| 2q24 | *IFIH1* | Exonic mutation | AGS, SLE |
| 3p14 | *DNASE1L3* | Exonic mutation | Early-onset SLE |
| 3p21 | *TREX1* | Exonic mutation | AGS, SLE |
| 5q31 | *TMEM173* | Exonic mutation | SAVI |
| 11q13 | *RNASEH2C* | Exonic mutation, intronic variant | AGS |
| 13q14 | *RNASEH2B* | Exonic mutation, intronic variant | AGS |
| 16p13 | *DNASE1* | Exonic mutation | SLE |
| 19p13 | *RNASEH2A* | Exonic mutation, intronic variant | AGS |
| 19p13 | *ACP5* | Exonic mutation | SPENCD |
| 20q11 | *SAMHD1* | Exonic mutation, intronic variant | AGS, SLE |
| **Lymphocyte Signaling** | | | |
| 1q24 | *FASLG* | Exonic mutation | ALPS, SLE with lymphadenopathy |
| 10q23 | *FAS* | Fas deficiency | ALPS |
| 10q25 | *SHOC2* | Exonic mutation | NSLAH, SLE |
| 11p12 | *RAG1.RAG2* | Exonic mutation | SCID, SLE, erosive arthritis |
| 12p12 | *KRAS* | Exonic mutation | NS, SLE |
| 12q24 | *PTPN11* | Exonic mutation | NS. SLE |

Gene name: *ACP5*, acid phosphatase 5 tartrate resistant; *ADAR*, adenosine deaminase RNA specific; *C1QA/ C1QB/C1QC*, complement C1q A chain, B chain, and C chain; *C1R/C1S*, complement C1r/C1s; *C2*, complement C2; *C3*, complement C3; *C4A/C4B*, complement C4A&B; *CYBB*, cytochrome b-245 beta chain; *DNASE1*, deoxyribonuclease 1; *DNASE1L3*, deoxyribonuclease 1 like 3; *FAS*, Fas cell surface death receptor; *FASLG*, Fas ligand; *IFIH1*, interferon induced with helicase C domain 1; *KRAS*, KRAS proto-oncogene GTPase; *NCF1*, neutrophil cytosolic factor 1; *PEPD*, peptidase D; *RAG1/2*, recombination activating 1 and 2; *PRKCD*, protein kinase C delta; *PTPN11*, protein tyrosine phosphatase nonreceptor type 11; *RNASEH2A/2B/2C*, ribonuclease H2 subunit A/B/C; *SAMHD1*, SAM and HD domain containing deoxynucleoside triphosphate triphosphohydrolase 1; *SHOC2*, SHOC2 leucine rich repeat scaffold protein; *TMEM173*, transmembrane protein 173; *TREX1*, three prime repair exonuclease 1. Abbreviations: AGS, Aicardi-Goutières syndrome; ALPS, autoimmune lymphoproliferative syndrome; AR-CGD, autosomal recessive chronic granulomatous disease; MPGN, membranoproliferative glomerulonephritis; NS, Noonan syndrome; NSLAH, Noonan syndrome with loose anagen hair; SAVI, STING-associated vasculopathy with onset in infancy; SCID, severe combined immunodeficiency; SPENCD, immuno-osseous dysplasia spondyloenchondrodysplasia; X-linked CGD, X-linked chronic granulomatous disease.

## OTHER LUPUS SUSCEPTIBILITY GENES

A variety of genes outside of the HLA system may predispose individuals to SLE. These include genes on mannose-binding protein, Fc receptor alleles, immunoglobulin G receptors, T-cell receptors, those involved with apoptosis, single-nucleotide polymorphisms (SNPs), and genetic polymorphisms associated with cytokines (particularly tumor necrosis factor alpha, apoptosis, interleukin-6, interleukin-10, interferon expression, C-reactive protein expression, and complement). Some of these are listed in Table 7.2.

**Table 7.2.** *SLE Susceptibility Genes with Common Variants Grouped by Pathways*

| Function/ Position | Gene | Population | Likely Causative Variant | Reference |
|---|---|---|---|---|
| **Innate/Adaptive Immune Response** | | | | |
| *TLR/IFN-I signaling* | | | | |
| 2q24 | IFIH1 | EU, AA | rs13023380 (A allele) results in decreased IFIH1 transcript levels; rs1990760 (A946T; A allele) and rs10930046 (H460R; A allele) confer increased apoptosis and elevated inflammation-related gene expression. | 17,2 I |
| 2q32 | STAT4 | EU, AS, AA, HS | | 17,24,2 >,27 |
| 5q34 | MIR146A | AS, EU | rs57095329 (G allele) conferring decreased Ets-1 binding is associated with reduced miR146a levels. | 17,29 |
| 7q32 | IRF5 | EU, AA, AS, HS | Four SNPs define risk haplotypes associated with increased expression of IRF5 and IFN-a. rs4728142 (A allele) tagging the promoter effect confers increased ZBTB3 binding and elevated IRF5 expression. | 27,30- Î1 |
| 9p24.1 | JAK2 | AS, EU | | 18 |
| 11p15 | IRF7 | EU, AA, AS | rs12805435 confers c/ s-eQTL effect on IRF7 expression and trans-eQTL effect on regulating type 11 FN responses in activated dendritic cells. | 17.32-: I3 |

**Table 7.2.** (continued)

| Function/ Position | Gene | Population | Likely Causative Variant | Reference |
|---|---|---|---|---|
| 11q13.1 | RNASEH2C | AS, EU | | 18.2Í |
| 12q24.32 | SLC15A4 | AS, EU | | 17,19,: 4 |
| 16q24.1 | IRF8 | EU, AS | | 24.34-Í 5 |
| 19p13.2 | TYK2 | EU, AS | | 17,34,5 6 |
| Xp22 | TLR7 | AS, EU, AA, HS | rs3853839 (G allele) confers increased TLR7 expression and IFN response. | 37–38 |
| Xq28 | TMEM187/ IRAK1 / MECP2 | EU, AS, AA, HS | rs1059702 (S196F; A allele) tagging a risk haplotype confers increased NFkB activity. | 17,24,29 |
| *NFkB signaling* | | | | |
| 5q33.1 | TNIP1 | AS, EU, AA, HS | | 16,24,27 40 |
| 6q23 | TNFAIP3 | EU, AS, AA | TT>A polymorphic dinucleotide (deletion T followed by A transversion) with decreased NFkB binding to the promoter attenuates TNFAIP3 expression. | 14,19 41–43 |
| 16p11.2 | PRKCB | AS, EU | | 44–45 |
| 22q11.21 | UBE2L3 | EU, AS, AA, HS | rs 140490 (T allele) tagging a risk haplotype amplifies NF-kB activation and promotes plasma cell development. | 17,24,46–47 |
| *T cell signaling* | | | | |
| 1q25 | TNFSF4 | EU, AS, AA, HS | | 17,24,48 |
| 3q13.33 | CD80 | AS | | 22,24 |
| 3q25.33 | IL12A | EU, AS | | 17.4S |
| 5q31.1 | TCF7 | EU, AS | | 17,24,49 |
| 5q33.3 | IL12B | AS | | |
| *TLR/IFN-I signaling/* | | | | |
| 2q24 | IFIH1 | EU, AA | rs 13023380 (A allele) results in decreased IFIH1 transcript levels; rs1990760 (A946T; A allele) and rs10930046 (H460R; A allele) confer increased apoptosis and elevated inflammation-related gene expression. | 17,21 |
| 2q32 | STAT4 | EU, AS, AA, HS | | 17,24,26, 27 |

(*continued*)

**Table 7.2.** (continued)

| Function/ Position | Gene | Population | Likely Causative Variant | Reference |
|---|---|---|---|---|
| 5q34 | MIR146A | AS, EU | rs57095329 (G allele) conferring decreased Ets-1 binding is associated with reduced miR146a levels. | 17,29 |
| 7q32 | IRF5 | EU, AA, AS, HS | | 27,30–31 |
| 9p24.1 | JAK2 | AS, EU | Four SNPs define risk haplotypes associated with increased expression of IRF5 and IFN-a. rs4728142 (A allele) tagging the promoter effect confers increased ZBTB3 binding and elevated IRF5 expression. | 18 |
| 11p15 | IRF7 | EU, AA, AS | | 17,32-13 |
| 11q13.1 | RNASEH2C | AS, EU | rs12805435 confers c/ s-eQTL effect on IRF7 expression and trans-eQTL effect on regulating type 11 FN responses in activated dendritic cells. | 18.2Í |
| 12q24.32 | SLC15A4 | AS, EU | | 17,19,24 |
| 16q24.1 | IRF8 | EU, AS | | 24,34–35 |
| 19p13.2 | TYK2 | EU, AS | | 17,34–36 |
| Xp22 | TLR7 | AS, EU, AA, HS | rs3853839 (G allele) confers increased TLR7 expression and IFN response. | 37-38 |
| Xq28 | TMEM187/ IRAK1 / MECP2 | EU, AS, AA, HS | rs1059702 (S196F; A allele) tagging a risk haplotype confers increased NFkB activity. | 17,24, 39 |
| *NFkB signaling* | | | | |
| 5q33.1 | TNIP1 | AS, EU, AA, HS | | 16,24,27,40 |
| 6q23 | TNFAIP3 | AS, EU | TT>A polymorphic dinucleotide (deletion T followed by A transversion) with decreased NFkB binding to the promoter attenuates TNFAIP3 expression. | 14,19, 41–43 |
| 16p11.2 | PRKCB | EU, AS, AA | | 44–45 |
| 22q11.21 | UBE2L3 | EU, AS, AA, HS | rs140490 (T allele) tagging a risk haplotype amplifies NF-kB activation and promotes plasma cell development. | 17,24, 46–47 |

**Table 7.2.** (continued)

| Function/ Position | Gene | Population | Likely Causative Variant | Reference |
|---|---|---|---|---|
| *T cell signaling* | | | | |
| 1q25 | TNFSF4 | EU, AS, AA, HS | | 17,24, 48 |
| 3q13.33 | CD80 | AS | | 22,24 |
| 3q25.33 | IL12A | EU, AS | | 17,49 |
| 5q31.1 | TCF7 | EU, AS | | 17,24,49 |
| 5q33.3 | IL12B | AS | | 24 |
| 15q24.1 | CSK | EU | | |
| 16q21 | CCL22 | AS | rs34933034 (A allele) is associated with increased CSK expression, Lyn phosphorylation, BCR-mediated activation of mature B cells and expansion of transitional B cells. | 17,65 23 |
| 15q21 | CCL72 | AS | | 25 |
| 17q21 | IKZF3 | EU, AS | | 17,65 |
| **Clearance Defects** | | | | |
| *Self-Antigen Clearance* | | | | |
| 1q25 | NCF2 | EU, AA, AS, HS | rs17849502 (H389Q; A allele) confers decreased NADPH oxidase activity and ROS production. | 67-68I |
| 6q21 | ATG5 | EU, AS | | 17,19 ' |
| 7q 11.23 | NCF1 | AS, EU, AA | rs201802880 (R90H;A allele) is associated with reduced ROS production. | 69 |
| 7q 11.23 | HIP1 | AS, EU | | 21,24,45 |
| 11q13.4 | ATG16L2 | AS | | 23–24 |
| 12p13.1 | CDKN1B | AS, EU | | 22,45 |
| 12q23.2 | DRAM1 | AS | | 22 |
| 16p13.13 | CLEC16A | AS, EU | | 17,24,70 |
| *IC Clearance* | | | | |
| 1q23 | FCGR2A | EU, AA, AS | rs1801274 (H166R; T allele) alters binding affinity of FcγRHa and affects IC clearance. | 17,26,71 |
| 16p11.2 | ITGAM | EU, AA, AS, HS | rs1143679 (R77H; A allele) impairs leukocyte phagocytosis and is associated with elevated IFN-I activity. | 17,26,27,72 |
| **Others** | | | | |
| *NMD* | SMG7 | EU | | 73/ |
| *Lysosome dysfuction* | LYST | EU | | 17 |

(*continued*)

**Table 7.2.** (continued)

| Function/Position | Gene | Population | Likely Causative Variant | Reference |
|---|---|---|---|---|
| *MAPK signaling* | SPRED2 | EU, AS | | 17,48 |
| *cell process,* | LBH | EU, AS | | 181 |
| *proliferation* | LPP | EU, AS | | 18/ |
| *and adhesion* | PRAG1/ CLDN23/ MFHAS1/ CTSB | EU | | 74 |
| | SIGLEC6 | AS | | 24 |
| DNA repair | RAD51B | EU | | 17 |
| **Unknown Immune Function** | | | | |
| 1q25 | NMNAT2 | EU, HS | | 73 |
| 1q25.3 | EDEM3 | EU | | 73 |
| 2p13 | TET3 | AS, EU | | 22,45 |
| 3p14.3 | ABHD6 | EU | | 17, 75 |
| 3q26.2 | MYNN | AS | | |
| 5p15.33 | TERT | AS | | 25,24 |
| 6p21 | UHRF1BP1 | EU, AS | | 17,77 |
| 6p21 | ANKS1A | AS | | 25¡ |
| 6p22.3 | ATXN1 | EU, AS | | 18 |
| 7p15 | JAZF1 | EU, HS | | 17,27 |
| 11p13 | PDHX/CD44 | EU, AS , AA | | 17,50 |
| 12q24 | SH2B3 | EU | | 17 |
| 16q22.1 | ZFP90 | AS, EU | | 18 |
| 18q22.2 | CD226 | AS, EU | | 24,51 |
| *B cell signaling* | | | | |
| 4q24 | BANK1 | EU, AS , AA | rs10516487 (R61H; G allele), rs3733197 (A383T; G allele) and rs17266594 (Tállele) are associated with alterations in peripheral B cell signaling and development. | 13,17,24,26 |
| 3p14.3 | PXK | EU | rs4681677 (G allele) tags a risk haplotype associted with decreased BCR internalization. | 15,17,5 I |
| 6q21 | PRDM1 | EU, AS | | 17,24 |
| 8p23 | BLK | EU, AS, AA | rs922483 (T allele) and tri-allelic SNP rs 1382568 (A, C alleles) reduce BLK promoter activity. | 17,24,53 |
| 8q12 | LYN | EU | | 15,54 |
| 10q21.2 | ARID5B | AS, EU | | 17,2 ! |
| 11q23.3 | CXCR5 | AS | | 55 |

**Table 7.2.** (continued)

| Function/ Position | Gene | Population | Likely Causative Variant | Reference |
|---|---|---|---|---|
| 13q33.3 | TNFSF13B | EU | GCTGT->A insertion-deletion variant (A allele) confers a short BAFF transcript and increased soluble BAFF production. | 56 |
| 16p13.13 | CIITA/SOCS1 | EU, AS | | 17,24 |
| *T&B cell signaling and interaction* | | | | |
| 1p13.2 | PTPN22 | EU, HS, AA, AS | rs2476601 (R620W; A allele) alters T cell receptor and B cell receptor signaling with enhanced B cell autoreactivity, and is associated with diminished type IIFN production in myeloid cells but enhanced functions in neutrophils. | 17,57–59 |
| 1q32.1 | IL10 | EU | rs3122605 (G allele) tags a risk haplotype associated with increased // .iOexpression by preferentially binding to Elk-1. | 16,60 |
| 1q31.3 | PTPRC | EU.AS | | 18 |
| 2p22.3 | RASGRP3 | AS.EU | | 24,61 |
| 2q34 | IKZF2 | EU | | 17 |
| 4q21 | AFF1 | AS.EU | | 21,4 5 |
| 6p21.3 | HLA Class II | EU, AS, HS | | 17,24,27,62 |
| 6p21.3 | HLA Class III | EU, AS, AA | | 17,24, 26 |
| 6p21.3 | DEF6 | AS | | 24 |
| 6q15 | BACH2 | EU, AS | | 18 |
| 7p12.2 | IKZF1 | AS, EU | rs4917014 (T allele) alters IKZF1 levels in cis and regulates expression of C1QB and five type I IFN response genes in trans. | 17,24 |
| 11q24.3 | ETS1 | AS, EU | rs6590330 (A allele) is associated with decreased ETS1 expression and increased STAT1 binding. | 17,20,24,63 |
| 13q14.11 | ELF1 | AS, EU | | 45,64 |
| 15q14 | RASGRP1 | AS | | 24 |

(*continued*)

**Table 7.2.** (continued)

| Function/ Position | Gene | Population | Likely Causative Variant | Reference |
|---|---|---|---|---|
| 8p23.1 | XKR6 | EU | | -<* 15 |
| 10q11.23 | WDFY4 | AS, EU | | 17,20,24 |
| 11q13.1 | PCNX3 | AS | | 24 |
| 11q13.4 | DHCR7/ NADSYN1 | EU | | 17 |
| 11q23.3 | PHLDB1 | AS | | 55 |
| 11q23.3 | DDX6íTREH | AS | | 19, 55 |
| 12q12 | PRICKLE1 | EU | | 45 |
| 15q14 | FAM98B | EU | | 75 |
| 17p13.2 | PLD2 | EU | | 17 |
| 22q13.1 | SYNGR1 | AS | | 24 |
| Xp21.2 | CXorf21 | EU | | 17' |
| Xp22.3 | PRPS2 | AS | | 78 |

These loci (yielding p<5><10^8 in at least one ancestry) are identified through genome-wide area studies, meta-analysis, fine-mapping, or replication studies. Gene name: *ABHD6*, abhydrolase domain containing 6; *AFF1*, AF4/FMR2 family member 1; *ANKS1A*, ankyrin repeat and sterile alpha motif domain containing 1A; *ARID5B*, AT-rich interaction domain 5B; *ATG5*, autophagy related 5; *ATG16L2*, autophagy related 16 like 2; *ATXN1*, ataxin 1; *BACH2*, BTB domain and CNC homolog 2; *BANK1*, B-cell scaffold protein with ankyrin repeats 1; *BLK*, BLK proto-oncogene, Src family tyrosine kinase; *CDKN1B*, cyclin dependent kinase inhibitor 1B; *CCL22*, C-C motif chemokine ligand 22; *CD44*, CD44 molecule; *CD80*, CD80 molecule; *CD226*, CD226 molecule; *CUTA*, class II major histocompatibility complex transactivator; *CLDN23*, claudin 23; *CLEC16A*, C-type lectin domain containing 16A; *CSK*, CSK nonreceptor tyrosine kinase; *CTSB*, cathepsin B; *CXCR5*, C-X-C motif chemokine receptor 5; *CXorf21*, chromosome X open reading frame 21; *DDX6*, DEAD-box helicase 6; *DEF6*, DEF6 guanine nucleotide exchange factor; *DHCR7*, 7-dehydrocholesterol reductase; *DRAM1*, DNA damage regulated autophagy modulator 1; *EDEM3*, ER degradation enhancing alpha-mannosidase like protein 3; *ELF1*, E74 tike ETS transcription factor 1; *ETS1*, ETS proto-oncogene 1 transcription factor; *FAM98B*, family with sequence similarity 98 member B; *FCGR2A*, Fc fragment of IgG receptor lia; *HIP1*, huntingtin interacting protein 1; *HLA class II*, major histocompatibility complex class II; *HLA class III*, major histocompatibility complex class III; *IFIH1*, interferon induced with helicase C domain 1; *IKZF1*, IKAROS family zinc finger 1; *IKZF2*, IKAROS family zinc finger 2; *IKZF3*, IKAROS family zinc finger 3; *IL10*, interleukin 10; *IL12A/B*, interleukin 12A/B; *IRAK1*, interleukin 1 receptor associated kinase 1; *IRF5*, interferon regulatory factor 5; *IRF7*, interferon regulatory factor 7; *IRF8*, interferon regulatory factor 8; *ITGAM*, integrin subunit alpha M; *JAK2*, Janus kinase 2; *JAZF1*, JAZF zinc finger 1; *LBH*, limb bud and heart development; *LPP*, LIM domain containing preferred translocation partner in lipoma; *LYN*, LYN proto-oncogene, Src family tyrosine kinase; *LYST*, lysosomal trafficking regulator; *MECP2*, methyl-CpG binding protein 2; *MFHAS1*, malignant fibrous histiocytoma amplified sequence 1; *MIR146A*, microRNA 146a; *MYNN*, myoneruin; *NADSYN1*, NAD synthetase 1; *NCF1*, neutrophil cytosolic factor 1; *NCF2*, neutrophil cytosolic factor 2; *NMNAT2*, nicotinamide nucleotide adenylyltransferase 2; *PCNX3*, pecanex homolog 3; *PDHX*, pyruvate dehydrogenase complex component X; *PHLDB1*, pleckstrin homology like domain family B member 1; *PLD2*, phospholipase D2; *PRAG1*, PEAK1-related kinase-activating pseudokinase 1; *PRDM1*, PR/SET domain 1; *PRICKLE1*, prickle planar cell polarity protein 1; *PRKCB*, protein kinase C beta; *PRPS2*, phosphoribosyl pyrophosphate synthetase 2; *PTPN22*, protein tyrosine phosphatase nonreceptor type 22; *PTPRC*, protein tyrosine phosphatase receptor type C; *PXK*, PX domain containing serine/threonine kinase like; *RAD51B*, RAD51 paralog B; *RASGRP1*, RAS guanyl releasing protein 1; *RASGRP3*, RAS guanyl releasing protein 3; *RNASEH2C*, ribonuclease H2 subunit C; *SH2B3*, SH2B adaptor protein 3; *SIGLEC6*, sialic acid binding Ig-like lectin 6; *SLC15A4*, solute carrier family 15 member 4; *SMG7*, SMG7 nonsense mediated mRNA decay factor; *SOCS1*, suppressor of cytokine signaling 1; *SPRED2*, sprout-related EVH1 domain containing 2; *STAT4*, signal transducer and activator of transcription 4; *SYNGR1*, synaptogyrin 1; *7CF7*, transcription factor 7; *TERT*, telomerase reverse transcriptase; *TET3*, tet methylcytosine dioxygenase 3; *TLR7*, toll-like receptor 7; *TMEM187*, transmembrane protein 187; *TNFAIP3*, TNF alpha-induced protein 3; *TNFSF4*, TNF superfamily member 4; *TNFSF13B*, TNF superfamily member 13b; *TNIP1*, TNFAIP3 interacting protein 1; *TREH*, trehalase; *TYK2*, tyrosine kinase 2; *UBE2L3*, ubiquitin conjugating enzyme E2L3; *UHRF1BP1*, UHRF1 binding protein 1; *WDFY4*, WDFY family member 4; *XKR6*, XK related 6; *ZFP90*, ZFP90 zinc finger protein. Abbreviations: AA, African American; AS, Asian; EU, European-derived; HS, Amerindian/Hispanic.

## WHAT IS BEING DONE TO ISOLATE THE GENES THAT CAUSE LUPUS?

Several consortia throughout the world have worked together to find ways to find the set of genes that bring on disease. Advances in the field have allowed the process of analyzing genetic markers to speed up dramatically. The efforts have proceeded along the following lines: linkage analysis (identifying genetic segments in families with two or more affected members), fine-mapping (where chromosome regions of interest are identified), candidate susceptibility genes (where a single gene is studied), and population whole-genome sequencing. Many candidate genes and regions of interest have been identified, even though the conclusions have often been contradictory. Nevertheless, it appears that in the next few years we will have a firm handle on the genes that cause lupus.

The work has shown the SLE-risk locus within or near genes encode products functioning in the clearance of immune complexes, type I interferon, and lymphocyte signaling.

## WHAT IS THE RISK THAT A MEMBER OF A LUPUS PATIENT'S FAMILY WILL DEVELOP LUPUS?

If you have lupus, members of your immediate family, or first-degree relatives (brothers, sisters, parents, and children), are at a slightly increased risk for developing it, too. Several surveys have estimated this risk at 10 percent for your daughter and 2 percent for your son. If you have lupus and have an identical twin, the chance that this sibling is similarly afflicted ranges from 26 percent to 70 percent. If your twin is fraternal, however, this figure is only 5 to 10 percent. Interestingly, the prevalence of SLE among all family members of lupus patients is 10 to 15 percent, whereas the chance of any of this group having autoimmune diseases (including lupus) is 20 to 30 percent. The most common other autoimmune disorders include autoimmune thyroiditis (also known as Graves's disease or Hashimoto's thyroiditis), rheumatoid arthritis, and scleroderma.

The body may also produce elevated levels of autoantibodies even though no specific immune disorder is present. For example, nearly half the first-degree relatives of my lupus patients may have a positive antinuclear antibody (ANA) blood test. However, ANA is only one of several criteria that must be present for SLE to be diagnosed. Whether the presence of ANA increases the chance of developing lupus isn't known; most ANA-positive family members of lupus patients feel well and have no symptoms.

Should children of lupus patients or family members be "typed" or screened for SLE? I don't recommend testing unless symptoms or signs point to some existing clinical problem. At this time there is nothing we can offer those who carry a lupus "gene" or autoantibody and have no symptoms. In other words, by testing them we would only make them anxious or worried. Only a small percentage of these individuals will ever develop the disease.

## THE FUTURE

It is very possible—indeed probable—that in the next 30 years we will be able to identify patients at risk for developing SLE by using HLA testing or other methods and that we'll then vaccinate them to prevent lupus. By that time, all lupus-causing genes will have been isolated and identified. Potentially this would allow us to manipulate these genes in patients with active SLE to turn off the disease process.

## FURTHER READING

1. Deng Y, Tsao BP. Updates in lupus genetics. Curr Rheumatol Rep. 2017;19(11):68.
2. Hiraki LT, Silverman ED. Genomics of systemic lupus erythematosus: insights gained by studying monogenic young-onset systemic lupus erythematosus. Rheum Dis Clin North Am. 2017;43(3):415–434.
3. Chen L, Morris DL, Vyse TJ. Genetic advances in systemic lupus erythematosus: an update. Curr Opin Rheumatol. 2017;29(5):423–433.

# 8
## *Environmental Villains*

Many of my newly diagnosed lupus patients examine everything they have done or experienced regarding travel, prescription medications, occupational activities, infections, and other factors in an effort to find a reason for their disease. In my experience, some individuals are convinced that they did something wrong and therefore became ill. This type of soul-searching represents a natural process that ultimately results in coming to terms with the diagnosis. Although the precise cause of lupus is not known in each case, there are indeed certain environmental factors that may occasionally play a role in initiating the disease or making it worse. How does this happen?

A few of these mechanisms are linked to environmental factors and may produce effects in a variety of ways. These include a virus, food, or a chemical acting as an antigen to which an antibody response is generated. Some of these agents in patients predisposed to lupus mimic antigens to which the body is sensitized, and the antibody response is wrongly directed against the environmental factor. Alternatively, an antigen or inciting factor such as ultraviolet sunlight can damage DNA and promote the production of anti-DNA as an immune response to the altered DNA.

Various medications may also play a role in inducing lupus. Drug-induced lupus is covered in the next chapter.

This chapter will review the concept of epigenetics and concern itself with four types of potentially inciting agents: (i) chemical factors, such as chemical agents, metals, and toxins; (ii) dietary factors, such as amino acids, fats, and caloric intake; (iii) ultraviolet radiation; and (iv) infectious agents, such as viruses and bacteria as well as their by-products. Table 8.1 summarizes important chemicals that may be associated with the development or aggravation of lupus.

## WHAT IS EPIGENETICS?

Why do only 28 percent of lupus patients with an identical twin both have lupus? The answer is being looked at through a discipline known as *epigenetics*. In this construct, the environment plays a major role. In other words, a person's

**Table 8.1.** *Environmental Susceptibility Factors That Can Predispose or Aggravate Lupus*

1. Definite associations
   Ultraviolet light
   L-tryptophan
   L-canavanine
   Anti-SSA
   Viruses (especially Epstein–Barr)
   Bacteria (including certain lupus microbiomes)
   Factors that increase oxidative stress
   Hormones
   Cytokine upregulation
   Aromatic amines
   Crystalline silica
   Tobacco smoke
2. Probable associations
   Agricultural or residential pesticides
   Aliphatic hydrocarbons
   Adulterated rapeseed oil
   Vaccines
   Cocaine and amphetamine containing substances
   Heavy metals

environment can trigger modifications in his or her DNA without any alterations in the basic sequence of the genetic code. Some of these modifications can actually then be inherited by the next generation. As an example, we all have a specific genetic make-up in our genome. In autoimmune patients, several inherited epigenetic changes involved in our development and differentiation have been identified and constitute the epigenome. Some of these include DNA methylation (which is responsible for the repair of damaged DNA), histone deacetylases (which can influence the rate of gene transcriptions), and microRNA (which can silence protein coding genes). A variety of environmental factors such as infection, smoking, aging, and diet can influence these factors.

The result of these epigenetic alterations in lupus is just beginning to be explored. For example, modifications relating to oxidative stress, inflammatory cytokine upregulation, and hormonal effects probably play a role.

## WHAT CHEMICAL FACTORS CAUSE LUPUS?

### Aromatic Amines

*Aromatic amines* are chemical agents that may induce or aggravate rheumatic disease. This class includes hair-coloring solutions, hydrazines (e.g., tobacco smoke), and tartrazines (e.g., food colorings or medication preservatives). Aromatic amines are broken down in the body by a process known as *acetylation*.

An increased incidence of drug-induced lupus has been observed after exposure to aromatic amines in patients who are *slow acetylators*, or those who metabolize aromatic amines slowly. About half of all Americans are slow acetylators. The mechanism by which aromatic amines may induce an immunologic reaction is poorly understood, and only a small percentage of people exposed to these chemicals ever develop clinical immune disease.

Hair-coloring solutions containing aromatic amines, specifically paraphenylenediamine, can reproduce features of autoimmune disease in experimental animals. Several large-scale epidemiologic surveys conducted to determine whether aromatic amines induce lupus or cancer have yielded conflicting results. Do I advise my lupus patients to avoid hair dyes? No, because I rarely see patients who report a flare-up because they used a hair-care product; also, they already have the disease when they visit me.

Hydrazines are present in hydralazine, a blood pressure medication known to induce lupus. In addition to their presence in medication, these substances are found in a variety of compounds used in agriculture and industry and occur naturally in tobacco smoke and mushrooms. A single published report tells of a pharmaceutical worker who was occupationally exposed to hydrazines, developed lupus, and had reproducible symptoms and signs upon repeated exposure to them.

*Tartrazines* are preservatives found in certain food dyes (such as FD&C yellow no. 5), in tattoos, and in some medicine tablets. Occasional well-documented reports of tartrazine-induced lupus have appeared.

## Silica and Silicone

One of the most ubiquitous elements in nature, silicon, has been the focus of numerous studies. Nearly 50 years have elapsed since the initial observations that sandblasters exposed to silica dust may develop an autoimmune type of reaction characterized by lung nodules and scarring as well as autoimmune-mediated lesions in the kidney.

The injection of *silicone*, a synthetic liquid form of silicon, under the skin has been similarly associated with autoimmune reactions. According to some scientists—but not all—silicone may be broken down into silica in the body. A few women who have undergone breast augmentation with encapsulated silicone gel implants have developed a lupuslike disease; this is probably coincidental.

## Other Chemicals

Some chemicals can produce lupuslike symptoms as part of other diseases. Scleroderma is a first cousin of lupus, and many overlapping features are present in both diseases. But the principal difference is that, with scleroderma, the inflammation heals with scarring and tightening of the skin. The development of diseases like scleroderma and perhaps lupus have been associated with a variety of chemicals, including polyvinylchloride, trichloroethylene, cocaine, appetite suppressant amphetamines, and adulterated cooking oils (e.g., an epidemic caused by denatured rapeseed oil—"toxic oil syndrome"—afflicted 15,000 people in Spain in the early 1980s, and several hundred of them died).

Autoimmune diseases resembling lupus have been found in animals exposed to certain metals, including mercuric chloride, gold, and cadmium. No similar reports on humans have appeared as yet. *Eosin* is a chemical contained in lipstick that may trigger sun-sensitivity rashes and allergic dermatitis. Other speculative lupus inducers include farm animals, residential and agricultural pesticides, nail polish, hair dyes, metal cleaning solvents, varnishes, paint strippers, and glutathione-S-transferase. As of this writing none of the chemicals listed in this paragraph meets the evidence-based definition for a "probable" association.

Cigarette smoking, hormones and use of alcohol are reviewed in Chapters 24.

## SHOULD LUPUS PATIENTS AVOID ANY FOODS OR SUPPLEMENTS? WHAT ABOUT THE MICROBIOME?

Foods are made up of three principal components: carbohydrates, proteins, and fat. Thus, dietary manipulations can include either altering these components or raising or lowering overall caloric intake. Studies conducted on mice with lupus have suggested that high-calorie diets may accelerate mouse kidney disease, but there is no evidence that this occurs in humans. On the other hand, while "starvation" low-calorie or low-fat regimens help mice with lupus, they can occasionally worsen the disease process in humans.

Until 1989, an amino acid dietary supplement known as *L-tryptophan* was commonly taken to help induce sleep. Amino acids are the building blocks of proteins. L-tryptophan was removed from the market when it was associated with the development of a sclerodermalike disorder known as *eosinophilic myalgic syndrome*, or EMS. The 1989 EMS epidemic was traced to impurities in the manufacture of L-tryptophan, but sporadic cases of a closely related disorder called *eosinophilic fasciitis* had appeared over a 20-year period. It turns out that some cases of EMS or eosinophilic fasciitis may be related to excessive L-tryptophan ingestion in patients who metabolize the drug through an uncommon chemical pathway, which provokes an autoimmune response.

Another amino acid, *L-canavanine*, is present in all legumes but highly concentrated in alfalfa sprouts. Immunologic testing has established that this amino acid is capable of causing or aggravating autoimmune responses (see Chapter 24 for more details). I generally advise my lupus patients to avoid alfalfa sprouts but in general do not limit the intake of legumes.

A polyunsaturated fat, *eicosapentaenoic acid*, is a major constituent of fish oil. Diets rich in this chemical ameliorate human rheumatoid arthritis and seem to help animals with lupus. But conflicting results were found when fish oil capsules were administered to humans with systemic lupus erythematosus (SLE).

One group has suggested that an autoantibody called anti-Sm (see Chapter 6), which is found in 20 to 30 percent of patients with SLE, may react with certain plant proteins in laboratory tests. This interaction theoretically implies that this autoantibody may be able to make human lupus worse, but it has not yet been studied.

The *microbiome* represents the aggregate of microorganisms that resides within any number of human tissues or biofluids and, for this discussion, our gut. Everybody has its own microbiome signature. It has been suggested, for example, that certain bacteria in our intestines may promote or suppress inflammation. Work in this area in patients with autoimmune disorders is just beginning to bear fruit. In the next 10 years, we might find that a "lupus diet" would be helpful in decreasing inflammatory activity.

## WHAT ABOUT SUN EXPOSURE OR RADIATION?

Although correlations between diet and lupus remain ambiguous, there is a strong connection between the disease and the sun's rays. The sun emits ultraviolet radiation in three bands known as A, B, and C. The first two, ultraviolet A (UVA) and ultraviolet B (UVB), are important for lupus patients. Some scientists have suggested that when these bands of ultraviolet light hit the skin, they may damage superficial deposits of DNA, which are the body's building blocks. This results in the release of by-products that induce the formation of anti-DNA, which is known to damage body tissues.

Other mechanisms, some involving altered apoptosis affected by sunlight in patients with autoantibodies known as anti-Ro (see Chapter 6), might also be harmful. The binding of these antibodies to skin cells turns on or accelerates the disease process. But not all light may be bad. For example, UVA light treatments, which generally make lupus (e.g., UVA-1) patients worse, are given to patients with psoriasis. Certain sub-bands of light seem to reduce inflammation. The role of sunlight and sun protection in lupus is discussed in detail in Chapter 24.

Cancer patients are frequently given radiation therapy. Despite some concerns that lupus patients could have their disease flare up when they receive radiation, this occurs very rarely and almost entirely in individuals with a scleroderma overlap.

## WHY DO LUPUS PATIENTS FEEL WORSE WHEN
## THEY HAVE A COLD?

Individuals who carry the lupus "gene" can have the process turned on by a virus, fungus, parasite, or bacteria. Some of the viruses implicated in SLE causation have fancy names; they include myxoviruses, reoviruses, measles, rubella, parainfluenza, mumps, Epstein–Barr, and type-C onco- or retroviruses. The evidence for this stems from the finding of elevated levels of viral antibodies in certain lupus patients, virus particles in lupus tissue, and documentation that microbes can mimic foreign substances or antigens that turn on autoimmunity. Moreover, rats injected with certain bacterial proteins develop a rheumatoidlike arthritis. Therefore, it is easy to see how patients with autoimmune disease can experience flare-ups when they develop infections. Proteins made by the infectious agents may also be found in the blood or tissue of autoimmune patients and document the presence of infection.

### "LUPUS CLUSTERS": HAS THERE EVER BEEN AN EPIDEMIC OF LUPUS?

Since nearly 1 woman in 500 has SLE, one might think that if several people in a neighborhood had the disease, this would constitute a "lupus cluster," or perhaps even an epidemic. Indeed, such clusters have been purported to occur in Moorpark, California; Newtown, Georgia; Boston, Massachusetts; and Nogales and Tucson, Arizona. Environmental pollution has been held to be the inciting source. However, careful scrutiny has shown that none of the claimed clusters actually exist. Several factors were responsible for these claims: (i) autoantibodies among related family members carrying lupus genes, (ii) occurrences in communities with large minority populations and greater than usual lupus prevalence, (iii) media advertising by litigation attorneys trying to suggest that somebody living in a neighborhood who feels unwell may have lupus, and (iv) well-meaning family doctors labeling a patient with a positive antinuclear antibody (ANA) as having lupus, which was not confirmed by a rheumatologist. Lupus clusters may exist; however, none have yet been confirmed using accepted field-testing methods.

### IS LUPUS CONTAGIOUS?

Beyond the issue of genetic transmission, there is no evidence that lupus can be spread from one individual to another. No cases of "contagious" lupus have ever been reported. However, several instances have been documented in which laboratory technicians handling large amounts of lupus blood samples developed positive ANAs and antibodies to lymphocytes without developing SLE. Similar claims concerning household contact between lupus patients and nonrelated individuals or the pets of lupus patients may be valid, but these reports are also not associated with the presence of disease.

### SUMMING UP

Our environment is full of chemicals and microbes that can induce or aggravate autoimmune diseases. In addition, sun exposure plays a role, as does diet. Only a small percentage of individuals exposed to "lupogenic" materials develop the disease, which suggests that certain genetic signatures greatly augment risk factors. The amount of lupogenic material necessary to bring on the disease is not known, and not everyone at risk becomes symptomatic. It is important to emphasize that if you are genetically at risk, prudent precautions to avoid unnecessary exposure are advised, but you should try not to become so fearful of the environment that you cannot function socially. Though a lupus patient may share certain genetic material with family members, our research confirms that lupus cannot be spread from one person to another, as if it were an infectious disease. It is important to keep in mind that both genetics and the environment play a role in inducing, easing, aggravating, or accelerating lupus.

## FURTHER READING

1. Barbhaiya M, Costenbader KH. Ultraviolet radiation and systemic lupus erythematosus. Lupus. 2014;23(6):588–595.
2. Cooper GS, Gilbert KM, Greidinger EL, et al. Recent advances and opportunities in research on lupus: environmental influences and mechanisms of disease. Environ Health Prospect. 2008;116(6):695–702.
3. Sarzi-Puttini P, Atenzi F, Iaccarino L, et al. Environment and systemic lupus erythematosus: an overview. Autoimmunity. 2005;38(7):465–472.

# 9
# Drugs That May Cause Lupus or Produce Flare-Ups

In 1945 Byron Hoffman reported that sulfa-containing antibiotics might provoke a lupuslike syndrome. Since that time more than 80 agents have been reported to bring on the disease. In addition, the administration of certain drugs has been found to cause a pre-existing lupus to flare up. This chapter reviews the mechanisms by which this process may occur. It also looks at published data on the most problematic drugs and discusses the treatment of drug-induced lupus.

## DRUGS THAT EXACERBATE LUPUS

Most drugs that cause pre-existing disease to flare up do so by acting as sun-sensitizing agents or by promoting hypersensitivity or allergylike reactions.

### Antibiotics

Susan was 20 years old when she began complaining of severe burning on urination. She had been diagnosed with systemic lupus erythematosus (SLE) 6 months earlier and had mild disease, in the form of skin rashes and joint aches. Susan's lupus was under excellent control with naproxen and Plaquenil. She decided to call her gynecologist about a bladder problem and was diagnosed as having a urinary tract infection. Her physician placed her on Bactrim DS. Within 2 days her mild cheek flush had become a bright red rash on her face, forearms, and neck. Her wrists and knees swelled up and she developed a temperature of 102°F. When she saw her rheumatologist the next day, he observed not only these physical signs but also that her white blood cell count and hemoglobin had substantially decreased. He stopped the antibiotic and put her on 40 milligrams of prednisone daily. She gradually responded to this regimen and managed to discontinue steroids within 2 weeks. She felt fine thereafter.

Like Susan, a disproportionate number of patients with lupus cannot tolerate arylamine *sulfa* derivatives. Sulfonamide-based antibiotics (e.g., sulfamethoxazole) are potent sun sensitizers. Drugs in this class include such commonly used brands as Bactrim, Septra, and Gantrisin, which are frequently prescribed to young women with urinary tract infections. Some antidiabetic drugs, sulfasalazine (used for ulcerative colitis and rheumatoid arthritis), and thia*zide* diuretics also contain sulfa. Even though these nonarylamine sulfas are generally well-tolerated, it is best to be cautious about using these drugs. A greater-than-expected number of lupus patients are unable to tolerate penicillin, and some tetracyclines are mildly sun sensitizing. Patients given minocycline for rheumatoidlike arthritis may flare if they really have lupus. I tend to avoid sulfa drugs unless no alternative treatment is available but do not restrict the use of any other antibiotics.

### Nonsteroidal Anti-Inflammatory Drugs (NSAIDs)

Nonsteroidal anti-inflammatory drugs (NSAIDs) are most frequently used to treat aches and pains, fevers, or pleurisy (see Chapter 26). NSAIDs run the gamut in potency from aspirin and ibuprofen to indomethacin. Though not approved by the Food and Drug Treatment to treat lupus, at least one of these preparations is used by over 90 percent of lupus patients at some point during their disease course.

Rarely, lupus patients taking ibuprofen (Advil, Motrin) complain of high fevers, mental confusion, and a stiff neck. This reversible noninfectious (*aseptic*) meningitis is practically seen only in SLE patients. Aseptic meningitis has been reported to occur with more than 10 NSAIDs, but 90 percent of the published cases implicate ibuprofen. Despite this, an individual's risk for aseptic meningitis with ibuprofen is probably less than 1 in 1,000. To be on the safe side, I tend to use other NSAIDs in treating lupus patients.

Certain NSAIDs sensitize users to sunlight, and toxic reactions have been reported in some cases. Extra care should be taken in prescribing piroxicam (Feldene). Although no longer commercially available in the United States, compounded phenylbutazone has been reported to cause a hypersensitivity reaction in lupus patients, which may lead to severe flare-ups.

### Hormones

Birth control pills for young women and estrogen replacement therapies after menopause as well as other hormonal preparations are frequently prescribed to lupus patients. Their use has been controversial, and this complex topic is covered in Chapter 17.

## DRUG-INDUCED LUPUS ERYTHEMATOSUS

Several thousand new cases of prescription drug-induced lupus are reported annually in the United States. First identified shortly after the introduction of hydralazine (Apresoline) for hypertension in 1951, drug-induced lupus erythematosus (DILE) is usually a benign, self-limited process. Although more than 70 agents have been implicated as inciters of drug-induced autoimmunity, most cases are associated with three products whose use has been decreasing: hydralazine, procainamide (Pronestyl), and methyldopa (Aldomet). If isoniazid (INH), chlorpromazine (Thorazine), TNF blockers, and D-penicillamine are added to the list, 99 percent of all clinically relevant cases can be accounted for. A more complete list of these drugs is given in Table 9.1.

**Table 9.1.** *Examples of Drugs Implicated in Provoking Lupus Erythematosus*

---

1. Drugs proven to induce clinical lupus in at least 1 out of 1,000 users
   Hydralazine (Apresoline)
   Methyldopa (Aldomet)
   Procainamide (Pronestyl)
   D-penicillamine
   TNF blockers (infliximab, adalimumab, etanercept)
   Terbinafine (Lamisil)
   Minocycline
2. Drugs proven to induce clinical lupus in at least 1 out of 10,000 users
   Isoniazid (INH)
   Phenothiazines (including Thorazine)
   Sulfasalazine (Azulfidine)
   Quinidine
   Carbamazepine (Tegretol)
   Griseofulvin (Fulvicin)
3. Drugs rarely associated with positive antinuclear antibodies (ANAs) and very rare clinical lupus
   Anticonvulsants (phenytoin, trimethadione, primidone, ethosuximide)
   Lithium carbonate
   Captopril (Capoten)
   Antithyroid preparation (propylthiouracil, methimazole)
   Beta-blockers (pracatolol, acebutolol, atenolol, labetalol, pindolol, timolol eyedrops)
   Lipid-lowering medicines ("statins")
   Prazosin (Minipress)
4. Drugs that can exacerbate lupus, produce subacute cutaneous rashes or allergic reactions
   Antibiotics (sulfa, tetracycline—rarely, penicillins or ciprofloxacins)
   Nonsteroidal anti-inflammatory agents (e.g., ibuprofen)
   Oral contraceptives and other hormones
   Sulfa diuretics and diabetic drugs (Dyazide, Aldactone)
   Cimetidine (Tagamet), alpha-interferon, and gold salts
Case reports have appeared implicating nearly 50 other drugs.

---

## Epidemiology of Drug-Induced Lupus

Some features distinguish DILE from SLE. First, unlike SLE, DILE affects the same number of men as it does women. Second, DILE is very rare among African Americans in the United States.

## A Note of Caution

If you are a lupus patient, how do you know if you have DILE? If you are prescribed a medication by your doctor and after several weeks to months start noticing a rash, fevers, pain on taking a deep breath, or swollen joints, consult your doctor immediately. Most DILE patients do not fulfill the criteria for systemic lupus. All the drugs implicated in DILE induce the formation of antinuclear antibody (ANA) to varying degrees, but the process is self-limited. In other words, once the drug is stopped, the formation of ANA stops as well.

Only a small percentage of these ANA-positive individuals ever develop clinical lupus. *A positive ANA does not constitute grounds to discontinue treatment with a useful drug.* Since DILE is completely reversible, the risks of not taking lifesaving heart or seizure medications, for example, are much more ominous. Moreover, there is no evidence that a lupus-causing drug administered to a patient who already has the disease will make the condition worse.

## How Do Drugs Cause Lupus?

An exciting research challenge is presented by DILE, because investigators might be able to use it as a model for understanding how lupus develops. Unfortunately, however, DILE may come about through different chemical processes unrelated to the evolution of the disease as it unfolds in most cases. Let's look at some proposed mechanisms by which drugs induce lupus.

For example, the drug can bind to a part of the cell that alters DNA. This altered DNA sets in motion an immunologic reaction, causing the body to make anti-DNA. Similarly, drugs can activate T or B lymphocytes and, as part of the immunologic response, lead to the formation of antibodies to white blood cells, or antilymphocyte antibodies—a common feature of lupus. Next, a drug can induce the hypomethylation of DNA, which results in altered DNA repair and autoantibody formation. Also, the drug may make your body so sun sensitive that, if you are genetically predisposed, it can turn on a lupus reaction. Finally, certain drugs are broken down into chemicals or by-products that promote the formation of autoantibodies—the antibodies that attack the body's own tissue.

Several genetic factors may also increase the risk of developing DILE. For example, the HLA-DR4 genetic marker is associated with hydralazine and D-penicillamine-induced lupus. If your liver cannot clear these breakdown products of drugs quickly, this slow clearance system is termed "slow acetylation." If you are a slow acetylator and are prescribed procainamide, hydralazine, or isoniazid and if you have a certain genetic make-up, there is an increased chance that you will develop DILE. Finally, the absence of certain HLA-derived complement genes also correlates with DILE.

## How Can We Tell DILE from SLE?

While taking a lupus-causing drug, the DILE patient displays many of the signs and symptoms seen in the patient with lupus. However, DILE patients rarely have symptoms involving the many organ systems of the body. (In other words, the central nervous system, heart, lung, and kidneys are not usually involved.) Antihistone antibodies are often found in these patients (in fact, they are found on blood testing in most with DILE; the problem is that 40 percent with SLE also develop these antibodies). The patient with DILE does not have the other typical lupus antibodies reviewed in Chapter 6. Normal complement levels are also present in DILE patients. Further, upon discontinuing the drug, DILE improves or resolves within days to weeks in these patients. Even though antihistone antibodies decrease, the ANA test may remain positive for years.

A doctor must differentiate DILE from bacterial or viral infections, polymyalgia rheumatica, SLE, rheumatoid arthritis, or Dressler's syndrome (fever with pericarditis in patients who have had a recent heart attack). Blood tests and cultures usually distinguish among these diseases.

## How Is DILE Treated?

If the offending drug is withdrawn as soon as DILE symptoms present themselves, no therapy may be necessary. Approximately one third of the time my patients have benefited from several weeks to months of aspirin or other NSAID medications (such as ibuprofen, naproxen, or indomethacin). If serious complications develop (e.g., pericardial tamponade or kidney disease) or the symptoms are severe (e.g., disabling arthritis, pleurisy with shortness of breath), I usually prescribe several weeks to months of moderate-dose steroids (less than 40 milligrams of prednisone daily).

Fewer than 5 percent of patients with DILE have a complicated or unfavorable course. A disproportionate number of these individuals were given minocycline, which is also associated with liver injury and an antibody associated with vasculitis, called ANCA. LUPUS PATIENTS SHOULD AVOID USING MINOCYCLINE. These circumstances arise when the inciting drug is not withdrawn despite several months of symptoms or the lupus-inducing drug is reintroduced after being stopped. If you are a lupus patient and you have had fevers, rashes, or joint aches that you or your doctor feel may be from taking a lupus-inducing drug, cease its use and *never* take the drug again.

## FURTHER READING

1. Alniemi DT, Gutierrez A, Drage IA, Wetter DA. Subacte cutaneous lupus erythematosus: clinical characterists, disease associations, treatments, and Outcomes in a series of 90 patients at May Clinic, 1996–2011. Mayo Clin Proc. 2017(3);92:406–414.
2. Szczęch J, Samotij D, Werth VP, Reich A. Trigger factors of cutaneous lupus erythematous: a review of current literature. Lupus. 2017;26(8):791–807.
3. Shovman O, Tamar S, Amital H, Watad A, Shoenfeld Y. Diverse patterns of anti TNF-alpha induced lupus: case series and review of the literature. Clin Rheumatol. 2017;37(2): 563–568.
4. Yung RL, Richardson B. Drug induced lupus. Rheum Dis Clin North Am. 1994;20(1):61–86.

# Part IV

# WHERE AND HOW CAN THE BODY BE AFFECTED BY LUPUS?

When rheumatologists evaluate an individual who might have lupus, they take a complete history, perform a physical examination, obtain appropriate blood tests, and order studies indicated by the patient's symptoms and signs. Once this information is compiled, diagnostic possibilities other than lupus must be considered and ruled out. The 14 chapters in this part take the reader through this diagnostic process using an approach that considers symptoms, signs, physical findings, and conditions affecting each organ, otherwise known as the *organ-system approach*. When the full evaluation is completed, the treating physician is able to formulate a comprehensive treatment plan.

# 10
## *History, Symptoms, and Signs*

### THE RHEUMATOLOGY CONSULTATION

A thorough medical evaluation is essential to make a diagnosis of lupus. This consultation should be performed by a rheumatologist or qualified internist. A rheumatologist is an internist (as are cardiologists, gastroenterologists, etc.) who has special expertise in diagnosing and managing diseases of the musculoskeletal and immune systems. The consultation includes several components, starting with a history of the patient's complaints. On the first visit to a consultant, it is helpful to present a summary of important symptoms and signs in a concise fashion, either by making a list of them or reviewing them mentally beforehand.

Proper preparation is essential, especially when a patient has only one visit with a qualified consultant to evaluate the possibility of lupus. Copies of outside records and previous tests or workups are also helpful. Lupus is not easy to diagnose; surveys have shown that the typical lupus patient consults three to five physicians before a correct diagnosis is made. In fact, studies have suggested that an average of 2 to 3 years elapse from the onset of symptoms until lupus is diagnosed. This interval may be as short as a few weeks to months in children, who usually display more obvious symptoms, but in patients over age 60, it can be up to 4 years before a firm diagnosis is assigned.

### THE HISTORY AND REVIEW OF SYSTEMS

The lupus consultation consists of a history, physical examination, and diagnostic laboratory tests, or imaging evaluations (X-rays, scans, etc.). A thorough initial interview is essential if the physician is to make a correct diagnosis and recommend proper treatment. After all the observations and tests are in, the doctor will discuss the findings, either at the time of the visit, by telephone after the initial meeting, or in a follow-up visit.

My physician interview begins by asking why the patient is there and how he or she feels. Once the patient's symptoms and history are heard, I conduct a "review of systems." As many as a hundred questions can be asked as part of this screening process. Positive responses may lead to an additional set of queries that clarify symptoms in a given area, such as how long the complaint has been present, what makes it better or worse, how it has been diagnostically evaluated and treated in the past, and what its current status is.

The patient will be asked about allergies and his or her and family members' history of rheumatic disease or other diseases. Other relevant facts include possible occupational exposures to allergic or toxic substances, level of education, and the patient's cohabitants. Unusual childhood diseases will be explored, as well as alcohol and tobacco use, previous hospitalizations and surgeries, and past and current prescriptions or frequently used over-the-counter medications. Not only do certain environmental and family histories predispose people to lupus, but this line of questioning forms the basis of a psychosocial profile that may be important in developing a productive doctor–patient relationship.

The rheumatic review of systems covers these 11 categories:

1. *Constitutional symptoms*, such as fevers, fatigue, malaise, or weight loss, are dealt with first. They refer to the patient's overall state and how he or she feels. This is followed by an organ system review that goes from head to toe.
2. The *head and neck* review includes inquiries about cataracts, glaucoma, dry eyes, dry mouth, eye pain, double vision, loss of vision, iritis, conjunctivitis, ringing in the ears, loss of hearing, frequent ear infections, frequent nosebleeds, smell abnormalities, frequent sinus infections, sores in the nose or mouth, dental problems, or fullness in the neck.
3. The *cardiopulmonary* area is covered next. I ask about asthma, bronchitis, emphysema, tuberculosis, pleurisy (pain on taking a deep breath), shortness of breath, pneumonia, high blood pressure, chest pains, rheumatic fever, heart murmur, heart attack, palpitations or irregular heartbeats, and the use of cardiac or hypertension medications.
4. The *gastrointestinal* system review includes an effort to find any evidence of swallowing difficulties, severe nausea or vomiting, diarrhea, constipation, unusual eating habits, hepatitis, ulcers, gallstones, blood in stool or vomit, diverticulitis, colitis, celiac or inflammatory bowel disease, or pancreatitis.
5. The *genito-urinary* area must be approached in a respectful, sensitive way. Aside from inquiring about frequent bladder infections, kidney stones, or blood or protein in the urine, I also review any history of venereal diseases (including false-positive syphilis tests) and, in women, the obstetric history, with special attention to miscarriages, breast disorders and surgeries (cosmetic and otherwise), and menstrual problems.
6. Next, *hematologic and immune* factors that the patient may be aware of include how easily he or she bruises, anemia, low white blood cell or platelet counts, swollen glands, or frequent infections.
7. A *neuropsychiatric* history takes into account headaches, seizures, numbness or tingling, fainting, dizziness, psychiatric or antidepressant interventions, substance abuse, difficulty sleeping, and—most important—what is called

*cognitive dysfunction*, a subtle sense of difficulty in thinking or articulating clearly.

8. *Musculoskeletal* features involve a history of joint pain, stiffness, rheumatoid arthritis or swelling; gout; muscle pains; or weakness.

9. The *endocrine* system review includes questions about thyroid disease, diabetes, or high cholesterol levels.

10. The *vascular* history may uncover prior episodes of phlebitis, clots, strokes, or Raynaud's phenomenon (fingers turning different colors in cold weather).

11. Finally, the *skin* is discussed. The skin is a major target organ in lupus, and evidence of sun sensitivity, hair loss, itching, mouth sores, the "butterfly rash," psoriasis, or other rashes is carefully reviewed.

In concluding the history taking, I always ask a patient whether there is anything I should know that was not covered. Ed Dubois, my mentor, dedicated his lupus textbook to "the patients, from whom we have learned." Physicians become better doctors when they listen to what patients have to say about things that the doctor may not have brought up. Occasionally, the patient hits on something in casual conversation that turns out to be quite important in shedding light on his or her disease.

## PHYSICAL EXAMINATION

The history and review of systems elucidate what physicians call symptoms; a physical examination reveals signs. Four methods known as *inspection* (looking at an area), *palpation* (feeling an area), *percussion* (gentle knocking against a surface such as the lung or liver to detect fullness), and *auscultation* (listening with a stethoscope to the heart, chest, carotid artery, etc.) are employed during the physical. The patient will be evaluated from head to toe.

First, *vital signs* are checked to ascertain weight, pulse, respiration, blood pressure, and temperature. The *head and neck* exam includes evaluation of the pupils' response to light, eye movements, cataracts, and the vessels of the eye. The ear exam searches for obstruction and inflammation. The oral cavity is screened for sores, poor dental hygiene, and dryness. I palpate the thyroid and the glands of the neck and also listen to the neck for abnormal murmurs or sounds (carotid artery bruits). The *chest* examination consists of inspection (e.g., for postural abnormalities), palpation for chest wall tenderness, percussion to evaluate fluid in the lungs, and auscultation (e.g., to rule out asthma and pneumonia). The *heart* is checked for murmurs, clicks, or irregular beats. The *abdomen* is inspected for obesity, distension, or scars; palpated for pain, a large aorta, or hernia; percussed to assess the size of the liver and spleen; and auscultated to rule out any obstruction or vascular sounds. This is followed by an *extremity* evaluation, which includes looking for swelling, color changes, inflamed joints, and deformities. Specific maneuvers allow me to assess range of motion, muscle strength, pulses, reflexes,

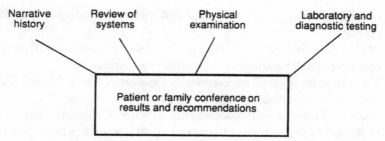

**Figure 10.1.** *The Rheumatology Consultation*

and muscle tone. If indicated, a *genito-urinary* evaluation is done. It includes a breast examination, rectal evaluation, pelvic examination, and—in women—pap smear. In rheumatology, a genito-urinary exam is necessary only if the patient has breast implants, complains of vaginal ulcers, or has other symptoms relevant to these areas. A *neurobehavioral* assessment that will reflect change in the nervous system is usually conducted as part of the ongoing conversation; neurologic deficits can be detected by observing the patient for tremor, gait abnormalities, or abnormal movements or reflexes. If necessary, a more formal mental status examination may be conducted. Finally, the *skin* is examined for rashes, pigment changes, tattoos, hair loss, Raynaud's, and skin breakdown or ulcerations.

The physical examination may include other steps as well, depending upon the problems reported and the nature of the consultation. A thorough physical examination conducted after a detailed interview allows the doctor to order the appropriate laboratory tests. Figure 10.1 summarizes the rheumatology consultation.

## THE CHIEF COMPLAINT AND CONSTITUTIONAL SYMPTOMS IN LUPUS

The most common initial complaint in early lupus is joint pain or swelling (in 50 percent of patients), followed by skin rashes (20 percent), and malaise or fatigue (10 percent). Certain constitutional symptoms and signs are not included in the following chapters because they do not fall into any specific organ system; they are therefore reviewed here. These generalized body complaints consist of fevers, weight loss, and fatigue. The most common symptoms, signs, and laboratory abnormalities in lupus are detailed in Table 10.1.

### Fever

Any inflammatory process is commonly associated with an elevated temperature. The official definition of a fever is 99.6°F or greater (most humans have 98.6°F as a normal temperature). Nevertheless, many patients have normal temperatures that are in the range of 96° to 97°, and what is normal for some individuals may

**Table 10.1.** *Approximate Prevalence (%) of Selected Symptoms, Signs, and Laboratory Abnormalities of Systemic Lupus Erythematosus during the Course of the Disease in the United States*

| Symptom | % |
|---|---|
| Positive antinuclear antibody | 97 |
| Malaise and fatigue | 90 |
| Arthralgia, myalgia | 90 |
| Sun sensitivity, skin changes | 70 |
| Cognitive dysfunction | 70 |
| Low C3 or C4 complement | 61 |
| Fever due to lupus | 57 |
| Antibodies to ds DNA | 50 |
| Arthritis | 50 |
| Leukopenia | 46 |
| Pleuritis | 44 |
| Anemia | 42 |
| Alopecia | 40 |
| Nephritis, proteinuria | 40 |
| Anticardiolipin antibody | 35 |
| Malar rash | 35 |
| Central nervous system | 32 |
| Increased gamma globulin | 32 |
| Weight loss due to lupus | 27 |
| Raynaud's | 25 |
| Hypertension | 25 |
| Sjögren's | 25 |
| Oral ulcerations (mouth, nose) | 20 |
| Discoid lesions | 20 |
| Central nervous system vasculitis | 15 |
| Adenopathy | 15 |
| Pleural effusion | 12 |
| Subacute cutaneous lupus | 10 |
| Myositis | 10 |
| Avascular necrosis | 10 |

Based on a summation of findings in diverse cohorts.

be a fever for others. Lupus surveys published in the 1950s documented low-grade fevers in 90 percent of patients. This number has decreased to 40 percent in recent reviews—a consequence of the widespread availability and use of nonsteroidal anti-inflammatory drugs (NSAIDs), especially those over-the-counter medications that can reduce fevers. These include aspirin, naproxen, and ibuprofen (e.g., Advil, Aleve); acetaminophen (e.g., Tylenol) can also decrease fever. Many lupus patients chronically run temperatures 1 to 2 degrees above normal without any symptoms. *The presence of a temperature above 99.6°F without obvious cause suggests an infectious or inflammatory process.*

At times I may find a normal temperature reading in a patient with a history of fevers and wonder whether a fever is really present. It may be helpful for certain patients to keep a fever logbook or to record temperature readings three times a day at the same hours for a week or two and to show the logbook to their physician. Fever curve patterns may suggest different disease processes.

A low-grade fever is not usually dangerous, except for its ability to cause the pulse to rise, which decreases stamina. In certain circumstances, fevers act as warning signs of infection and suggest the need for cultures, specific testing, or antibiotics. If the temperature rises above 104°F, precautions should be taken to prevent seizures or dehydration. This might include alternating between aspirin and ibuprofen or acetaminophen every 2 hours, sponging down the head and body to lower the fever, having the patient take plenty of fluids, or admitting the patient to the hospital. *The presence of a significant fever in any patient taking steroids (e.g., prednisone) or chemotherapy drugs should be taken very seriously* and is often a reason for hospitalization. Steroids usually suppress fevers and can mask infections.

### Anorexia, Weight Loss, and Weight Gain

Half of all patients with lupus have a loss of appetite (anorexia), with resulting weight loss. The loss of more than 10 percent of body weight over a 3-month period is rare and indicates a serious condition. Usually noted in the early stages of lupus, anorexia and weight loss are associated with disease activity. Evidence of active lupus often results in the administration of corticosteroids (e.g., prednisone), with subsequent weight gain. If your doctor has detected large amounts of protein in your urine, you have what is termed "nephrotic syndrome." Seen in up to 15 percent of those with lupus, this also results in weight gain.

### Malaise and Fatigue

*Malaise* is the sense of not feeling right. It conveys a message of aching, loss of stamina, and the "blahs." Loss of stamina or decreased endurance associated with a tendency to be tired is known as *fatigue*. Malaise and fatigue are observed in 80 percent of systemic lupus erythematosus patients at some point during the course of their disease; in half of these, it can be disabling. Evidence of active disease or inflammation as well as infection, depression, anemia, hormonal problems, and stress may also be associated with malaise and fatigue. The management of malaise and fatigue is discussed in more detail in Chapter 25.

### SUMMING UP

Before physicians can treat lupus, they must take a detailed history, perform a physical examination, and order proper laboratory tests. An accurate diagnosis encompassing all symptoms and physical signs is the goal of a consultation. The patient may have more than one process going on at the same time, and these frequently benefit from different approaches. Both patient and doctor should be flexible in how they understand the concept of disease and allow themselves to consider differing viewpoints as to what might be responsible for a specific medical complaint. Many things may contribute to fatigue, for example. And as we've seen all along, lupus is a complex disease that can be difficult to diagnose.

## FURTHER READING

1. Mahieu MA, Ramsey-Goldman R. Candidate biomarkers for fatigue in systemic lupus erythematosus: a critical review. Curr Rheumatol Rev. 2017;13(2):103–112.
2. Jung JY, Suh CH. Infection in lupus erythematosus, similarities and differences with lupus flare. Korean J Intern Med. 2017;32(3):429–438.

# 11
## *Must We Draw Blood?*

Unfortunately, the history and physical examination are not enough to diagnose or manage lupus, so yes, we must draw blood. Blood testing can make a difference. It is essential to diagnose a disease correctly and to gauge the patient's response to therapy. And specific tests are employed to monitor the safety of medications that might be used to treat the disease. Finally, some lupus patients have specific complications that can be diagnosed only by blood testing. This chapter offers an overview of the tests doctors order and why.

### WHAT IS CONSIDERED "ROUTINE" LAB WORK?

When a patient arrives at an internist's or primary care doctor's office for a general medical evaluation, this usually calls for what doctors refer to as "screening laboratory tests." In other words, by obtaining a blood count, urine test, and blood chemistry panel, abnormalities can be detected in 90 percent of individuals with serious medical problems. This is the starting point of the workup. All the studies listed in this chapter are inexpensive and mostly automated; they can be performed within a matter of hours and do not require special expertise. Most large medical offices are equipped to perform these tests on the premises.

A *complete blood count* (*CBC*) is the most commonly performed laboratory test in the United States. It analyzes red cells, white cells, and platelets. Patients with systemic lupus erythematosus (SLE) can have low red blood cell counts or be anemic as a result of chronic disease, bleeding from lupus medication, auto-immune hemolytic anemia (breakdown of red blood cells due to antibodies), or a vitamin deficiency. The white blood cell count can be high due to steroid therapy or inflammation, or low from active lupus or a virus. Platelets are decreased when antibodies attack platelets or when the bone marrow is not making enough of them. Most patients with active SLE have an abnormal CBC.

*Blood chemistry* panels consist of anywhere from 7 to 25 tests that evaluate a variety of parameters, including blood sugar, kidney function (blood urea nitrogen [BUN], creatinine), liver function (aspartate aminotransferase [AST], alanine aminotransferase [ALT], bilirubin, alkaline phosphatase, γ-glutamyltransferase

[GGT]), electrolytes (sodium, potassium, chloride, bicarbonate, calcium, phosphorus, magnesium), lipids (cholesterol, triglycerides, high-density lipoproteins [HDL], low-density lipoproteins [LDL]), proteins (albumin, total protein), thyroid function (T3, T4, thyroid stimulating hormone [TSH]), and gout (uric acid). Occasionally, chemistry panels include additional studies (amylase for pancreatic function, LDH for hemolysis, iron levels, etc.), which are also inexpensive and can be done by request. Any of these tests may be abnormal in SLE patients; readers are referred to the index to find specific discussions that address their questions.

*Urinalysis* is a useful screen for kidney involvement and urinary tract infections. All but 1 percent of lupus patients with clinically significant renal disease will have an abnormal urinalysis.

Several additional blood tests relevant to SLE also are inexpensive, readily available, and commonly ordered by rheumatologists. These consist of the *creatine phosphokinase (CPK)*, which screens for muscle inflammation; a *Westergren sedimentation rate* or *C-reactive protein (CRP)*, which quantitates levels of inflammation; and the *prothrombin time (PT)* or *partial thromboplastin time (PTT)*, which are clotting tests and may be prolonged in those who have the lupus anticoagulant.

## ROUTINE ANTIBODY PANELS AND SCREENS

Very few doctors' offices are equipped to do reliable antibody screening. Most community and hospital laboratories are capable of performing these tests, but the lack of a national standard, inexperienced technicians, and failure to double- and triple-check results impair their accuracy. Autoantibodies can be tested for anywhere, but if the results are positive they should be confirmed in a reliable rheumatology laboratory. Such facilities include university-based teaching medical centers, private facilities with a national reputation for special expertise in rheumatology (e.g., Exagen), and certain large national lab networks (e.g., Mayo Clinic Laboratories). The reader is referred to Chapter 6 for a detailed discussion of all the tests listed in this chapter.

What does autoantibody screening consist of and how does your doctor interpret these results? Most of the previously listed centers have what is called a "reflex panel." Simply stated, a doctor orders an antinuclear antibody (ANA) test, and if it is positive, another 8 to 10 antibody and immune determinations are automatically obtained.

The *ANA* test is the cornerstone of rheumatic disease screening. As mentioned earlier, some 10 million Americans have a positive ANA of 1:80 or greater, but fewer than 1 million have SLE. Patients with other rheumatic diseases such as rheumatoid arthritis and scleroderma, as well as healthy relatives of patients with autoimmune diseases, can have a positive ANA. The ANA can also become positive with aging, certain viral infections, or as a result of taking specific prescription drugs. However, less than 3 percent of patients with SLE are ANA negative.

Practically speaking, interpretation of the ANA test is guided by a few principles. First, high levels of this antibody (greater than 1:1,280 or greater than 30 International Units) are usually associated with a real rheumatic disease. Second, whereas rimmed patterns are specific for lupus, homogenous ANA patterns generally correlate with SLE, and speckled patterns are seen in SLE and with other autoimmune processes. Even though ANA levels decrease with clinical improvement, this correlation is weak at best and not a reliable gauge of the disease process. Also, different laboratories use varying standards for ANA. Therefore, a reading of 1:640 from one laboratory may be the same as 1:320 from another.

*Anti-double-stranded DNA* antibodies are rarely present in patients who do not have SLE. They are found in half of those with the disease and represent one of the more specific parameters for diagnosis and for following severe inflammation or organ involvement. Occasionally, healthy patients have low-level positive tests. If performed by a Farr or ELISA method, anti-DNA can be quantitated, and its values reflect clinical disease activity; the values are higher with flares, and they decrease with improvement.

Serum *complement* measures levels of a protein that is consumed during the inflammatory process. Along with anti-DNA, complement components C3, C4, or CH50 are the most reliable parameters for following serious disease activity. Low complement levels imply active inflammation. A few patients with genetic complement deficiencies always have low complements, and in them these determinations are not useful in following disease activity. Antibodies to C1q and complement activation products may be an excellent correlate with disease activity.

Levels of *anti-Ro (SSA)* or *anti-La (SSB)* are of no value in following disease activity. These tests are either positive or negative. Positive tests confirm the presence of an autoimmune problem that may not even be symptomatic and suggest that the doctor look for Sjögren's syndrome and subacute cutaneous lupus rashes while also asking the patient about severe sun sensitivity. Young women with these antibodies should be warned about the possibility of having a baby with neonatal lupus or congenital heart block (see Chapters 22 and 30). Similarly, levels of *anti-Sm* or *anti-RNP* are of little value in following patients. These tests are also either positive or negative. Anti-Sm is of no importance in following disease activity but is extremely specific and useful in confirming the diagnosis of SLE. Anti-RNP in high levels suggests that the patient may have mixed connective tissue disease (MCTD) and at low levels supports the diagnosis of SLE. The levels rarely change.

Because one third of patients with lupus have antiphospholipid antibodies that may lead to blood clots, miscarriages, and strokes, most rheumatologists screen for these antibodies. As discussed in Chapter 21, the antiphospholipid antibodies can be tricky to detect, and a given patient may have only one of several possible autoantibodies. The most commonly ordered screen consists of an *RPR* or *VDRL* (syphilis test), *anticardiolipin antibody*, and the *lupus anticoagulant*. Further testing is necessary only if the patient's history includes a blood clot and these initial screenings are negative.

I usually test for *serum protein electrophoresis,* which breaks down our body's protein fractions into albumin and globulins. The globulins include alpha 1 and 2 globulins which may be increased with inflammation and gamma globulin fractions. Up to 20 percent with SLE have increases in this component, which is called a polyclonal gammopathy.

Additional tests that are frequently done are screening for the rheumatoid factor and serum protein electrophoresis. The *rheumatoid factor* test is positive in 80 percent of rheumatoid arthritis patients and in 20 to 30 percent of those with SLE. High levels of rheumatoid factor with low levels of ANA suggest that a diagnosis of rheumatoid arthritis should be considered as opposed to SLE. *Anticyclic citrullinated peptide (CCP)* antibodies, if present, are fairly specific for rheumatoid arthritis and are only present in 5–10 percent with SLE. *Serum protein electrophoresis* is an inexpensive test for blood protein abnormalities; if a broad band of gamma globulin is found, it confirms an autoimmune process.

## ADDITIONAL ANTIBODY SCREENS AND TESTS

Occasionally, additional blood testing is indicated to sort out peculiar or unusual symptoms. These tests are expensive, take longer to perform, and should be sent only to laboratories that have special immunologic expertise.

*Antihistone antibodies* are found in nearly all patients with drug-induced lupus but are not specific, because at least half of all lupus patients have them. *Antineuronal antibodies* in the spinal fluid are usually specific for central nervous system lupus. In the blood, these antibodies are positive in 20 percent of all patients with lupus, but high levels are found in 70 percent with nervous system activity. *Antiribosomal P* antibody may be positive in central nervous system disease and may correlate with SLE psychosis. *Coombs' antibody* testing screens for autoimmune hemolytic anemia, a serious blood complication of SLE.

The workup of antiphospholipid antibodies in patients with unusual manifestations of the syndrome includes obtaining *protein C, protein S, antithrombin 3, Factor V Leiden mutation, anti-β-2 glycoprotein-1 antibodies, platelet antibody tests,* and *noncardiolipin antiphospholipid antibodies.* Sludging of the blood—which leads to dizziness, difficulty concentrating, and a sense of fullness—is evaluated by testing for *cryoglobulin* and *viscosity,* which, if present, imply that the blood is too thick. Systemic vasculitis atypical for lupus can be assessed with *anti-neutrophilic cytoplasmic antibody (ANCA)* testing. Similarly, lupuslike diseases such as rheumatoid arthritis scleroderma or autoimmune myositis are characterized by the presence of numerous autoantibodies rarely seen in SLE, such as *anti-PM-1, anti-Jo, anti-Scl-70, antisynthetase,* or *anticentromere antibodies.* Lupus patients with high levels of the amino acid *homocysteine* may be at risk for cardiac disease and benefit from folic acid therapy.

## FURTHER READING

1. Olsen NJ, Choi MY, Fritzler MJ. Emerging technologies in autoantibody testing for rheumatic diseases. *Arthritis Res Ther.* 2017;19(1):172.
2. Pisetsky DS. Antinuclear antibody testing—misunderstood or misbegotten? *Nat Rev Rheumatol.* 2017;13(8):495–502.
3. Donald F, Ward MM. Evaluative laboratory testing practices of United States rheumatologists. *Arthritis Rheum.* 1998;41(4):725–729.

# 12

# *Reactions of the Skin: Rashes and Cutaneous Lupus*

The skin is often an affected area in lupus, with 60 to 70 percent of lupus patients reporting some skin complaint. And there is a wide range of such complaints. This chapter discusses how the skin is damaged in lupus and what it looks like under the microscope. It reviews the classifications of skin disorders in lupus as well as their principal dermatologic features. A complete discussion of remedies used for skin disorders in lupus can be found in Part V, but specific interventions that are appropriate under special circumstances are mentioned here.

## HOW IS THE SKIN DAMAGED IN LUPUS?

The sun emits ultraviolet radiation in three bands known as A, B, and C. Only the first two, ultraviolet A (UVA) and ultraviolet B (UVB), are directly harmful in lupus and are probably harmful to most of us with the exception of a some of the UVA-1 band. When these bands of ultraviolet light hit the skin of lupus patients, they damage deposits of DNA near the surface of the skin. In some mouse lupus models, radiation to the top (epidermal) layer of the skin has resulted in the generation of denatured or altered DNA, which researchers have found can lead to the formation of anti-DNA and result in tissue damage. Also, ultraviolet light can induce the production of other antibodies—anti-Ro (SSA), anti-La (SSB), and anti-RNP—partly through altered apoptosis in a skin cell known as a kera-tinocyte. Most patients who test positive for the anti-Ro (SSA) antibody are very sun sensitive.

## CLASSIFICATION OF CUTANEOUS LUPUS

*Cutaneous* (relating to the skin) lupus can be broken down into three general categories:

1. *Acute cutaneous lupus erythematosus.* Almost all of these patients have active systemic lupus with skin inflammation.
2. *Subacute cutaneous lupus erythematosus* (SCLE). This is a nonscarring rash that can coexist with both discoid and systemic lupus.
3. *Chronic cutaneous lupus erythematosus,* also known as *discoid lupus erythematosus* (DLE). Patients with SCLE or SLE may also have discoid lesions. See Table 12.1.

The cutaneous features of lupus include *mucosal ulcerations*—sores in the mouth, nose, or vagina; *alopecia*—hair loss; *malar rash*—butterfly rash on the cheeks; *discoid lesions*—thick, scarring, plaquelike rashes; *pigment changes*— both loss of pigment and more pigment in different places; *erythema*—reddening of lesions, *urticaria*—hives or welts; and *cutaneous vascular* features involving the blood vessels. Included in this category are *Raynaud's phenomenon*—when the fingertips turn red, white, and blue in reaction to cold temperatures; *livedo reticularis*—a red mottling or lacelike appearance under the skin; *purpura*—which appears like a bruise or black-and-blue mark; *cutaneous vasculitis*—breakdown of the skin due to inflammation of the superficial vessels, which can lead to *ulcers* or *gangrene*—a breakdown of the skin due to inflammation of the deep vessels or a blood clot. Sometimes *calcinosis*, or calcium deposits under the skin, can be found. See Table 12.2.

There are other conditions not usually seen in lupus patients that involve the skin and require attention. One condition is *panniculitis*—which involves inflammation of the dermis of the skin. *Bullous lupus*, another condition, produces fluid-filled blisters or a rash similar to that of chickenpox. Complications from the use of steroids as a treatment for lupus can also induce skin damage such as

---

**Table 12.1.** *Types of Rashes Noted in Lupus*

Acute cutaneous
Subacute cutaneous
Chronic (discoid) cutaneous
Lupus profundus
Hypertrophic lupus
Lupus tumidus
Lupus pernio (chilblains)
Bullous lupus

**Table 12.2.** *Some Skin Manifestations of Lupus*

---

A. **Cutaneous**
    Sun sensitivity
    Mouth sores
    Nasal sores
    Genital ulcerations
    Butterfly rash
    Hair loss or thinning
    Changes in pigmentation
    Hives or welts
    Telangiectasias
    Calcinosis
B. **Cutaneo-vascular**
    Cutaneous vasculitis
    Cryoglobulinemic vasculitis
    Raynaud's
    Livedo reticularis
    Erythromelalgia
    Ulceration/gangrene
    Purpura

---

*ecchymoses*, or black-and-blue marks, as well as *skin atrophy*, which results in paper-thin skin.

## DISCOID LUPUS ERYTHEMATOSUS

*Chronic cutaneous lupus erythematosus* is commonly known as DLE. It is diagnosed when a patient with a discoid lupus rash (confirmed by skin biopsy) does not fulfill the American College of Rheumatology criteria for systemic lupus (see Chapter 2); 10 percent of all lupus patients have DLE. Remember, discoid lesions may be a feature of SLE.

In the United States, 70 percent of patients with DLE are women, and 75 percent are Caucasian, with the mean age of onset in the 30s. Discoid lesions appear on sun-exposed surfaces but, in rare cases, can also be found on non-sun-exposed areas. Such lesions generally do not itch. They appear as thick and scaly; under the microscope, one sees plugging of hair follicles, thickening of the epidermis, and atrophy or thinning of the *dermis* (the part of the skin under the epidermis, which is the topmost layer of skin). Signs of inflammation are also present.

Aching joints and other constitutional symptoms are found in 10 to 20 percent of patients with DLE. Blood testing shows a positive antinuclear antibody (ANA) test in about half of the cases; other autoantibodies are seen in less than 10 percent. Anemia may be observed in 20 percent of the patients, and a low white blood cell count in half.

Discoid lupus can appear similar to other skin lesions. For example, rosacea, fungal infections, sarcoidosis, seborrhea, dermatomyositis, and a sun-sensitive rash called polymorphous light eruption can be ruled out by a simple skin biopsy and blood tests before diagnosing DLE.

Without treatment, discoid lesions may progress. After many years, some may turn into skin cancer. *Localized DLE* was a term coined at the Mayo Clinic in the 1930s to describe discoid lesions appearing only above the neck. They rarely evolve into systemic lupus and are treated with antimalarial drugs or local remedies. *Generalized DLE* implies lesions above and below the neck. This form has a 10 percent chance of developing into systemic lupus. Discoid lupus is managed by avoiding the sun and by using sunscreens, antimalarial drugs, and topical anti-inflammatories. Sometimes steroid injections are helpful with these lesions. In rare cases, severe resistant lesions may require antileprosy drugs, such as thalidomide or dapsone, oral corticosteroids, azathioprine, or nitrogen mustard ointment. See Part V of this book for a review of these treatments.

## SUBACUTE CUTANEOUS LUPUS ERYTHEMATOSUS

Subacute cutaneous lupus erythematosus (SCLE) is a rash seen in about 9 percent of lupus patients; 20 percent of individuals with SCLE also have lesions typical of discoid lupus. Unlike DLE, SCLE does not scar the skin. Under the microscope, the inflammation is mild and diffuse, not thick and scaly. The lesions in SCLE, like those in systemic lupus, also do not usually itch. The rash may look similar to that of psoriasis but primarily affects the dermis as opposed to the epidermis.

Among SCLE patients, 70 percent are women and 85 percent are Caucasian. The mean age of onset is in the early 40s. Half of these patients fulfill the American College of Rheumatology criteria for systemic lupus. Among the SCLE cases, 75 percent are sun sensitive and 65 percent have joint aches, but less than 10 percent develop organ complications (in which the heart, lungs, kidneys, or liver are involved).

We know little about the causes of SCLE, but certain drugs such as thiazide diuretics (e.g., Dyazide) and proton pump inhibitors have been known to bring it on. Two thirds of SCLE patients have a positive ANA and 90 percent have anti-Ro (SSA) tests. Nearly all have the HLA-DR3 marker.

The lesions of SCLE are notoriously resistant to the usual drug therapies. Skin creams and antimalarials sometimes provide only modest results. But retinoid (Vitamin A) derivatives have been helpful and are important in the management of acute SCLE.

## CUTANEOUS FEATURES OF LUPUS

### Photosensitive Rashes

When lupus patients are queried, approximately two thirds report that they are sun sensitive. If a doctor actually tries to induce a rash in these circumstances, it is a success about half of the time. These rashes are usually limited to areas exposed to ultraviolet light from the sun. Sometimes systemic symptoms such as fevers, swollen glands, aching, and fatigue are noted by patients who have acute sun exposure.

### Mouth or Nose Sores (Mucosal Ulcerations)

Mouth sores are seen in 20 percent of patients with systemic or discoid lupus. Occasionally, nose ulcerations are noted, which may result in nasal septal perforation. In rare cases, women may develop recurrent vaginal sores. Oral ulcers must be differentiated from herpes lesions or cold sores seen in lupus patients, especially those who are on steroids or are receiving chemotherapy. The sores may be solitary or appear as crops of lesions. They may be found on the tongue or any part of the mouth, especially on the hard palate or buccal mucosa. Patients with other autoimmune disorders such as reactive arthritis, Behçet's disease, celiac disease, Wegener's granulomatosis, and Crohn's disease also can have mucosal ulcers.

Oral ulcers look like lupus under the microscope. They are managed conservatively with old-fashioned remedies such as buttermilk gargles or hydrogen peroxide diluted in a few ounces of water, gargled and spit out several times a day. A local steroid, triamcinolone, which can be found in a dental gel (e.g., Kenalog in Orabase), can be applied to the lesions and usually brings about prompt healing. Antimalarial drugs and systemic steroids are also helpful. Nasal ulcers sometimes respond to a petroleum jelly such as Vaseline.

### Hair Loss (Alopecia)

There are many reasons why lupus may lead to hair loss. First, active disease is associated with the plugging of hair follicles, which results in clumps of hair simply falling out after being combed or washed (*lupus hair*). Patients with discoid lupus can experience mild, generalized hair loss, bald spots (*alopecia areata*), or even total baldness. Steroids may induce hair loss in the male pattern of baldness—in the temples and on top of the head. Also, infections, chemotherapy, emotional stress, and hormonal imbalances are associated with hair loss. All told, about 30 percent of patients with SLE and DLE report significant hair loss.

The treatment of alopecia depends on its cause. For example, discoid lesions respond to local scalp injections with steroid preparations. If these areas form thick scars, hair may not regrow. Tapering off steroid use eliminates the balding pattern. Antimalarials and corticosteroids promote hair growth. *Minoxidil* (Rogaine) solution is a blood pressure preparation that promotes hair growth in balding men. It promotes hair growth in male and female lupus patients but does not decrease hair loss.

### Butterfly (Malar) Rash

The term "lupus" was derived from the Latin word for "wolf" in an effort to describe one of the disease's most recognizable features. About 35 percent of patients with systemic or discoid lupus report a butterfly rash on their cheeks that suggests a wolflike appearance. The rash reflects the angle at which the ultraviolet radiation from the sun hits the skin. Rosacea, a sun-sensitive rash called "polymorphous light eruption," and other disorders can be associated with butterfly rashes, and many patients referred to me with a malar rash and a suspected diagnosis of lupus turn out to have one of these conditions and not lupus. Again, lesions in lupus generally do not itch and are identified as lupus under the microscope. One differentiating tip is that the nasolabial folds (where the outer parts of the nose and cheek meet the upper lip) are usually not affected in lupus. Occasionally, patients with a malar rash ignore their doctor's advice and apply a great deal of fluorinated (e.g., triamcinolone, clobetasol) steroid salve for weeks or months. This results in thinning and wasting of the skin, which makes the condition look like a severe malar rash. The reason for this is that capillaries (blood vessels) near the skin become more visible and mislead the patient into believing that the lupus has worsened. Malar rashes from lupus are treated with the judicious use of steroid ointments or gels, topical calcineurins (e.g., pinecrolimus, tacrolimus), sun avoidance, and management of lupus activity in other parts of the body.

### Changes in Pigmentation

Increased or decreased pigmentation of the skin is present in 10 percent of those with DLE or SLE. In other words, these patients may have areas of skin that are darker or lighter than expected. As inflammation heals, patients may note increases or decreases in pigment. Also, steroid deficiency (a decrease in the steroids made by the adrenal gland) can increase pigmentation, as may antimalarial drugs. *Vitiligo* is an autoimmune skin condition associated with depigmentation; it may be more common in those who have lupus. No systemic drug is helpful for the pigmentation abnormalities of lupus, but some dermatologic preparations applied to affected skin areas can improve the patient's appearance.

## Hives or Welts (Urticaria)

At some point in the course of their disease, 10 percent of patients with systemic lupus will develop hives. This is one of the few skin rashes of lupus that itch. Most cases are related to coincidental allergic reactions, but an uncommon form of lupus may be associated with lupus urticaria. Most of these patients have deficiencies in certain blood complement components. For unclear reasons, lupus patients have an increased incidence of allergies in general (see Chapter 29). Lupus urticaria is managed with antihistamines—H1 blockers such as hydroxyzine (Atarax, Zyrtec, Claritin, Benadryl) and H2 blockers such as cimetidine (Tagamet, Zantac)—antiserotonin drugs (Periactin), cyclosporin (Neoral), omalizumab (Xolair), and steroids.

## VASCULAR RASHES

*Vasculitis* refers to inflammation of blood vessels, and such inflammation can lead to features detectable in the skin. Lupus usually involves the medium- and small-sized blood vessels. Small arteries and capillaries under the skin can be deprived of oxygen because of inflammation, abnormal vascular tone (which controls whether a vessel dilates or constricts), or blood clots. A variety of lesions associated with lupus stem from vascular problems.

## Raynaud's Phenomenon

One third of patients with systemic lupus exhibit an unusual sign, referred to as *Raynaud's phenomenon*, in which their fingers turn a patriotic red, white, and blue in response to stress, cold, or vibratory stimuli (e.g., jackhammers, pneumatic drills). This usually reflects a dysfunction of the sympathetic nervous system's ability to regulate the tone of the small blood vessels of the hand (whether they dilate or constrict). At times, Raynaud's may be observed in the feet, tongue, the tip of the nose, or on the outsides of the ears. There are many other causes of Raynaud's, and it can be seen in most other rheumatic autoimmune diseases. In fact, several surveys have shown that only about 9 percent of all Raynaud's is found among lupus patients. Raynaud's can exist by itself (as *Raynaud's disease*), but a minority of these patients develop an autoimmune disease over a 10-year observation period, and some cases evolve into lupus. Infrequently, Raynaud's becomes so severe that the skin ulcerates from lack of oxygen and gangrene may develop. Raynaud's activity is usually independent of lupus activity. (In other words, active SLE does not necessarily appear at the same time as active Raynaud's, and vice versa.)

Raynaud's is managed with preventive measures. These include wearing gloves or mittens, avoiding cold environments, not smoking, and using hand warmers. Medication such as beta-blockers, decongestants, and ergots given for migraine headaches should be avoided or used sparingly. A variety of medications that increase the flow of blood to the hands may be prescribed, including nitroglycerine ointment, calcium channel blockers (diltiazem [Cardizem], nifedipine [Procardia], nicardipine [Cardene], amlodipine [Norvasc]), sildenafil (Viagra), tadalafil (Cialis), bosentan (Tracleer), and other vasodilators such as Losartan. Severe ulcerations of the fingers or gangrene can be treated with intravenous preparations such as prostaglandin. As a last-ditch effort to save a finger, sympathetic blocks or *digital sympathectomies* (cutting the autonomic nerves to the hand) are occasionally performed. Ulcers limited to one finger can be differentiated from a lupus anticoagulant-derived clot (treated with blood thinners; see Chapter 21) or cholesterol clots called emboli (treated by lowering cholesterol levels). Blood testing and studies of the blood vessels are used to determine the exact nature of such ulcers.

### Livedo Reticularis

Some 20 to 30 percent of all lupus patients have a red mottling or lacelike appearance, or *livedo reticularis*, under the skin. Causing no symptoms, it indicates a disordered flow in blood vessels near the skin due to dysregulation of the autonomic nervous system. Even though normal individuals may demonstrate livedo reticularis and no treatment is ever required, recent work has associated this condition with a secondary fibromyalgia, with the circulating lupus anticoagulant or with anticardiolipin antibody. Livedo reticularis on rare occasions can lead to *livedoid vasculitis*, a condition that involves superficial skin breakage. This complication may be treated with steroids or colchicine.

### Cutaneous Vasculitis, Ulcers, and Gangrene

Inflammation of the superficial blood vessels (those near the skin) is known as *cutaneous vasculitis*. Seen in up to 70 percent of patients with lupus during the course of their disease, this finding is a reminder that more aggressive management may be required in some individuals. These lesions often appear as red or black dots or hard spots and are frequently painful. If untreated, cutaneous vasculitis can result in ulceration, or breakdown of the skin. This may lead to gangrene, or dead, black skin. Gangrene from systemic vasculitis can be a limb- and life-threatening emergency. Such a condition is usually the result of a clot from the circulating lupus anticoagulant or vasculitis of a deep middle-sized artery; a prompt workup is vital to determine whether steroids, blood-thinning agents, or both are warranted. Cutaneous vasculitis is treated less urgently with colchicine, medicines that dilate blood vessels, immune modulators, and corticosteroids. As with Raynaud's, sometimes prostaglandin infusions are used. Vasculitic lesions are not limited to the fingertips or ends of the toes; systemic vasculitis may produce ulcers on the trunk of the body or on the extremities. Occasionally, they may be associated with a cold-precipitating protein known as *cryoglobulin*.

## Black-and-Blue Marks (Purpura and Ecchymoses)

Black-and-blue marks that appear as blotches under the skin may result from abnormal blood coagulation in patients with active lupus. *Purpura* is the term for this phenomenon. If the purpura is small and "palpable" (feels markedly different from normal skin when touched without looking), this may be a warning sign of active systemic vasculitis (see the previous section, Cutaneous Vasculitis, Ulcers, and Gangrene) or low platelet counts (called *thrombocytopenic purpura*). On the other hand, black-and-blue marks that cannot be felt may result from the use of nonsteroidal anti-inflammatory agents (e.g., aspirin, naproxen) or corticosteroids. Nonsteroidals can prolong bleeding times; corticosteroids promote thinning and atrophy of the skin, which can lead to the rupture of superficial skin capillaries (*ecchymoses*).

This condition is not serious and is managed by reassuring the patient that it does not represent a systemic disease process.

## OTHER SKIN DISORDERS IN LUPUS PATIENTS

Unusual forms of cutaneous lupus may occur that are not necessarily associated with any other aspect of lupus activity. Most are extremely rare, and a few are briefly mentioned here.

### Lupus Panniculitis (Profundus)

One out of 200 patients with lupus develops lumps under the skin and no obvious rash. The ANA test of these patients is often negative, and the criteria for systemic lupus are not fulfilled. Under the microscope, biopsy of the skin reveals inflamed fat pads in the dermis with characteristic features of lupus. If untreated, the skin feels lumpier and atrophies. Known as *lupus panniculitis* or *profundus*, this rare disorder responds to antimalarials, antileprosy drugs (dapsone), mycophenolate mofetil (CellCept), oral corticosteroids, and steroid injections into the lumps.

### Blisters (Bullous Lupus)

For every 500 patients with lupus, 1 has *bullous lesions*. Looking like fluid-filled blisters or blebs (large chickenpox marks), this complicated rash can be further divided into several different subsets. Resembling another skin disease called pemphigus, bullous lupus is also called *pemphigoid lupus*. A biopsy of the skin is essential, because treatment depends on which of the three types of bullous rashes are present. Bullous lupus can be quite serious and on occasion constitutes a medical emergency, because widespread oozing from the skin can lead to dehydration and even shock. Systemic corticosteroids are frequently prescribed for this condition, as are antileprosy drugs such as dapsone.

## Rare Variants

Exaggerated thick skin is termed *hypertrophic lupus erythematosus*; mucous-like containing patches, *tumid lupus*; and red-purple patches that appear in cold weather, *lupus pernio* in chilblains.

## WHAT IS THE LUPUS BAND TEST?

Since 1963 skin biopsies have been improved by our ability to determine whether a rash is mediated by the activity of the immune system, which is detected by the presence of what are called *immune deposits*. At the junction of the epidermis (top of the skin) and the dermis (the layer below the skin), we can now see whether immune complexes (see Chapter 6) have been deposited. Most patients with immune disorders will have these immune complexes at the dermal–epidermal junction. Lupus is one of the few diseases in which the deposits are "confluent" (i.e., once stained with a fluorescent dye, the skin of lupus patients will reveal a continuous line).

To perform a *lupus band test*, as this procedure is called, a dermatologist takes a skin biopsy from both a sun-exposed area (e.g., forearm) and an area never exposed to the sun (e.g., buttocks). These biopsies are then frozen and transported in liquid nitrogen and stained to detect specific immune reactants (IgG, IgM, IgA, complement 3 [C3], and fibrinogen) at a pathology laboratory. The biopsy is relatively painless and leaves a small scar.

A confluent stain with all five reactants or proteins implies a greater than 99 percent probability of having systemic lupus; if four proteins are present, there is a 95 percent probability; three proteins, an 86 percent probability; and two proteins, a 60 percent probability provided that IgG is one of the proteins. In discoid lupus, only lesions (areas with rashes) display these proteins. In systemic lupus, most sun-exposed areas and some non-sun-exposed areas will display these proteins.

**Table 12.3.** *Results of the Lupus Band Test*

| Diagnosis | Positive Tests in Lesions (%) | Positive Tests in Normal-Appearing Skin (%) |
|---|---|---|
| Systemic lupus patients | 90 | 50 |
| Discoid lupus patients | 90 | 0–25 |
| Normal patients, sun-exposed skin | NA | 0–20 |
| Normal patients, non-sun-exposed skin | NA | 0 |

NA, not applicable.

Lupus band tests are performed for two reasons. First, the test can confirm that a rash is part of an immune complex–mediated reaction, which would indicate the need for anti-inflammatory therapy. Second, the test is performed when a patient with a positive ANA test but nonspecific symptoms does not fulfill all the criteria for systemic lupus but the physician feels strongly that a diagnosis must be made one way or the other to initiate treatment. Table 12.3 summarizes the results of the lupus band test for groups of patients.

## FURTHER READING

1. Haber JS, Merola JF, Werth VP. Classifying discoid lupus erythematous: background, gaps and difficulties. *Int J Womens Dermatol*. 2017;3(suppl 1):S62–S66.
2. Gronhagen CM, Gunnarsson I, Svenungsson E, et al. Cutaneous manifestations and serologic findings in 260 patients with systemic lupus erythematosus. *Lupus*. 2010;19:1187–1194.
3. Sanders CJ, van Weelden H, Kazaaz GA, et al. Photosensivity in patients with SLE: a clinical and photobiological study of 100 patients using a prolonged phototest protocol. *Brit J Dermatol*. 2003;149:131–137.

# 13

## *Why the Aches? Arthritis, Muscles, and Bone*

The musculoskeletal system is the most common area of complaint in lupus patients. This system involves different types of tissues: the joints, muscles, bone, soft tissues, and supporting structures of joints such as tendons, ligaments, or bursae. The reader may wish to refer to Figure 13.1 as these areas are discussed.

### JOINTS AND SOFT TISSUES

*Arthralgia* is used to describe the pain experienced in a joint; *arthritis* implies visible inflammation in a joint. Although there are over 100 joints in the human body, only those joints that are lined by synovium can become involved in lupus. *Synovium* is a thin membrane consisting of several layers of loose connective tissue that line certain joint spaces, as in the knees, hands, or hips. It is not found in the spine except in the upper neck area. In active lupus, synovium grows and thickens as part of the inflammatory response. This results in the release of various chemicals that are capable of eroding bone or destroying cartilage. Inflammatory synovitis is commonly observed in rheumatoid arthritis but occurs less frequently and is less severe in systemic lupus.

Surveys have suggested that 80 to 90 percent of patients with systemic lupus complain of arthralgias; arthritis is seen in less than half of these cases. Deforming joint abnormalities characteristic of rheumatoid arthritis are observed in only 10 percent of patients with lupus. The most common symptoms of arthritis in lupus patients are stiffness and aching. Most frequently noted in the hands, wrists, and feet, the symptoms tend to worsen upon rising in the morning but improve as the day goes on. As the disease evolves, other areas (particularly the shoulders, knees, and ankles) may also become affected. Non-lupus forms of arthritis such as osteoarthritis, gout, and joint infections can be seen in systemic lupus erythematosus and are approached differently.

Synovium also lines the tendons and bursae. *Tendons* attach muscle to bone; *bursae* are sacs of synovial fluid between muscles, tendons, and bones that promote easier movement. These are the supporting structures of our joints and are

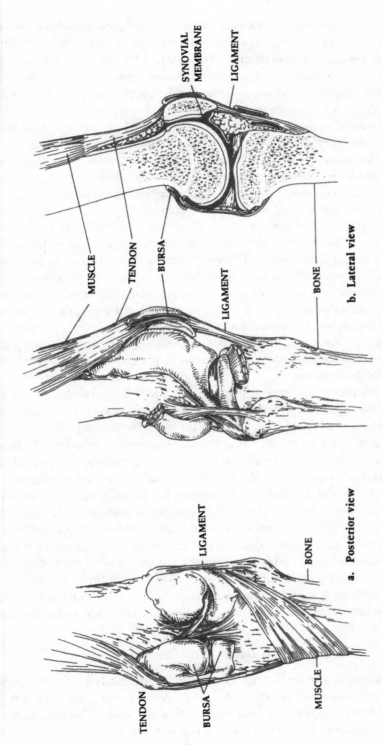

**Figure 13.1.** *Anatomy of the Knee Joint*

SYNOVIAL MEMBRANE

LIGAMENT

MUSCLE

TENDON

BURSA

LIGAMENT

BONE

b. Lateral view

TENDON

BURSA

LIGAMENT

MUSCLE

BONE

a. Posterior view

responsible for ensuring the structural integrity of each joint. In addition, bursae contain sacs of joint fluid that act as shock absorbers, protecting us from traumatic injury. Inflammation of these structures may lead to deformity if *ligaments* (tethers that attach bone to bone) or tendons rupture. *Trigger fingers, carpal tunnel syndrome*, and *Baker's cyst* (all described later in this chapter) are examples of what can result from inflammation in these areas.

Occasionally, cysts of synovial fluid may form. These feel like little balls of gelatin and are called *synovial cysts*. When a joint or bursa is swollen, it is often useful to aspirate or drain fluid from the area to ensure good joint function. When viewed under the microscope, *synovial fluid* (fluid made by synovial tissue) provides a great deal of diagnostic information. Its analysis usually focuses on red and white blood cell counts, crystal analysis (e.g., for gout), and culture (e.g., for bacteria). White blood cell counts of 5,000 to 10,000 are common in active lupus; counts above 50,000 suggest an infection; counts below 1,000 suggest local trauma or osteoarthritis. Normal joint fluid contains zero to 200 white blood cells. Crystals of uric acid (as in gout) or calcium pyrophosphate (as in pseudogout) are occasionally observed in lupus patients and necessitate specific treatment modifications. Joint fluid may also be cultured for bacteria. Viruses are rarely, if ever, tested for when cultures are taken (they grow poorly in cultures), but because viruses, fungi, parasites, or foreign bodies may complicate lupus, the analysis of synovial tissue obtained at synovial biopsy may be required in addition to synovial fluid cultures.

If no evidence of infection is present when a joint is aspirated, I usually inject a steroid derivative with an anesthetic (e.g., lidocaine). This often provides prompt symptomatic relief and successfully treats the swelling. Occasionally, one joint may remain swollen despite anti-inflammatory measures. In these situations, *arthroscopy* (looking at the joint with an operating microscope) along with a synovial biopsy may be diagnostically useful. A persistent *monoarticular arthritis* (arthritis in one joint only) implies either an infection, the presence of crystals, or internal damage (structural abnormalities) in the joint. The presence of *oligoarthritis* (inflammation of two to five joints) and *polyarthritis* (inflammation of more than five joints) suggests a systemic process. Joints are often imaged via ultrasound before or during any diagnostic procedures are performed to make sure that no other process is being missed and also to confirm the anatomy of the area involved. A magnetic resonance image (MRI) can detect stress fractures, dead bone (avascular necrosis), as well as ligamentous, meniscal, or tendon tears.

### Joints and Soft Tissues Often Involved in Lupus

Any joint lined with synovium may be affected by systemic lupus. Starting at the top, the *temporomandibular joint* (TMJ, or jaw joint) can produce symptoms in up to one third of lupus patients. Manifesting itself as jaw pain, TMJ inflammation is often confused with *myofascial pain* (a regional form of fibromyalgia), which consists of tense facial muscles. Fibromyalgia (see the next section, The Muscles in Lupus Patients) affects 20 percent of lupus patients.

The upper *cervical spine* is the only part of the spinal column lined with enough synovium to produce significant inflammation. Inflammation of this area in lupus patients is usually mild and produces pain in the back of the head. Patients who have been treated with steroids for many years can develop instability in the ligaments supporting the neck, so I may recommend that these patients use a collar when driving a car. Again, myofascial problems in the neck and upper back area are much more common than synovitis of the upper cervical spine. Myofascial pain is managed with heat, traction, cervical pillows, muscle relaxants, pain killers, and remedies that improve sleep habits.

*Shoulder* inflammation is not uncommon in lupus patients and often, when arms are raised over the head, feels the way a "bursitis" pain does. Such inflammation responds to anti-inflammatory medications or a local injection.

*Elbows* are occasionally affected in lupus patients. About 10 percent of patients may have *rheumatoidlike nodules* in this area, which feel like little peas. These nodules are much smaller than those seen in rheumatoid arthritis and are of little clinical importance except that they may cause the area below the elbow to fill up with fluid when they break down.

The *hands and wrists* are affected in most lupus patients, with swelling occurring in up to 50 percent of those with systemic lupus. Symptoms of stiffness and aching are frequently experienced in the morning hours. Because it is used more often, the dominant hand is usually more inflamed. In other words, because most people are right-handed, the knuckles of the right hand are larger than those in the left. With chronic inflammation, an "ulnar drift," or outward movement of the knuckles away from the body, is observed. Inflammation of the tendons of the hand may result in *trigger fingers* (locking) or deformities in the form of *contractures* (shortening of the tendon) or tendon ruptures. *Carpal tunnel syndrome* has received a lot of attention in the media as a result of "repetitive strain syndrome," suffered by certain workers such as machine and computer operators. In lupus, it results from chronic swelling in the wrist, which compresses the nerves running through the wrist to the hand. Occasionally, the soft tissues show evidence of *calcinosis*, or calcium deposits under the skin. More commonly seen in scleroderma than systemic lupus, these deposits may cause occasional pain or may break through the skin, ooze, and drain.

*Costochondral margin* irritation, or *costochondritis*, produces chest pain that may mimic a heart attack. The costochondral margin is defined as the place where the sternum (breastbone) meets the ribs. Also known as *Tietze's syndrome*, costochondritis is frequently observed in lupus but is also found in many healthy young women.

Even though the lower spine is not involved in lupus, some of my patients complain of back pain, because their *hips and sacroiliac* joints are lined with synovium. About one third complain of discomfort in this area, but destructive changes are unusual. *Knee* pain, on the other hand, is quite common in lupus patients, but because most lupus patients are young, internal damage to the knee as a consequence of athletic endeavors must also be ruled out.

The *ankle and feet* are common focuses of joint involvement. Ankles can be swollen because of fluid retention, poor circulation, or proteins that have leaked from the kidneys. In addition, swelling can occur from direct joint inflammation or altered gait as a result of foot abnormalities or deformities. *Metatarsals* are the foot bones in our soles that bear the brunt of our weight when we walk. In systemic lupus, the supporting ligaments of the toes loosen and produce bunions and calluses. This may evolve to the point where patients must walk on their metatarsal heads (a normally straight bone), often causing severe foot pain. If the problem is determined to be a local one, I prescribe anti-inflammatory agents and special footwear. Local injections may be used, and occasionally surgery is necessary.

## THE MUSCLES IN LUPUS PATIENTS

Two thirds of my lupus patients complain of muscle aches, which are called *myalgias*. Most frequently located in the muscles between the elbow and neck and the knee and hip, myalgias are rarely associated with weakness. Inflammation of the muscles, or *myositis*, is observed in 15 percent of patients with systemic lupus. Established by blood elevations of the muscle enzyme CPK (creatine phosphokinase), a diagnosis of myositis necessitates steroid therapy because muscle inflammation may cause permanent muscle weakness and atrophy if not treated. Occasionally, an electromyogram (EMG) or "cardiogram" of the muscles is needed to confirm the presence of an inflammatory process. Muscle biopsies are rarely necessary. In addition to physical inactivity, another cause of muscle weakness (not pain) is chronic, long-term steroid use for inflammation, which paradoxically induces muscle atrophy and wasting. In rare cases, high doses of antimalarial agents for many years can cause muscle weakness.

A number of my lupus patients have aching muscles in the neck and upper back areas as well as tenderness in the buttocks, but these aches do not respond to steroids or anti-inflammatories. *Fibromyalgia* consists of amplified pain in what are known as "tender points" (in areas we have already discussed, among others). About 6 million Americans have fibromyalgia. Associated with trauma, infections, and inflammation, fibromyalgia brings on fatigue, sleep disorders, and skin that is painful to the touch and is aggravated by stress and anxiety. Lowering steroid doses can also temporarily aggravate fibromyalgia ("steroid withdrawal syndrome"). I manage fibromyalgia with tricyclic antidepressants—which can relax muscles, induce restful sleep, and raise pain thresholds—along with other non-anti-inflammatory interventions. It can be difficult to differentiate lupus flare-ups from aggravated fibromyalgia. (See Chapter 23 for a complete discussion.)

## BONES IN LUPUS PATIENTS

### Osteoporosis

*Osteoporosis*, or thinning of the bones as a result of lost calcium, may be observed in systemic lupus. A complete discussion of this disease is found in Chapter 29.

### Avascular Necrosis

Penelope went to her doctor with a sudden onset of severe pain in her right hip. She had a 5-year history of lupus, which involved her skin and joints, and had experienced recurrent bouts of pleural effusions (fluid in her lungs). Her disease was well controlled with 20 milligrams of prednisone a day. An X-ray of her hip was normal, but because Penelope rarely complained, Dr. Smith ordered an MRI scan, which revealed avascular necrosis (see the following paragraph for definition). The pain did not respond to any anti-in-flammatory medications, and only an aspirin with codeine preparation provided temporary relief. Dr. Smith referred Penelope to an orthopedist, who put in an artificial hip joint. She is feeling fine now.

One of the more feared consequences of steroid therapy in lupus patients is a condition known as *avascular* (or *aseptic*) *necrosis*. Experienced as a localized pain, avascular necrosis begins when fat clots produced by steroids clog up the blood supply to bone and deprive it of oxygen. This results in dead bone tissue, which, in turn, produces a tremendous amount of pain and ultimately the destruction of bone. About 10 percent of avascular necrosis is not the result of steroids but derives from clots in the blood supply to the bone in patients with the circulating lupus anticoagulant or antiphospholipid antibodies or in those with active inflammation of blood vessels (vasculitis), which obstructs blood flow to the bone. Even though avascular necrosis is seen in 5 to 10 percent of those with systemic lupus, signs of the affliction may not appear on plain X-rays for many months. Early cases may be identified by MRI. The most common target areas are the hip, shoulder, and knee. Crutches may be helpful, and medications may alleviate symptoms somewhat. Limited surgical procedures including revascularization grafts or core decompression are beneficial if performed early in selected joints, but the overwhelming majority of patients ultimately require surgery for joint replacement.

## SUMMING UP

Most lupus patients complain of joint aches, but only a minority demonstrate in-flammatory arthritis, and only 10 percent develop deformities. Inflamed synovium can cause pain and swelling in joints, tendons, and bursae. The small joints of the hands and feet are most frequently involved. Muscles aches are also present in most patients with systemic lupus, but inflammatory muscle disease (myositis) is observed in only 15 percent during the course of their disease. To provide optimal management, arthritis, myalgias, and myositis due to lupus must be differentiated from avascular necrosis, fibromyalgia, and the adverse effects of lupus medications.

## FURTHER READING

1. Alarcon-Segovia D, Abud-Mendoza C, Diaz-Jouanen E, et al. Deforming arthropathy of the hands in systemic lupus erythematosus. *J Rheumatol.* 1998;57:540–544.
2. Van Vugt R, Derksen R, Kater L, et al. Deforming arthropathy or lupus or rhupus hands in systemic lupus erythematosus. *Ann Rheum Dis.* 1998;57(9):540–544.
3. Navarra SV, Torralba TP. The musculoskeletal system and bone metabolism. In Wallace DJ, Hahn BH, eds. *Dubois' Lupus Erythematosus.* 9th ed. Philadelphia: Elsevier, 2018: 3–340.

# 14

## *Pants and Pulses: The Lungs and Heart*

Every grammar school child learns that the heart and lungs are the engine that runs the human body. If you suffer from chest pains or notice shortness of breath, you are reminded of the importance of these two organs. And for those of us treating lupus patients, studying the effect of systemic lupus on the heart and lungs is critical. Most lupus patients have complaints pertaining to the chest. This chapter will review the pulmonary and cardiac manifestations of lupus. Figures 14.1 and 14.2 depict the principal anatomic areas in the lungs and heart that are relevant to our discussion.

### THE LUNGS

When the lungs are working perfectly, they exchange oxygen for carbon dioxide effortlessly. When lupus affects the lungs, or *pulmonary system*, as many as eight different problems can arise that impede the ability to breathe easily. Doctors can diagnose such problems fairly accurately and quickly by using a variety of tests, including chest X-rays, pulmonary function tests, lung scans, heart ultrasounds, biopsies, drainage of lung fluid, and analysis of lung cells derived through bronchoscopy.

### The Pulmonary Workup

Surprisingly, patients may not think of mentioning their lung complaints during an interview. I make a point of asking about shortness of breath, chest pains, pain on taking a deep breath, dry cough, coughing up blood, fever, and rapid breathing. I also inquire about tobacco use and take a job history to see if there has been exposure to toxins. For example, contact with coal or asbestos can certainly damage the lungs.

In addition to a physician listening to the patient's lungs, the first diagnostic tool used in evaluation is the *chest X-ray*. It is inexpensive, quick, and widely available, and it can detect nearly all the important syndromes discussed in this chapter. Should additional testing be necessary, a *computed tomography (CT) scan*

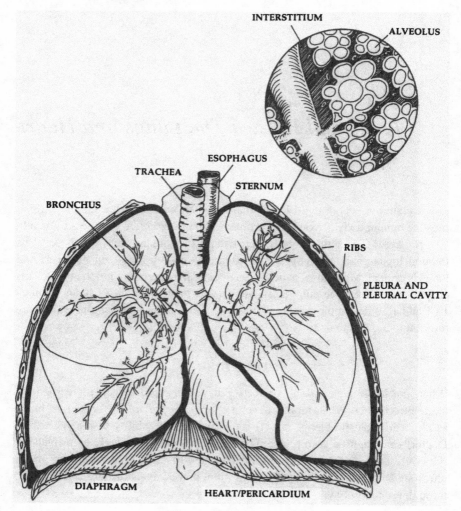

**Figure 14.1.** *The Lung*

or *magnetic resonance imaging (MRI )* may demonstrate structural abnormalities in the chest cavity and pleura. (The CT scan is a modified X-ray, whereas the MRI scanner uses magnets to create an image and releases no radiation.) *Ultrasound* machines employ sound waves to create an image and are used to evaluate pleural disorders. Measurement of *arterial blood gases* (taking blood from the artery instead of a vein) demonstrates how much oxygen is flowing through a patient's arteries, and *pulse oximetry* is a simple, noninvasive measurement of how well the body is saturating oxygen when a patient breathes. By asking the patient to breathe in and out of a balloon (i.e., performing a *pulmonary function test*), the doctor can help to determine whether an asthmatic or bronchospastic component

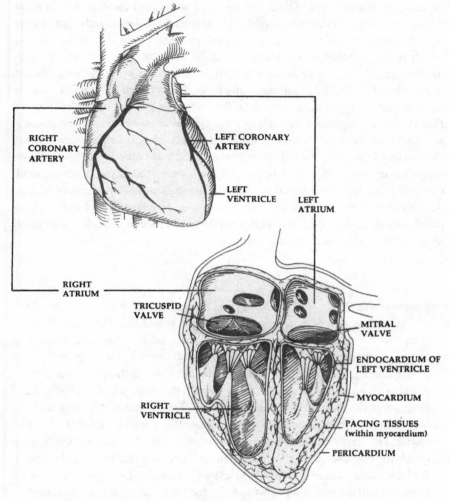

**Figure 14.2.** *The Heart*

is present, assess lung breathing capacities, and evaluate interstitial lung function. The *interstitium* is tissue that provides general support to the lung and facilitates the exchange of oxygen and carbon dioxide when a person breathes. Interstitial lung function is tested by the diffusing capacity, which, if low, suggests a defect in the exchange of oxygen for carbon dioxide in the lung tissue rather than in the air sac.

*Lung scans* are also used. They are painless, noninvasive nuclear medicine studies that can diagnose pulmonary artery blood clots called *emboli*, infection, or inflammation of the interstitium. A ventilation/perfusion scan is used to detect pulmonary emboli; an indium or gallium scan is used to detect inflammation of the interstitium. Sometimes *D-Dimers* are elevated with blood clots, as well as in active systemic lupus erythematosus (SLE). If an infection is suspected or a diagnosis of active lupus needs confirmation, doctors sometimes perform a *thoracentesis*, which is the removal of the pleural fluid for analysis. *Bronchoscopy* permits the removal of lung tissue through a flexible, thin tube for diagnostic purposes. A washing of cells obtained through this procedure is called *bronchoalveolar lavage*; it enables physicians to analyze the cell types present in the lung tissue. *Pulmonary angiograms* (whereby dye is injected into the pulmonary arteries) are the "gold standard" for diagnosing pulmonary emboli and a *video-assisted thoracoscopic surgery (VATS)* procedure permits more lung tissue to be microscopically examined. A *2-D Doppler echocardiogram* is a simple, noninvasive ultrasound procedure that enables doctors to estimate pulmonary pressures in most patients with significant pulmonary hypertension. As a last resort for diagnosing pulmonary disease, doctors can perform a surgical procedure known as an *open-lung biopsy*, but this is rarely necessary.

## Pleurisy

John was a healthy young man until one day, upon taking a deep breath, he felt an odd sensation in his chest. Thinking it would pass, he ignored this symptom for several months. Finally, he measured his pulse and found it to be fast. John consulted his family doctor, who obtained a temperature of 99.8°F and a pulse of 120. Although he did not hear anything unusual upon listening to John's chest, a chest X-ray showed that there was fluid lining the lungs on both sides. At this point, an ultrasound estimated that John had a liter of fluid on his right side (around his lung). Because John felt well otherwise, Dr. Smith called in a pulmonary consultant, who removed the fluid. Under the microscope, the fluid showed an elevated white blood cell count. A blood antinuclear antibody (ANA) test was ordered, which came back positive, and a diagnosis of lupus was made. John was started on 20 milligrams of prednisone (a steroid) a day along with naproxen (an anti-inflammatory drug) at 500 milligrams every 12 hours. Within 10 days John was off steroids and holding his own with naproxen. Plaquenil (an antimalarial drug) was then initiated, and John was able to stop naproxen 3 months later.

## What Is Pleurisy?

The principal symptom of pleurisy is pain on taking a deep breath. The thin membrane sac enveloping the lung is known as the *pleura*. When it is inflamed, the term *pleuritis* is used. If fluid forms and seeps out of this membrane, there is a *pleural effusion*. The pleura does not contain lung tissue, so there should be no fear of lung disease.

Pleuritic discomfort (with or without effusions) is evident in 40 to 60 percent of patients with systemic lupus. Effusions are found in about 20 to 30 percent of patients, and for 2 to 3 percent of patients pleurisy is the initial manifestation of lupus. The pain can be on either side or both sides of the rib cage, or it can be felt as front or back chest pain. At autopsy, more than 90 percent of lupus patients show pleural abnormalities resulting from the disease. The lining of the lungs looks similar to the lining of the heart (*pericardium*) and the lining of the abdominal cavity (*peritoneum*). Under a microscope, the pleural membranes normally consist of a few layers of loose connective tissue, but in lupus, the tissue drastically thickens and shows signs of inflammation. Chemicals that the body makes as part of the inflammatory process irritate the lung and pleura and can eventually form scars and adhesions, resulting in further pain. Effusions are usually visible on a chest X-ray. Occasionally, their presence is confirmed when the patient is lying down and the fluid can be observed spreading into other body cavities. Pleural fluid moves much like water in a glass that has been turned on its side. An ultrasound or CT scan can also confirm the presence of fluid.

### What Can Be Learned from Looking at Pleural Fluid?

The fluid made by an irritated pleura can be clear, a *transudate*, or cloudy, an *exudate*. Transudates, associated with simultaneous irritation of the pericardium and pleura, are observed clinically when the abdomen swells (a condition known as *ascites*), when massive amounts of protein leak from the kidney (a condition called *nephrosis*), or when the kidney fails.

Exudates suggest three possibilities: active lupus in the organs, an infectious process, or a malignancy. By performing a *thoracentesis*, a procedure by which pleural fluid is withdrawn from the lung at the bedside and analyzed under the microscope, a doctor can diagnose exudative effusions. Because lupus patients are susceptible to infections, pleural fluid is usually cultured.

### How Is Pleurisy Treated?

In addition to infection, pleural-like pain is also observed in lupus patients who have rib fractures because of osteoporosis, trauma, or steroid use. Because 20 percent of patients with systemic lupus have fibromyalgia (see Chapter 23), the physician must distinguish fibromyalgia from pleurisy, two conditions that share certain symptoms (e.g., chest wall tenderness, for example).

If pleuritic pain is present but a pleural effusion is not, the doctor may try a higher dose of a nonsteroidal anti-inflammatory drug (e.g., naproxen). Prednisone given in doses up to 40 milligrams daily is also effective but is not always necessary. Radiographically evident effusions usually necessitate corticosteroid therapy. A group of anti-inflammatory drugs known as antimalarials (e.g., Plaquenil) decrease pleural inflammation over a period of several months. Rare instances of recurrent pleural effusions may call for removal of the pleura, a procedure known as *pleurectomy*, or for the introduction of irritating materials (such as talc, tetracycline, or quinacrine) into the pleural lining to prevent fluid from forming.

### Acute Lupus Pneumonitis

Over a 2-day period, Anastasia noticed a temperature of 101°F; a dry, hacking cough; and shortness of breath. She was taking 30 milligrams of prednisone and 100 milligrams of azathioprine (Imuran) a day for systemic lupus that involved autoimmune hemolytic anemia and low platelet counts. She called her family doctor, who was unable to see her and who prescribed azithromycin over the telephone. Three days later, when she was still not better, Dr. Matthews obtained a chest X-ray that showed an infiltrate in the interstitial tissues. As an internist, he knew that these infiltrates are most frequently associated with mycoplasmal pneumonia; therefore, he hospitalized her for intravenous antibiotics. Three days later, Anastasia was still so short of breath that she had to be transferred to the intensive care unit. A pulmonary specialist and her rheumatologist were called to see her in consultation. A bronchoscopy failed to show any evidence of infection. The rheumatologist started her on high-dose intravenous steroids, and after a few days her breathing improved.

Occasionally, lupus patients develop shortness of breath, a dry cough, pleuritic pain, and a blood-tinged sputum. More often than not, this signifies a bronchial infection or pneumonia. However, as in Anastasia's case, lupus itself can inflame the lungs and produce a condition known as *acute lupus pneumonitis* (ALP). Seen in 1 to 9 percent of lupus patients during the course of their disease, ALP affects the lung's interstitium (its supporting tissue), which becomes inflamed. ALP is easily observed on a chest X-ray. Most physicians are cued to look for ALP when their patients' symptoms do not clear up with antibiotics and the chest X-ray remains abnormal. When a bronchoscope is used to take a tissue biopsy of the lung, the physician will observe the interstitial areas of the lung filled with lymphocytes. Clots or vasculitis is rarely noted. Under a immunofluorescent stain, lung tissue is stained to determine the presence of immune complexes, complement, and immunoglobulin.

If it is promptly managed with high doses of steroids, ALP can be completely reversible. Drugs that decrease steroid requirements, such as azathioprine, mycophenolate mofetil (CellCept), or cyclophosphamide, are sometimes added. Despite this, it is unfortunate that up to 50 percent of patients with ALP die within months, often due to a delay in diagnosis.

## Diffuse Interstitial Lung Disease

Florence was diagnosed with lupus 10 years ago and had only mild aching along with sun sensitivity. She also complained of dry, gritty eyes, and her ophthalmologist recommended that she use artificial tears. Over the next several months, Florence began having a dry, hacking cough with only occasional shortness of breath. She consulted a pulmonary specialist, who obtained a chest X-ray showing increased interstitial markings. Pulmonary function tests demonstrated mild restrictive abnormalities. Dr. Hughes ordered a high-resolution CT scan that suggested the presence of lung inflammation. This indicated that the interstitial changes were reversible. She was started on a moderate dose of steroids and now feels a lot better.

When the symptoms described for ALP evolve over a period of several years, it is called diffuse *interstitial lung disease* (ILD). This is a common complication of scleroderma, Sjögren's syndrome, mixed connective tissue disease, and rheumatoid arthritis. It is seen in 10 to 20 percent of patients with systemic lupus. Florence's case is not atypical. Indeed, the symptoms can be so subtle that patients may not even tell their doctors about it at first. Most cases are finally identified after about 10 years of disease.

Chest X-rays along with a restrictive defect on pulmonary function testing help diagnose ILD. A specialized imaging study known as a high-resolution CT scan or a gallium scan frequently sheds light on the degree and nature of pulmonary involvement. Lung biopsies of ILD are occasionally necessary and appear similar to those of ALP, though they are more chronic and less aggressive.

If identified early, ILD is responsive to treatment with steroids and immunosuppressive therapies. After years of the disease, the inflammation diminishes and heals with scars. At this point, treatment is not helpful, because scars do not respond to anti-inflammatory medication. Although ILD rarely leads to respiratory failure, it does lead to rapid, shallow breathing with decreased stamina in its chronic phase. For patients to be treated properly, ILD must be differentiated from *chronic aspiration* (swallowed material going down the wrong pipe), adverse reactions to medication, interstitial lung infections such as pneumocystis pneumonia, and environmental irritants.

## Pulmonary Embolism

Gertrude noticed that her right leg was swollen and tender. This had never happened before, and her lupus was in remission. Her friend, a nurse's aide, told Gertrude that it might be phlebitis and that she should see her doctor. Her life was hectic and Gertrude couldn't spare the time to have it checked out. Three days later, Gertrude suddenly complained of severe chest pain on the right side and couldn't breathe. It was so severe that her sister had to drive her to the nearest emergency room. Her oxygen saturation was low and D dimers were high, which confirmed the presence of a pulmonary embolus. It turned out that a clot from the phlebitis in her leg had broken off and traveled to the lung. Her serum anticardiolipin antibodies were positive, suggesting a predisposition to form blood clots. Gertrude was given heparin and was very lucky to be alive.

One-third of lupus patients have antiphospholipid antibodies such as anticardiolipin (see Chapter 21), and one-third of these patients have a clot or thromboembolic episode during the course of their disease. One-third of these episodes consist of clots that travel through the blood and settle in the vessels of the lung; once there, they are called *pulmonary emboli*. Even though blood clots can be caused by something other than lupus, surveys have reported that 5 to 10 percent of patients with systemic lupus will sustain a pulmonary embolus at some time in their lives.

A patient with a pulmonary embolus will complain of acute shortness of breath and chest pains. The diagnosis is confirmed if the patient exhibits a combination of low levels of oxygen saturation in the blood and a lung scan that shows a mismatched defect (oxygen not being exchanged for carbon dioxide in the blood vessels). Characteristic changes can be found on an electrocardiogram (ECG; which will show right-heart strain), and through blood tests (which will reveal elevation of D-Dimers and LDH). The chest X-rays may look normal at first, but after several days most show a pattern of infarction (dead tissue) with a wedge-shaped defect representing collapsed, unoxygenated lung tissue.

For lupus-mediated pulmonary emboli, treatment is threefold: a patient initially gets an intravenous injectable or oral anticoagulant (heparin) followed by oral medication, warfarin (Coumadin or heparin) for at least several months, and then often a daily low dose of aspirin. Some patients with very certain types and levels of antiphospholipid antibodies or those who have recurrent emboli on low-dose aspirin are treated with oral anticoagulants.

## Pulmonary Hemorrhage

Less than 1 percent of patients with systemic lupus sustain bleeding or hemorrhage into the air sacs of their lungs *(pulmonary hemorrhage)*, but up to 10 percent of the deaths from all forms of active lupus are associated with such an event. Manifested by coughing up blood, pulmonary hemorrhage usually occurs early in the course of the disease, and children are unusually susceptible. Pulmonary hemorrhage may look like ALP, but it progresses more rapidly and targets the air sacs *(alveoli)* of the lungs. The chest X-ray in a patient with pulmonary hemorrhage will reveal fluffy alveolar infiltrates; in addition, active multisystem organ disease is often present. *Bronchoscopy* (whereby a narrow tube with a telescope is placed in the airways through the mouth) will reveal *hemosiderin* (blood pigment) and stained macrophages, but vasculitis is rare. Immune complexes, blood complement, and immunoglobulin can be detected through characteristic stains. How blood gets into the air sacs is unknown, but the process can be triggered by active lupus or a concurrent infection. Pulmonary hemorrhage is often fatal, but a patient may be saved by aggressive, quick management that combines high-dose steroids and a chemotherapy known as cyclophosphamide with or without a blood-filtering treatment know as *apheresis*, in which antibodies and other chemicals that promote inflammation are removed.

### Pulmonary Hypertension

George was mildly short of breath and light-headed. After waiting about a year, he finally consulted his family doctor. He had been diagnosed with discoid lupus 20 years earlier and had occasional aches, Raynaud's, and puffy hands, but otherwise he felt well and worked full time. His doctor obtained a normal chest X-ray but was concerned enough to order pulmonary function tests. These were only mildly abnormal. A pulmonary consultation was requested, which resulted in ordering a 2-D Doppler echocardiogram. It showed elevated, twice-normal pulmonary pressures. His 6-minute walk time was prolonged. Further blood testing for antiphospholipid antibodies was negative. By now, George was winded on minimal exertion and had to stop working. He was given a combination of drugs that included vasodilators, calcium channel blockers, phosphodiesterase inhibitors, and prostaglandin antagonists and is improving.

Along with pulmonary hemorrhage, pulmonary hypertension is one of the most feared complications of systemic lupus. Mildly increased pressure in the pulmonary arteries is observed in 8 to 15 percent of patients with lupus and is generally without symptoms, but significant rises (above 50 millimeters of mercury) can be life threatening. Many lupus patients with pulmonary hypertension have a positive anti-RNP as well as overlapping features with scleroderma and polymyositis. Active inflammation can infrequently raise pulmonary pressures. Like George, most patients feel well at first; later they start experiencing mild shortness of breath or light-headedness. Higher pressures are often associated with a sense of breathlessness, but chest X-rays are surprisingly normal and reveal pulmonary function tests with only mildly restrictive changes. Under certain circumstances, pressures are measured by a 2-D Doppler echocardiogram and more accurately but invasively by use of a *Swan-Ganz catheter*, a pressure gauge that is wedged into the pulmonary artery. If a patient experiences a rise in pressure because of pulmonary emboli, the condition may reverse itself with the administration of anticoagulant drugs. However, pulmonary hypertension of greater than 50 millimeters of mercury in patients without antiphospholipid antibodies (see Chapter 21) can be fatal within months to years if not aggressively managed.

**Table 14.1.** *Drugs Used to Manage Pulmonary Hypertension in Patients with Systemic Lupus Erythematosus*

| Drugs | Examples |
|---|---|
| 1. Nitrates (vasodilators) | isosorbide (Isordil) |
| 2. Calcium channel blockers | nifedipine |
| 3. Diuretics | |
| 4. Anticoagulants | warfarin |
| 5. Phosphodiesterase inhibitors | sildenafil (Viagra, Revatio), tadalafil (Adcirca, Cialis) |
| 6. Endothelin antagonists | bosentan (Tracleer), ambrisentan (Letaris) |
| 7. Prostaglandin antagonists | epoprostenol (Flonan), inhaled iloprost (Ventavis), treprostinil (Remodulin) |

Other causes of pulmonary hypertension include a cardiac shunt between chambers, or severe inflammation that responds to anti-inflammatory regimens. A 6-minute walk time is commonly used to measure response to medication. Very elevated pressures are treated with endothelin receptor antagonists, which reverse a substance that causes vessels to constrict or phosphodiesterase type-5 inhibitors). Resistant cases may respond to prostacyclin analogues that are given by inhalation or infusion. Occasionally, lung transplantation is advised. The cause of antiphospholipid antibody-negative pulmonary hypertension in patients with systemic lupus is not known, but it probably has something to do with the lining of pulmonary arteries of the lung being sensitive to a variety of chemicals. See Table 14.1.

## The "Shrinking Lung" Syndrome

An uncommon complication of systemic lupus is manifested by a sense of breathlessness and decreased chest expansion in patients who have elevated diaphragms on chest X-rays. This is known as the "shrinking lung" syndrome. The diaphragm is a muscle that weakens as a result of pleural scarring or other proposed mechanisms. The shrinking lung syndrome may respond to steroid therapy, but it is usually a benign, nonprogressive process.

## Adverse Reactions to Medications Used in Lupus

A small but significant group of individuals are sensitive to aspirin or other salicylates (aspirin products) and develop wheezing (bronchospasm) when they take salicylates. Similar reactions can also occur, to a lesser extent, with other nonsteroidal anti-inflammatory drugs (e.g., ibuprofen, naproxen). Drugs used to treat autoimmune disease—such as methotrexate—can induce ILD and occasionally provoke acute asthma. Steroids and chemotherapy drugs can also make a lupus patient more susceptible to pulmonary infections. These possibilities must be ruled out before any of the lung conditions previously discussed are considered.

## Summing Up

If you suffer from lupus, are short of breath or it hurts to take a deep breath, have a dry cough, cough up blood, wheeze, or have chest pain, your lungs are probably involved. Inflammation of the pleura is common and usually not serious. ILD (which involves the supporting structures of the lungs) and pulmonary emboli are the second and third most frequently observed lung complications in systemic lupus. They can be managed with steroids and drugs that thin the blood and prevent clots. ALP, pulmonary hemorrhage, and pulmonary hypertension are very serious conditions and are difficult to treat, even in the most experienced hands. Infections, malignancies, allergic reactions, and other processes must be ruled out before a diagnosis of lupus-related lung disease can be arrived at successfully; a variety of well-understood diagnostic tests are available to do this.

## THE HEART

Abnormalities of the heart can also significantly undermine the lupus patient's quality of life, and like lung diseases associated with lupus, heart disease can be serious. The major cardiac symptom, chest pain, is reviewed in detail here, along with heart diseases in lupus patients. Unfortunately, blood testing is not particularly useful in looking for active heart disease. Instead, there are many sophisticated tools that allow physicians to assess and manage the cardiac manifestations of lupus.

## Why Do Lupus Patients Get Chest Pains?

Esther had systemic lupus with symptoms of occasional pleurisy, a mild anemia, and swollen wrists. Her disease was adequately controlled with ibuprofen and Plaquenil. One evening, while reading in bed, she experienced the sudden onset of severe chest pressure. She told her husband, who thought it might be a heart attack, and he took her to the emergency room. Esther's chest X-ray and ECG were normal. She saw her family doctor the next day, who ordered a 2-D Doppler echocardiogram to look for evidence of a *pericardial effusion* (fluid around the heart sac). This turned out to be negative. Eventually, an upper gastrointestinal endoscopy examination was performed, which showed an erosive gastritis from ibuprofen with evidence of esophageal reflux (whereby food is pushed back up into the esophagus from the stomach). She was started on an antireflux and antiulcer regimen consisting of omeprazole (Prilosec) and told not to lie down right after eating a big meal. Ibuprofen was discontinued, and Esther was much better within a week.

Chest pain is a common but potentially misunderstood feature of systemic lupus. Fortunately, it only rarely indicates heart disease, but it can be traced to many causes, each requiring its own method of management. I find it important to exercise patience and have an open mind when I am interviewing patients with chest pain because of the complexity of its diagnosis and treatment.

The most frequent cause of noncardiac chest pain in lupus is *esophageal.* The movement of acid made by the stomach backward into the esophagus, termed *reflux esophagitis,* and a digestive disorder involving the movement of food have been reported in half of those with the disease (GERD, or gastroesophageal reflux disease). Autoimmune diseases and anti-inflammatory medications used to treat them may also induce esophageal pain. (The diseases, because of altered motility and the medications, can erode or ulcerate tissue lining.) This type of pain is managed with antacids and medications that improve the movement of food and block acid release, both of which are reviewed in detail in Chapter 18.

The second most common type of chest pain is *chest wall pain.* This is easily diagnosed: the patient feels extreme discomfort when pressure is applied to the breastbone or, more technically, the costochondral margins of the sternum. It can be a symptom of fibromyalgia or a syndrome known as costochondritis (also called Tietze's syndrome). Aspirin, local moist heat, and occasional injections into tender points are the treatments of choice.

Fluid that settles around the sac of the heart, or *pericardium,* can also produce a central chest pain that occurs when the patient is at rest, which is relieved by leaning forward. *Angina pectoris,* or decreased blood flow to the coronary arteries with pain resulting from lack of oxygen, is just as likely—if not more likely—to occur in lupus patients as in anybody else. Spasms of the coronary arteries, termed *microvascular angina,* and can occur with normal coronary arteries. However, it often has an earlier onset in patients on a long-term steroid course that can be a sign of coronary vasculitis or myocarditis as well as atherosclerosis of the coronary arteries (discussed later in this chapter). Chest pain of *pulmonary origin* is common with pneumonia or a pulmonary clot (embolus) and may have nothing to do with lupus.

**Other Cardiac Symptoms**

A persistently rapid heartbeat, called *tachycardia,* is a feature of active lupus resulting from inflammation or fevers. Other causes of tachycardia, such as infections or an overactive thyroid gland, must be considered. Rapid heartbeats are treated with anti-inflammatory medications and occasionally beta-blockers (e.g., atenolol). *Irregular heartbeats* are noted when the *myocardium* (heart muscle) or pacing system of the heart is inflamed or scarred. *Shortness of breath* can be due to lung disease (such as asthma) or a failing heart muscle that cannot provide adequate cardiac output.

## CARDIAC DISORDERS

### What Is the Pericardium?

Heather was recently diagnosed with lupus on the basis of skin rashes, fatigue, and a positive ANA test. She began experiencing chest pressure, a low-grade fever, and a rapid pulse associated with shortness of breath. The chest pain diminished in intensity when she leaned forward. Her doctor obtained a chest X-ray, which showed an enlarged heart shadow as well as small pleural effusions. An ECG revealed inflammation of the pericardium, and the diagnosis of pericarditis was made. When a 2-D Doppler echocardiogram showed a moderate amount of fluid in the pericardium, a diagnosis of *lupus serositis* was also made (fluid in both the pleura and pericardium), and Heather was started on 40 milligrams of prednisone daily. Shortly thereafter, three Aleve twice a day was added to her treatment. Within 3 weeks, she was able to discontinue the steroids, but she had to take colchicine twice a day for another month. Plaquenil (an antimalarial also known as hydroxychloroquine) was also begun, and a year later she has yet to have a recurrence.

The term *pericardial effusion* is used to describe fluid around the sac of the heart. Present in 50 percent of patients with lupus who have undergone 2-D echocardiography, the condition is usually without symptoms and may not require any specific measures. During the course of their disease, 25 percent of my patients, like Heather, complain of chest pains below the breastbone, which are frequently relieved by bending forward. The pain correlates with abnormalities in what are called "ST segments" on an ECG. These individuals have *pericarditis*, or inflammation of the pericardium, the sac surrounding the heart. Evidence of prior pericarditis is found microscopically in 60 percent of autopsied lupus patients. In pericarditis, the pericardial fluid contains several thousand white blood cells, and areas of the sac show that lymphocytes and plasma cells are present in pericardial tissue. By listening through a stethoscope, a doctor can hear a harsh rubbing sound, or *pericardial rub*, in up to 20 percent of those with acute pericarditis. Pericarditis does not imply an organ-threatening disease, because the heart tissue is not involved. If the pericardial fluid does not show evidence of infection, acute pericarditis is managed with an anti-inflammatory known as colchicine, as well as high-dose nonsteroidal anti-inflammatory drugs (e.g., indomethacin) and, if needed, with a short course of moderate-dose corticosteroids.

On rare occasions, pericarditis is complicated by *pericardial tamponade* or *constrictive pericarditis*. Tamponade occurs when so much fluid is formed that the heart muscle is prevented from pumping blood adequately. This life-threatening complication necessitates immediate removal of the fluid, or "windowing," to allow the fluid an outlet. Chronic inflammation can promote adhesions and scars in the pericardial lining, which can result in signs similar to those of tamponade.

*Constrictive pericarditis*, as this process is called, is cured surgically by stripping or removing the affected pericardial tissue, a procedure known as a *pericardiectomy*.

## What Is Myocarditis?

Shanna was 20 years old and had already had lupus for 8 years. Her course had been very rocky and was complicated by kidney involvement and one attack of seizures from central nervous system vasculitis. At this point, Shanna became concerned about her appearance and was reluctant to take the steroid dose her doctors recommended; she "forgot" to take it two to three times a week. One morning she began experiencing low-grade fevers, a rapid pulse, and a dull chest pressure. Her ECG showed nonspecific abnormalities with an elevated blood *creatine phosphokinase* (CPK; a muscle enzyme released during a heart attack or with muscle inflammation). A *myocardial infarction* (heart attack) was ruled out, but her continued symptoms warranted admission to the coronary care unit. A cardiologist was called to see her in consultation, and because her clinical status was unclear, he recommended a cardiac catheterization. When it was performed the next day, a myocardial biopsy was also obtained. Shanna was diagnosed with lupus myocarditis. High doses of intravenous steroids were administered immediately, and a rapid improvement in Shanna's condition was noted.

Underneath the pericardium lies the *myocardium*, which is the body's heart muscle. Each time this pump contracts, a person experiences a heartbeat. The blood supply to this muscle is provided by the *coronary arteries*. Ten percent of lupus patients eventually experience *myocarditis*, or inflammation of the heart muscle. In fact, at autopsy, 40 percent of patients with systemic lupus show evidence of prior myocardial involvement. The symptoms of myocarditis usually include a rapid pulse and chest pains and frequently coexist with active, systemic lupus. Chest X-rays frequently show an enlarged heart, and signs of congestive heart failure may be evident. Infections, particularly viruses, can also induce myocarditis. It is important to remember that lupus patients are very susceptible to a variety of infections. Creatine phosphokinase (a muscle enzyme that is released with trauma, inflammation, and heart attacks) or troponin levels are often elevated when the blood is tested. Because it may not be possible to differentiate a heart attack from lupus myocarditis or viral myocarditis, a specialized coronary CT scan may be taken or a heart catheterization administered. Inflamed heart muscles can decrease blood flow through coronary arteries. *Catheterization* consists of injecting dye into the coronary arteries to determine how open they are and whether the heart is receiving enough oxygen. The procedure may also include an *endomyocardial biopsy*, in which a tissue sample of the myocardium is taken. Under the microscope, lupus myocarditis reveals the presence of plasma cells and lymphocytes.

Because myocarditis is a serious complication of systemic lupus, the condition is treated with high doses of corticosteroids for at least several weeks. Other measures include medications that alleviate heart failure and coronary artery insufficiency.

### Congestive Heart Failure and Myocardial Dysfunction

Raphael was 50 years old and his lupus had been in remission for over 10 years. Nevertheless, when he was in his 20s and 30s, his disease had been quite active and he had taken moderate doses of steroids for quite a while. During this time, he developed high blood pressure and elevated cholesterol levels. His blood sugars were borderline high. As long as he watched his diet, limited his salt intake, and walked for a half-hour twice daily, Raphael felt well. He was on a mild blood pressure medication. When his daughter graduated from college in Boston, he flew from the West Coast with his wife to attend the ceremony. Unfortunately, he forgot to take his medicine with him, and when he called his clinic on a weekend to have them call it in to a Boston pharmacy, he was unable to get an immediate response. That evening he went to a seaside restaurant and splurged. After consuming a 3-pound lobster in drawn butter with French fries, Raphael began wheezing and complaining of shortness of breath. Within 3 hours, he couldn't breathe and had to be taken to an emergency room. His blood pressure was 200/130 and his chest X-ray showed *pulmonary edema* (water in the air sacs). Diuretics were administered intravenously. Within an hour, he had urinated over 800 milliliters and felt much better.

A failing heart muscle cannot pump enough blood into the arteries and tissues to maintain normal body functioning. *Congestive heart failure* results when either the left or right side of the heart fails to pump enough blood. In right-sided heart failure, fluid accumulates in the ankles, the liver enlarges, and the neck veins become fuller. A failing left heart, as in Raphael's case, pushes fluid back into the lungs, which may lead to pulmonary edema. In the past, 5 to 10 percent of lupus patients developed congestive heart failure, although recent surveys suggest that—as a result of general medical advances and improvements in lifestyle and diet—its incidence is decreasing. The B-type natriuretic peptide (BNP) is a reliable measure of heart failure.

Failure can be brought on or aggravated by the long-term administration of corticosteroids, anemia, hypertension, serositis, fevers, or disorders of the heart valves. To minimize heart failure, patients are advised to restrict salt in their diets. Alternatively, they might be prescribed diuretics (drugs that reduce pressure on the heart muscle), digitalis (a drug that makes the heart pump more efficiently), beta blockers, or other agents that dilate blood vessels.

Two-D Doppler echocardiograms and studies of wall motion have shown that many patients with active lupus have subtle abnormalities in the left side of the heart that affect filling and pumping, but they show no evidence of congestive heart failure. Termed *myocardial dysfunction*, these abnormalities reflect a low-grade myocarditis or inflammation-induced stress on the heart muscle. These abnormalities usually disappear when lupus is in remission.

## Libman-Sacks Endocarditis and Other Valve Disorders

Eliza had three miscarriages before her physician found the presence of antiphospholipid antibodies upon blood testing. Her doctor diagnosed her as having a very mild case of lupus that did not require treatment. Several weeks later, after she had had several teeth repaired and root canal work done, Eliza complained of feeling lethargic. Her doctor detected a low-grade fever of which Eliza was not aware, but he also obtained a blood count that revealed anemia, and this needed attention. When the fevers persisted and became more pronounced, blood cultures were obtained that were positive for a bacterium called *streptococcus*. A diagnosis of subacute bacterial endocarditis was made when her 2-D Doppler echocardiogram showed a bacterial growth, known as a vegetation, on her aortic valve. Eliza was hospitalized and treated with intravenous antibiotics for 3 weeks, but she became increasingly short of breath. A cardiac catheterization was performed that suggested severe impairment of an aortic valve. She was taken to surgery, where her aortic valve was replaced. At surgery, evidence for Libman-Sacks endocarditis was found, with the complication of an infected vegetation.

The inner surfaces of the heart, particularly those that line the four heart valves, are known as the *endocardium*. Materials such as cellular debris, proliferating cells, and immune complexes that may average 1 to 4 millimeters in diameter, which may be found on the endocardium in lupus patients, are called *vegetations*. Originally described by doctors Emanuel Libman and Benjamin Sacks in 1923, *Libman-Sacks endocarditis* is almost exclusively found in patients with antiphospholipid antibodies (see Chapter 21). Clinically manifested as a heart murmur, the vegetations are usually so small that they are detectable by a 2-D Doppler echocardiogram only 30 percent of the time. A *transesophageal echocardiogram* (an ultrasound performed after a tiny tubelike camera is swallowed to rest in the esophagus) increases detectability to about 60 percent.

Although they alter the dynamics of the heart only 1 to 2 percent of the time, Libman-Sacks vegetations have two potentially serious complications. First, they are prone to become infected, which leads to what is called *subacute bacterial endocarditis*, where the vegetation is a growth site for bacteria. This condition has a high mortality rate and may necessitate a cardiac valve replacement. As in Eliza's case, a vegetation can become infected after a visit to the dentist. *Hence, I advise all patients with antiphospholipid antibodies to take prophylactic antibiotics before and after any dental procedure to prevent the valve from receiving infected materials swallowed during surgery to the mouth.* Second, portions of the vegetations that flake off and travel into the brain through the carotid artery may cause a cerebral clot or stroke. *Therefore, I advise all patients with established vegetations that they should be treated prophylactically with low-dose aspirin or other drugs that reduce the ability of platelets to promote clotting or initiate anticoagulation therapy.*

Damage to the mitral, aortic, pulmonic, or tricuspid heart valves is found only slightly more often in patients with lupus than in the general population. Pulmonary hypertension in these patients is associated with damage to the tricuspid valve, which results in a condition known as tricuspid regurgitation (see Figure 14.2).

For unclear reasons, a floppy mitral valve, or *mitral valve prolapse*, is probably more prevalent among lupus patients. Palpitations, chest pains, and fibromyalgia are also associated with this syndrome, which is managed with beta blockers (e.g., atenolol), antibiotics for dental or surgical procedures, and a decrease in caffeine intake.

### Coronary Artery Disease and Myocardial Infarction (Heart Attack)

Bonnie was 38 years old and had been treated for lupus since she was 20. For the last 3 years she had been maintained on dialysis. Prior to that she had taken high doses of steroids along with chemotherapy for active systemic lupus. While on vacation, she developed sudden pressure in her chest and visited the local emergency room. The attending doctor told her she was too young to have heart disease, gave her antacids, and sent her home after obtaining a normal ECG. When the pain persisted several hours later, she returned to the hospital. This time, her ECG showed an elevated troponin level, suggestive of an evolving heart attack. She was admitted and had a coronary angiogram.

*Atherosclerotic heart disease* (hardening of the arteries) has become the third most common cause of death in lupus patients, following complications of kidney disease and infection. Because more young women are surviving other early organ-threatening complications of lupus, heart complications are now becoming more prevalent after 10 to 20 years of disease. The side effects of long-term use of moderate- to high-dose steroids include hypertension, diabetes, hyperlipidemia (e.g., high cholesterol), and ultimately premature atherosclerosis. Many healthy-appearing patients of mine in their 30s and 40s, such as Bonnie, have developed angina or sustained myocardial infarctions.

In rare circumstances, active lupus is associated with chest pains (angina pectoris) from inflammation or vasculitis of the coronary arteries, or *coronary arteritis.* A coronary angiogram shows the characteristic narrowing of arteries in this unusual condition. It is treated with corticosteroids to prevent a heart attack. Interestingly, children as young as 5 years of age have been reported to develop acute reversible coronary arteritis.

## Microvascular Angina

Surveys have suggested that 10 to 20 percent of lupus patients have chest discomfort significant enough to report it to their physician. Sometimes it can be difficult to pinpoint the cause of this pain, especially when pleurisy, pericarditis, costochondritis, and esophageal reflux are ruled out. Recently, our group at Cedars-Sinai Medical Center demonstrated that myocardial ischemia (angina) in the absence of obstructive coronary disease may account for chest pains. A form of small vessel disease with coronary spasm, this "Raynaud's of the heart" is measured by adenosine stress cardiac magnetic resonance perfusion scanning. Most patients respond to beta-blockers, nitrates, and vasodilators, but some require the addition of anti-inflammatory regimens.

## Hypertension

Monitoring blood pressure during each office visit is a good medical practice. *Hypertension,* defined as a blood pressure greater than 140/90, is observed in 25 to 30 percent of patients with systemic lupus. The most common causes are kidney disease and long-term steroid use. There are no special considerations unique to managing hypertension in lupus patients, because it usually responds to conventional regimens. Untreated or inadequately treated blood pressure can minimally cause headaches, but hypertension can also lead to stroke, cardiac failure, and heart attack.

## The Electrocardiogram and Conduction Defects

The ECG is an inexpensive, harmless, and readily available tool that provides the doctor with numerous clues in screening for heart problems. An ECG detects the heart rate, rhythm, anatomic orientation, and heart chamber size. Moreover, it can suggest whether the lining of the heart (pericardium) or heart muscle (myocardium) is inflamed and whether the coronary arteries are damaged or in danger. Although one-third of lupus patients may display abnormalities on an ECG, a normal ECG does not rule out heart disease.

An ECG can also assess the heart's pacing system, which may be abnormal in lupus patients. Ten percent of patients with systemic lupus have pacing abnormalities or electrical conduction defects that lead to palpitations or missed beats as a result of inflammation or scarring of the heart tissue. The heart's electrical or pacing mechanism travels through this damaged tissue, and these abnormalities result when electrical signals are interrupted.

Lupus present at birth (*neonatal lupus*) can be characterized by varying degrees of heart blockage, because autoantibodies (e.g., anti-Ro) cross the placenta and can damage fetal pacing tissues. Conduction abnormalities in the heart may be treated with drugs that control the resulting arrhythmia, but insertion of a pacemaker is occasionally required. (See Chapter 22 for a more complete discussion of neonatal lupus.)

## Accelerated Atherogenesis

Patients with lupus develop more hypertension, elevated lipid and blood sugar levels, coronary artery disease, heart attacks, strokes, and hardening of the arteries than healthy individuals for their age. For many years, this was assumed to be due to the use of corticosteroids. However, it has since been demonstrated that young lupus patients are at greater risk for these events even if steroids were never prescribed. Systemic lupus itself is associated with defective good cholesterol ("pro-inflammatory HDL") and a process that accelerates inflammatory changes seen with atherosclerosis. Cardiac screening in SLE includes lipid levels, plasma homocystine, blood pressure monitoring, duplex scanning of the carotid arteries, echocardiography, stress testing, or CT scanning of the coronary arteries.

## SUMMING UP

Lupus patients frequently complain of chest pain that may or may not be related to heart disease. The sources of true cardiac pain most frequently involve the lining of the heart, which rarely points to a serious disorder. Myocardial disease, which involves the heart muscle, is often serious and may include inflammation in the form of myocarditis or heart muscle dysfunction, which occasionally produces congestive heart failure. In patients with antiphospholipid antibodies or the circulating lupus anticoagulant, the inner surface of the heart is predisposed to developing vegetations. This may lead to valve damage or stroke. Coronary artery disease and high blood pressure appear prematurely in patients taking steroids for the long-term treatment of lupus. It is essential that doctors take complaints of chest pain seriously and establish its source in order to treat it properly. Finally, the pacing mechanism of the heart can be impaired by scarring from previous inflammation or by the presence of autoantibodies that preferentially settle in pacing tissue.

## FURTHER READING

1. Ticani A, Rabaioli CB, Taglietti M, et al. Heart involvement in systemic lupus and antiphospholipid syndrome and neonatal lupus. *Rheumatology* (Oxford). 2006;45(suppl 4):8–13.

2. Keane MP, Lynch JP. Pleuropulmonary manifestations of systemic lupus erythematosus. *Thorax.* 2000;55(2):159–166.
3. Kamen DL, Strange C. Pulmonary manifestations of systemic lupus erythematosus. *Clin Chest Med.* 2010;31(3):479–488.
4. Appenzeller S, Pineau C, Clarke A. Acute lupus myocarditis: clinical features and outcome. *Lupus.* 2011;20(9):981–988.

# 15

## *Heady Connections: The Nervous System and Behavioral Changes*

When my patients tell me they feel as though their brains had been fried, I have to know what is going on to help them. For many reasons, the central nervous system (CNS) and its related behavioral changes in lupus are the most misunderstood and mismanaged aspects of the disease. The numerous signs and symptoms that are found may indicate any of the clinical and behavioral syndromes associated with systemic lupus. Because all of these syndromes are managed differently, your doctor's carefully honed diagnostic skills will be important. Working together, patients, allied health professionals, and physicians can optimize the management of nervous system lupus.

### HISTORICAL NOTES

Neurologic involvement in lupus patients was first mentioned in 1875 by Moriz Kaposi, who described altered mental status and coma in a terminal patient. Sir William Osler, often called the father of modern medicine, described several patients with CNS lupus at the turn of the twentieth century. The first modern study appeared in 1945, and most of the reports through the 1960s dealt with *CNS vasculitis*, or inflammation of the blood vessels in the brain. A landmark report from the Massachusetts General Hospital in 1968 reviewed brain sections at autopsy in 24 individuals with lupus and surprisingly concluded that vasculitis in the brain was quite rare. As a result, for nearly 20 years there was a great deal of confusion regarding the classification of CNS lupus. In the early 1980s Graham Hughes and his colleagues described an antiphospholipid antibody known as anticardiolipin and were able to show that as many as one third of all acute CNS events were due to clots traveling to the brain or formed within the brain and not due to active lupus. This was followed by the description of cognitive dysfunction as a unique complication of systemic lupus by Judah Denburg and his colleagues in the early 1980s. New classification systems of neurologic lupus have been proposed. We review the relevant findings here.

## WHAT ARE THE MAJOR NEUROLOGIC MANIFESTATIONS OF LUPUS?

The principal neurologic manifestations of lupus are shown in Table 15.1. Most are present in several of the syndromes associated with CNS lupus.

The most common symptom of CNS involvement is *cognitive dysfunction*. Characterized by confusion, fatigue, memory impairment, and difficulty in articulating thoughts, it may be present by itself (discussed in its own section; see Cognitive Dysfunction) or as a part of active lupus. Cognitive dysfunction may also appear as a component of vasculitis, lupus headache, and organic brain syndrome, among other syndromes.

*Headaches* are a feature of the "lupus headache" syndrome (discussed in the section Lupus Headache), but they can also be a manifestation of cognitive dysfunction, CNS vasculitis, hypertension, or fibromyalgia.

*Seizures* result from acute brain inflammation, scarring from prior vasculitis, acute strokes, or reactions to medications used to treat the disease, such as corticosteroids or high-dose antimalarials.

*Altered consciousness*—such as stupor, excessive sleepiness, or coma—is observed with CNS vasculitis, but it can be induced by medication or an infectious process.

*Aseptic meningitis* is an acute condition that involves inflammation of the lining of the spinal cord (meningitis), but in which spinal fluid cultures do not

---

**Table 15.1.** *Neuropsychiatric Syndromes in Systemic Lupus Erythematosus as Defined by the American College of Rheumatology Research Committee*

1. Central
   a. Aseptic meningitis
   b. Cardiovascular disease
   c. Demyelinating syndrome
   d. Headache
   e. Movement disorder
   f. Myelopathy
   g. Seizure disorders
   h. Acute confusional state (stupor coma)
   i. Anxiety disorder
   j. Cognitive dysfunction (not thinking clearly)
   k. Mood disorder
   l. Psychosis
2. Peripheral
   a. Guillain-Barré syndrome
   b. Autonomic neuropathy (flushing, mottled skin)
   c. Mononeuropathy (numbness, burning, tingling)
   d. Myasthenia gravis
   e. Cranial neuropathy
   f. Plexopathy
   g. Polyneuropathy

grow out bacteria, viruses, or fungi. This usually indicates either CNS vasculitis or a reaction to ibuprofen (Motrin, Advil).

On occasion, a patient may develop *paralysis*. The most common causes range from strokes related to lupus anticoagulant clots or paralysis due to clots induced by antiphospholipid antibody. Vasculitis of the covering of the spinal cord, infection, or bleeding can also induce paralysis.

*Movement disorders* such as tremor, writhing motions termed *chorea*, and balance deficits (known as *ataxia*) imply disease in areas of the brain containing the basal ganglia or cerebellum. Almost any of the 12 syndromes discussed in this chapter can be responsible for movement disorders.

*Altered behavior* includes psychosis (e.g., losing touch with reality), organic brain syndrome (e.g., including a demented mental state), depression, and confusion. This behavior is differentiated from cognitive dysfunction in that these alterations are obvious to physicians and family, whereas the cognitive changes are usually subtle and often noticed only by the patient. Chemical imbalances, active disease, infection, or reaction to medication may cause altered behavior, whereas cognitive dysfunction without other symptoms usually derives from a blood flow abnormality.

When *strokes* are due to lupus, they result from high blood pressure, low platelet counts, antiphospholipid antibodies, and long-term use of steroids with premature atherosclerosis or active vasculitis.

*Visual changes* may be caused by inflammation of the optic nerve, clots resulting from antiphospholipid antibodies, medication such as steroids or antimalarials, or an uncommon condition known as pseudotumor cerebri (which involves swelling of the optic nerve).

Finally, *peripheral* or *autonomic nerves* may produce numbness, tingling, or local nerve palsies (e.g., inability to lift up the wrist).

A careful history and thorough physical examination are critical components of the diagnostic evaluation, which allows physicians to determine which syndrome they are dealing with. These syndromes are discussed below.

## LUPUS SYNDROMES OF THE NERVOUS SYSTEM

The manifestations of lupus discussed above can be part of numerous syndromes. This section examines how they appear clinically and reviews the management of the 12 principal CNS syndromes due to lupus.

### Central Nervous System Vasculitis

Elyse developed a rash while sunbathing with her high school friends. When it did not go away, her mom took her to see their family doctor, who ultimately diagnosed lupus. She was slightly anemic and had a small amount of protein in her urine. Upon taking 20 milligrams of prednisone daily, her tests started to improve and her rash disappeared. Three weeks later, she caught a flu that was going around and, within a few days, began noticing difficulty concentrating and connecting her thoughts. She had a low-grade fever that quickly rose to 104°F. Dr. Baker started her on antibiotics and a decongestant. However, Elyse developed severe headaches and a stiff neck; she also started convulsing. She was admitted to the hospital. A rheumatologist and neurologist were called in to see her in consultation. Magnetic resonance imaging of the brain was normal, but her spinal tap was consistent with CNS vasculitis based on an elevated protein and cell count as well as large amounts of antibodies to nerve cells. No evidence for infection was found. Elyse was transferred to intensive care and given high doses of intravenous steroids. She worsened for several days and became practically comatose but eventually began to respond. She was discharged 3 weeks later and, after convalescing for a month at home, finally returned to school on 20 milligrams of prednisone a day.

Vasculitis of the CNS is an inflammation of the brain's blood vessels due to lupus activity. The most serious of the CNS syndromes associated with lupus, it was the first to be described. Vasculitis of the CNS usually occurs early in the disease course; over 80 percent of episodes take place within 5 years of diagnosis. The typical patient experiences high fevers, seizures, and meningitislike stiffness of the neck, and he or she may manifest psychotic or bizarre behavior. Ten percent of lupus patients develop CNS vasculitis. Untreated, their course rapidly deteriorates into stupor and ultimately coma.

### How Is CNS Vasculitis Diagnosed?

The most helpful diagnostic studies are obtained using a spinal tap. There is no need to fear this procedure. Also known as a lumbar puncture, it sounds scarier than it is. Spinal taps are usually only minimally uncomfortable. It is, however, important to lie flat in bed for at least 8 hours afterward to avoid a post–spinal tap headache. The spinal fluid obtained from a spinal tap may indicate increased white blood cells or protein. I usually order a test known as an MS panel, so called because it was originally used to diagnose multiple sclerosis. This panel may show data suggesting an immune reaction (e.g., elevations in immunoglobin G (IgG) synthesis rates, IgG levels, or the presence of oligoclonal bands) in the CNS. Antineuronal antibodies are often present but it may take 1 to 2 weeks to be processed.

Vasculitis of the CNS can also be diagnosed in several ways. The physician may order a conventional angiogram (an X-ray study of the vessels of the brain after injecting them with dye now rarely performed), a magnetic resonance angiogram, tests to detect of antineuronal antibodies in the serum, a brain biopsy, single photon emission computerized tomography (SPECT), or positron emission tomography (PET) imaging. These tests may be negative in CNS vasculitis, but, if positive, they usually correlate with evidence from blood testing for active lupus (elevated sedimentation rates, low complements, high anti-DNA, etc.).

### How Is CNS Vasculitis Treated?

CNS vasculitis is treated with high doses of corticosteroids, which are often given intravenously. Very high doses or pulse dosing of steroids (Chapter 27) may be instituted. If improvement is not noted fairly quickly, cyclophosphamide is given intravenously with or without a blood-filtering treatment known as apheresis (Chapters 27 and 28). Sometimes an intravenous biologic known as rituximab is used. The mortality rate of CNS lupus has decreased over the last 30 years as a result of improved diagnostic testing and greater awareness of this syndrome. In the 1950s, the majority of patients with acute episodes did not have a good chance of surviving; today 80 percent of patients recover from such episodes. Unfortunately, doctors sometimes treat a condition that is not present because CNS vasculitis mimics various syndromes, some of which we address in the following discussion.

### The Antiphospholipid Syndrome

Monica thought she had licked lupus. Ten years into the disease, she was off all medication, felt well, and was working full time as a designer. Glad to be off Plaquenil and ibuprofen, Monica had lots of plans for the future. One day, while braiding her niece's hair, Monica suddenly found herself unable to move her right arm. She saw a doctor at the clinic she attended and was told that she had had a stroke. A brain magnetic resonance imaging (MRI) was ordered, which showed several small defects pointing to prior CNS episodes. The neurologist Monica was referred to confirmed the diagnosis of stroke and, in view of her history of lupus, started her on 60 milligrams of prednisone daily to rule out CNS vasculitis. However, the spinal tap results were negative, as were all blood tests for lupus activity. Monica then decided to see her rheumatologist in the next town, who stopped her prednisone and detected, through blood tests, the presence of antiphospholipid antibodies. Monica's right arm began to return to normal after several months and, as a long-term preventive measure, her rheumatologist placed her on lifelong low-dose aspirin.

Anyone who has antiphospholipid antibodies (Chapter 21) has an added risk of developing blood clots that can travel to and settle in the brain. Whether from a Libman-Sacks endocarditis (Chapter 14) or other sources, clots to the arteries or veins (called *arterial emboli* or *venous thromboses*) account for 10 to 35 percent of all sudden CNS complications in lupus. The disease does not have to be active; sedimentation rates, blood complements, and anti-DNA levels may all be normal.

Blood clots (called *thromboembolic events*) to the brain usually occur suddenly and are not associated with pain. Patients may find themselves unable to move an arm or leg, or they may develop slurred speech or acute weakness in a particular part of the body. Eventually, MRI and computed tomography (CT) show a focal defect in the affected area of the brain. Spinal fluid is usually normal. Some patients are fortunate in having warnings of these events, which may disappear after seconds, minutes, or hours and are called *transient ischemic attacks*, or *TIAs*.

I recommend that all my patients with certain types of antiphospholipid antibodies take low-dose aspirin on a continuous basis to try to prevent clots. I treat clotting episodes aggressively with anticoagulant medications (warfarin or heparin) or drugs that inhibit certain actions of blood platelets that are responsible for clotting blood, and I avoid using steroids unless lupus activity is present.

## Other Coagulation and Flow Abnormalities

Complications in the CNS may arise when one's blood becomes too thick or too thin or when it clots too easily. Sjögren's syndrome is found in up to one third of patients. Patients with Sjögren's complain of dry eyes, dry mouth, and arthritis. These patients have particularly high autoantibody levels on blood testing. Very large amounts of antibody, particularly immunoglobin M antibodies with or without Sjögren's, can increase the viscosity (thickness) of blood.

Several autoimmune disorders, including lupus, may be complicated by a condition known as *hyperviscosity syndrome*, in which blood takes on the quality of sludge and is accompanied by symptoms of confusion, dizziness, and mental clouding. Occurring as a result of an excessively large number of autoantibodies, it is treated with chemotherapy and blood filtering (*apheresis*). Similarly, a circulating protein that becomes solid in cold temperatures known as *cryoglobulin* is occasionally found in systemic lupus erythematosus (SLE). Because it "clogs up the works," this disorder, known as *cryoglobulinemia*, is very similar to hyperviscosity syndrome, sharing many of its symptoms. Often associated with the hepatitis C virus, cryoglobulinemia is more common than hyperviscosity syndrome and is usually investigated when the skin is ulcerated, has a mottled appearance, or shows vasculitic skin lesions. Cryoglobulinemia may respond to chemotherapy intravenous immune globulin, and, if needed, apheresis.

Alterations in blood clotting, which can lead to bleeding from blood vessels in the brain and therefore can mimic strokes, are observed when platelet counts become very low. Two examples of this are *idiopathic thrombocytopenic purpura* and *thrombotic thrombocytopenic purpura*. The reader is referred to Chapter 20 for more details.

## Lupus Headache

Naomi had suffered from headaches for years, but this was the headache from hell. Her lupus was responding fairly well to treatments and seemed under control. And even though she told her parents not to worry all the time, Naomi was a chronic overachiever and her parents couldn't help but be concerned. In the past, Fioricet (acetaminophen with caffeine and butalbutol) or an occasional aspirin with codeine preparation had stopped Naomi's headaches. Also, she found that when she lowered her stress level and practiced biofeedback, her headaches lessened. But neither medication nor relaxation helped this time. Her doctor gave her an injection of sumatriptan (Imitrex), which gave Naomi some temporary relief. When she was in his office, he drew blood and was puzzled to find her lupus to be more active than usual. Upon seeing these results, Dr. Metzger prescribed 20 milligrams of prednisone daily for a week, and the headache finally disappeared.

At least once a week one of my patients calls me and complains that his or her head is going to "split open." Compared with the general population, lupus patients are perhaps twice as likely to suffer from migrainelike headaches. These headaches seem to coincide with dilation of the cerebral blood vessels, but we still don't know their cause. Many patients also have antiphospholipid antibodies, whereas others display Raynaud's phenomenon (see Chapter 12), which, interestingly, is caused by restriction of the blood supply to the hands and feet. This instability in the tone (ability to dilate or constrict) of the blood vessels, which allows them to be easily altered, may result from a defect in local autonomic nervous system control.

The diagnosis of lupus headache involves a careful consideration and ruling out of other causes of headache, including high blood pressure, osteoarthritis of the neck, fibromyalgia-associated muscular tension headaches, lupus medications that can cause headaches (e.g., methotrexate, omeprazole, indomethacin), brain infections, or other cerebral pathology, such as an aneurysm, tumor, or malformation of brain vessels present from birth. The physician can rule out these possibilities by taking a history, performing a physical examination, and, if necessary, ordering an MRI scan of the brain.

Lupus headache is managed much like conventional migraine in that pain killers (analgesics) such as Fioricet, sumatriptan (Imitrex) injections, triptans, anti-inflammatories like naproxen (Naprosyn, Aleve), and/or vasoconstrictors such as ergot derivatives are used for acute attacks. Beta-blockers, anticonvulsants (Depakote, Keppra), tricyclic antidepressants, or calcium channel blockers offer a degree of prevention and may sometimes be taken all the time. Lupus headache may dramatically respond to a 1-week trial of 20 to 60 milligrams of prednisone daily, which is occasionally useful to migraine sufferers. Any lupus patient with a headache that does not respond to routine measures deserves a neurologic workup.

## Lupus Myelitis and Neuromyelitis Optica

This rare but serious complication of lupus can include paralysis or weakness that ranges from difficulty in moving one limb to quadriplegia. In lupus myelitis, the sac encasing the spinal cord is inflamed or blood clots are formed in the spinal arteries. Half of all lupus myelitis stems from antiphospholipid antibodies, and half is from active vasculitis. The physician will probably first administer steroids to treat any possible inflammation. Anticoagulant drugs, such as heparin, are frequently added. *Chronic inflammatory demyelinating polyneuropathy,* or CIDP, and post-infectious Guillain-Barré have an increased prevalence in SLE and may be responsive to intravenous immunoglobulin (gamma globulin) therapy.

Neuromyelitis optica (also known as Devic's syndrome) is a heterogeneous condition consisting of the simultaneous inflammation and demyelination of the optic nerve (optic neuritis) and the spinal cord (myelitis). Mostly seen in patients who are anti-SSA positive and difficulty to distinguish at times from multiple sclerosis, it can be seen infrequently with SLE.

## Fibromyalgia

Angela was a shy woman without a great deal of self-confidence. When she was diagnosed with systemic lupus, her self-esteem plummeted to an all-time low, and she had a terrible time coping. Angela read everything she could about lupus and was almost obsessive in her desire to control her disease. She consulted four rheumatologists before she found one who was responsive to her needs. She called or emailed Dr. Jones three times a day about every new development she thought he should know about. Her most troubling complaint was memory loss. Over the past few months, Angela had had difficulty remembering dates and suffered from severe headaches and muscle spasms. She read in medical textbooks about severe CNS disorders and became convinced that she had vasculitis. On the basis of her symptoms, Dr. Jones ran a blood panel that revealed a minimally elevated sedimentation rate and a slight increase in DNA antibody. He then prescribed 40 milligrams of prednisone a day, and she felt a bit better the first week. In time, however, her skin became so sensitive that it could not be touched. Also, Angela gained 20 pounds over the next few weeks. Her sister, who worked in a medical office, insisted that Angela see a physician who had treated her earlier in the year.

At this office visit, Dr. Wolfe explained the difference between CNS vasculitis and lupus with fibromyalgia, which he had diagnosed a year earlier. He showed how fibromyalgia can mimic inflammatory (or vasculitic) symptoms and explained that steroids make fibromyalgia worse. Angela was started on pregabalin (Lyrica) for fibromyalgia, and she was quickly tapered off the steroids.

Many of my lupus patients may complain of difficulty sleeping and cognitive problems (e.g., decreased ability to concentrate) similar to those observed in chronic fatigue syndrome as well as lack of stamina and chronic muscle-tension headaches. Fibromyalgia is a syndrome that makes a person very sensitive to pain; it afflicts 6 million Americans. Fifteen to 30 percent of patients with systemic lupus have a concurrent fibromyalgia syndrome characterized by at least 11 of 18 specific tender points throughout the body and increased pain in the soft tissues. The administration of steroids, with an adjustment of their doses, induces most of the fibromyalgia I see in lupus patients, although poor coping mechanisms, anxiety, and untreated inflammation leading to a secondary fibromyalgia are also, less commonly, causes of the syndrome.

Because medications used to treat lupus do not help fibromyalgia and corticosteroids can worsen its symptoms, I make an effort to rule out active lupus before assuming that fibromyalgia is causing these symptoms. This can be tricky and difficult. Tricyclic antidepressants, muscle relaxants, and drugs that boost chemicals in the brain such as norepinephrine, dopamine, or serotonin are used to treat the syndrome, which is reviewed in depth in Chapter 23.

## The Peripheral Nervous System

Sarah was an accomplished artist when she was told she had lupus. Fortunately, it was relatively mild and controlled with antimalarial drugs. One day, having recently gotten over a cold, she was sitting at her easel in a sunny spot outdoors. When she tried to stand up, however, she could not raise her left foot above her ankle. For the past few weeks, Sarah had noticed intermittent symptoms of numbness and tingling in her left leg and foot, but she thought nothing of it. Upon this episode she was sent to a neurologist, who performed a muscle study called an electromyogram (EMG) along with a nerve conduction study. Her "foot drop" turned out to be consistent with mononeuritis multiplex resulting from active lupus. Sarah was started on high doses of steroids for a few weeks and made a complete recovery.

I occasionally come across patients with symptoms of numbness and tingling with or without a burning sensation or an inability to move part of the body. These problems fall into the domain of the peripheral nervous system, which consists of the 12 cranial nerves that are found in the face as well as nerves emanating from the cervical, thoracic, lumbar, and sacral spine. These nerves are divided into motor and sensory roots. Impairment of motor nerves leads to problems with movement, ranging from Bell's palsy in the face to a wrist or foot drop in the extremities. Sensory defects produce numbness and tingling. The CNS includes the spinal cord and brain and is distinguished from the peripheral nervous system for purposes of diagnosis and treatment.

Between 10 and 20 percent of patients with lupus exhibit inflammation of the peripheral nervous system at some point. Peripheral neuropathies can result from inflammation of the nerves, a consequence of lupus (which is also called *mononeuritis multiplex*), or compressed nerves, which can result from lupus synovitis, as in carpal tunnel syndrome. Many other conditions are associated with peripheral neuropathies and must be considered in what physicians term a "differential diagnosis." These include fibromyalgia-induced numbness and tingling (which produces normal EMGs and nerve conduction studies), diabetes, kidney failure, neuropathy, or a herniated disc.

Inflammation in peripheral nerves is managed with short courses of moderate-to high-dose corticosteroids, and compressed nerves may respond to anti-inflammatories, local injections, splinting, or surgical decompression. A minority of lupus patients with Sjogren's syndrome or cryogloublinemia develop a chronic inflammatory polyneuropathy with widespread lower extremity burning and tingling. In addition to corticosteroids, rituximab or intravenous immune globulin may be helpful.

## The Autonomic Nervous System

When you sweat, urinate, or have palpitations, your autonomic nervous system is at work. These are the body functions we rarely think about and over which we have some control—like breathing and the heart rate. The autonomic nervous system is our "fight or flight" response to any form of stress. This system regulates adrenalin release, the tone of local blood vessels (with labile blood pressure), and muscular contractions. Rapid or slow pulse rates, sweating, feelings of hot and cold, speed of bladder and bowel transit, and burning sensations are counted among our autonomic responses. Although inadequately studied in lupus, the autonomic nervous system may also be impaired in many patients. Table 15.2 provides examples of autonomic-related complaints reported by some lupus patients.

**Table 15.2.** *Examples of Autonomic Nervous Dysfunction in Lupus*

1. *Raynaud's phenomenon:* Fingers turn different colors in cold weather
2. *Lupus headache:* A migrainelike headache from dilation of blood vessels
3. *Cognitive impairment:* Constriction of brain blood vessels decreases oxygen flow
4. *Livedo reticularis* and *palmar erythema:* Lacelike, checkerboard mottling of skin due to altered autonomic signals to superficial capillaries and increased flow through small, superficial arteries
5. *Mitral valve prolapse:* Palpitations due to release of adrenalin, which increases heart rates
6. *Numbness, burning, tingling:* Abnormal vascular tone on nerves, which activates their sensors; nerve inflammation, or tingling from nerve compression from synovitis, needs to be ruled out

## NERVOUS SYSTEM SYNDROMES THAT AFFECT BEHAVIOR

### Cognitive Dysfunction

Neil was an accountant with a large firm, and nobody knew he had lupus. Since having been treated successfully for pleurisy and joint swelling a year before, Neil would not even think about his illness, and his general practitioner had him on no treatment other than occasional aspirin. Over the past month, Neil had encountered difficulty in remembering the names of his secretary's husband, the postman, and the parking attendant. If he tried hard enough, the names came to him, but it took a few minutes. Neil was surprised to find that none of his coworkers noticed his poor recall; it was so bad that he had to look at his smart phone every hour to remember what to do next. He returned to the consulting rheumatologist, who initiated a neurologic workup that uncovered nothing unusual. However, when Neil was given some psychological tests for memory and other thinking abilities, some odd results turned up. Neil denied depression or fibrositic pain. His rheumatologist placed him on Plaquenil and 3 months later added Lexapro to reduce anxiety. Although Neil showed a 70 percent improvement, he still had to take it easy and pace himself to function well at work.

I frequently encounter lupus patients who complain of confusion as well as profound fatigue, difficulty in articulating thoughts, and memory impairment. Blood testing may confirm evidence of systemic lupus, but other tests may be normal. Conventional spinal fluid evaluations and brain imaging frequently show no abnormalities, and these individuals often look well. A superficial examination of mental function will detect no deficiencies, leaving the physician puzzled. When this occurs, some well-meaning physicians may explain to their patients that they are depressed, stressed, or having difficulty coping. They may have lupus, but the disease could not be causing their symptoms.

### How Can I Convince My Doctor This Really Exists?

Even though this scenario is still all too common, studies began to appear in the early 1980s showing that lupus could be responsible for a whole host of subtle cognitive difficulties. Behavioral testing of lupus patients revealed that up to 70 percent at times had decreased ability to focus, deficits in attention span and task completion, altered memory, and decreased problem-solving capabilities. Only 20 percent of control subjects had similar difficulties.

The cause of cognitive dysfunction is not known, but it is probably mediated by two factors. First, circulating chemicals such as cytokines (Chapter 5) may induce the syndrome. Some of these cytokines work differently in lupus patients, particularly interleukin-1, interleukin-6, and the interferons, and they have been shown to cause cognitive dysfunction when they are administered to patients and can also be found in increased amounts in the spinal fluid. However, the symptoms of cognitive dysfunction are often intermittent.

Recent work has suggested that blood-flow abnormalities (termed *hypoperfusion*) may play a role. For example, on utilizing forms of brain imaging known as positron emission tomography (PET), functional MRI (fMRI), or SPECT scanning, lupus patients with cognitive dysfunction display specific areas of the brain that do not receive enough oxygen, and this correlates with their symptoms.

Cognitive dysfunction must be differentiated from depression, fibromyalgia, and behavioral alterations due to medication, infections, strokes, or other brain disorders. In certain patients with cognitive symptoms, we sometimes find increased antibody levels that react to nerve cells in the spinal fluid and evidence of active lupus on blood testing.

## Can Anything Help Cognitive Dysfunction?

The treatment of cognitive dysfunction, which may come and go on its own, is often unsatisfactory. Emotional support and reassurance are important. Corticosteroids are a two-edged sword, and there is little evidence that these drugs alleviate the syndrome when other evidence for active lupus is not also present. I prescribe antimalarial drugs, particularly hydroxychloroquine (Plaquenil), for active lupus and quinacrine for profound fatigue. Cognitive-behavioral therapy mindfulness and regular biofeedback are quite useful. Tricyclic antidepressants or specific serotonin reuptake inhibitors (e.g., Prozac, Zoloft, Lexapro), modafanil (Provigil), amphetamine (Adderall), or vitamin derivatives may also be useful. Dehydroepiandrosterane (DHEA), St. John's wort, counseling, and gingko biloba are complementary medicine alternatives.

## Organic Brain Syndrome

Charlene barely survived an episode of CNS vasculitis when she was 20. At that time, she had high fevers, seizures, and psychotic behavior, and she lapsed into a coma for 3 weeks. Charlene is slightly mentally underdeveloped and picks up supplies for Goodwill Industries, and she is now 40 years of age. Her lupus has not been active in over 10 years. Charlene moved to the country to be with her boyfriend. She had not had a seizure in 2 years; therefore, when her epilepsy prescription lapsed, Charlene figured that it was no longer necessary. Last week Charlene had a grand mal seizure at the Goodwill loading dock. Her new doctor looked at her chart and noticed a long-standing history of lupus. He placed her on 60 milligrams of prednisone a day for presumed CNS vasculitis with seizures, but Charlene immediately became agitated and displayed psychotic tendencies. Her old rheumatologist was called, and he explained to her doctor that she had a chronic organic brain syndrome and probably had a seizure due to scarring in brain tissue because of the earlier episode of CNS vasculitis. Charlene was taken off prednisone and resumed her anticonvulsant medication.

In patients who have had a previous stroke because of antiphospholipid antibodies and in those with a history of CNS vasculitis, brain lesions heal with scarring. This results in permanent motor and mental deficits as well as seizures. These patients have what is called *organic brain syndrome* or clots. They do not have active lupus but have scars from previous inflammation related to lupus. Therefore, steroids do not help them and will only increase brain atrophy. Because blood tests and spinal fluid usually reveal that the lupus is inactive, a patient's history is very important. Organic brain syndrome is managed with emotional support and, if needed, psychotropic medications or anticonvulsants.

### Psychosis

Sometimes lupus patients may demonstrate symptoms of psychosis. *Psychosis* is defined as an inability to judge reality, marked by disordered thinking and bizarre ideas, often including delusions and hallucinations. It usually results in an inability to carry out the ordinary demands of living. The incidence of acute (and, fortunately, temporary) psychosis is between 10 percent and 15 percent during the course of systemic lupus.

Most psychotic episodes occur with CNS vasculitis, but others occur as a result of steroid therapy, water intoxication with low blood levels of sodium, seizures, inadequate antidiuretic hormone secretion, central hyperventilation, or antimalarial therapy. Psychosis may, however, be evident without CNS vasculitis.

Psychosis is managed with corticosteroids when active lupus is evident. I attempt to take a careful history to ascertain the exact use of prescription drugs, over-the-counter medications, street drugs, and herbal or vitamin remedies to assess any possible interactions. Antipsychotic preparations (phenothiazines such as Thorazine and Haldol or Risperedal; atypical antipsychotics such as Abilify) are usually used to treat this syndrome. (The management of steroid-related behavior problems is discussed in Chapter 27.)

### Functional Behavioral Syndromes

Depression and anxiety are present in at least half of all lupus patients as a consequence of stress, inflammation (which induces a rapid pulse), cytokines (which may alter mood and behavior), generalized pain (which may result from fibromyalgia), other sources of nonrestorative sleep because of medication or steroids, or inadequate coping mechanisms. These behavioral features of lupus as well as their management are discussed fully in Chapter 25.

## OTHER CENTRAL NERVOUS SYSTEM ABNORMALITIES THAT MAY ACCOMPANY LUPUS

### Complications of Medications Used to Treat Lupus

Agents used to treat lupus can cause CNS symptoms that must be distinguished from what has been described here as CNS lupus. *Nonsteroidal anti-inflammatory drugs* are infrequently the cause of headaches and may induce dizziness. Headache and confusion have been reported by 5 to 15 percent of patients taking indomethacin or methotrexate. Ibuprofen has, on rare occasions, been associated with aseptic meningitis.

Very high doses of the *antimalarials* (chloroquine, hydroxychloroquine, and quinacrine) have been associated with manic behavior, seizures, and psychosis, whereas *corticosteroids* can produce agitation, confusion, mood swings, depression, and psychosis. Certain drugs that treat *hypertension* may cause a loss of sexual desire as well as depression. Nearly every prescription medication can affect the CNS.

### CNS Syndromes Associated with SLE

*Posterior reversible encephalopathy syndrome (PRES)* has been found in an increasing number of SLE patients as well as patients with other disorders who are receiving chemotherapy. Defined by a characteristic abnormality in the white matter on MRI scanning, patients present with headache, altered mental status, and very high blood pressure. It does not represent a lupus flare and does not respond to corticosteroids but instead is reversed by vigorous control of blood pressure and monitoring of fluid intake and kidney function.

A rare form of CNS vasculitis, *acute disseminated encephalomyelitis,* can be fulminant and involves all types of brain tissue.

*Benign intracranial hypertension (pseudotumor cerebri)* is much more frequent among SLE patients than in the general population. The main symptoms are headache, nausea, vomiting, double vision, and ringing in the ears. It is diagnosed by elevated spinal fluid pressures at a lumbar puncture or swelling of the optic nerve on an ophthalmologic examination. The treatment includes the removal of spinal fluid, and corticosteroids may be prescribed as well.

### Abnormalities Not Related to Lupus Activity

Michelle had severe active multisystem lupus. Maintained on high doses of prednisone and mycophenolate, she still had rashes, fevers, swelling, pleurisy, and advanced kidney disease. One day her fever rose higher than usual, and she began experiencing seizures as well as headaches and a stiff neck. Her doctors hospitalized Michelle for presumptive CNS lupus. An MRI of her brain, however, suggested an abscess. Her spinal tap showed evidence of *Cryptococcus*, which is a fungus not usually seen in healthy people. She was started on antifungal medication, and mycohphenolate was discontinued to facilitate the medication's ability to kill the microbes. However, Michelle still required her steroids.

*Infections* of the CNS mimic CNS lupus; they must be carefully considered and ruled out, because lupus patients are especially susceptible to infection. The most common infectious agents include *Mycobacterium tuberculosis, Meningococcus, Salmonella, Shigella, Staphylococcus*, and *Streptococcus*. Opportunistic organisms are microbes that cause infection only in immunologically compromised individuals, such as those with cancer, patients taking chemotherapy and high doses of steroids, or those who have AIDS. In these people, unusual forms of bacteria, viruses, and fungi can be present. Brain imaging and spinal taps can usually allow doctors to make a definitive diagnosis.

Lupus patients develop *strokes, hypertension, psychiatric disorders, malignancies, aneurysms*, and *Parkinson's disease* at the same or greater frequency as healthy people. However, an established diagnosis of lupus clues the physician into considering other possibilities in evaluating the CNS.

Autoimmune disorders that affect the CNS include myasthenia gravis and multiple sclerosis; they have an increased incidence among lupus patients. *Myasthenia gravis* is characterized by rapid muscle fatigue with repetitive tasks, whereas *multiple sclerosis* causes blurred vision, loss of bladder and bowel control, and difficulty walking. What may add to the confusion is that one third of multiple sclerosis patients have a positive antinuclear antibody (ANA) test. Brain imaging and spinal fluid evaluations usually help differentiate multiple sclerosis from systemic lupus.

Table 15.3 summarizes the clinical, laboratory, and therapeutic features of some of the important CNS syndromes.

## NEURODIAGNOSTIC TESTING

A neurologic workup includes a lot more than blood tests and X-rays. Many of the diagnostic techniques used are unique to the CNS. Neurologic testing in lupus patients is divided into several categories, including blood tests, spinal fluid evaluations, brain imaging, electrical studies, and neuropsychological tests.

### Blood Testing

Blood testing is often helpful yet frequently unsatisfactory. It enables physicians to confirm whether lupus is present or active outside the CNS. Inflammation of the brain's blood vessels (called *cerebral vasculitis*) is usually associated with elevated sedimentation rates, low blood complement levels, and high values for

**Table 15.3.** *Major Central Nervous System Syndromes and Their Management*

| Syndrome | Incidence in Lupus (%) | Treatment |
|---|---|---|
| Cerebral vasculitis | 10 | High-dose intravenous steroids, immunosuppressives |
| Antiphospholipid syndrome with brain clots | 5 to 10 | Platelet inhibitors, anticoagulants |
| Lupus headache | 15 | Migraine therapy, steroids |
| Cognitive dysfunction | 50 | Antimalarials, psychotropics, sometimes steroids, emotional support |
| Chronic organic brain syndrome | 5 | Emotional support, seizure prevention if needed |
| Fibromyalgia | 10 to 30 | Nonsteroidals, counseling, antidepressants, physical therapy |
| CNS infection | 1 | Antibiotics/antimicrobials |
| Cryoglobulinenemia or hyperviscosity | 1 | Steroids, apheresis, chemotherapy |
| Bleed due to low platelet counts | 2 | Steroids, apheresis, chemotherapy, factor replacement, transfusion |

CNS, central nervous system.

anti-DNA. The presence of antiphospholipid antibodies along with a focal neurologic deficit suggests the antiphospholipid syndrome. Platelet counts should be checked to rule out sources of bleeding. Blood cultures should be obtained if fevers are present. On occasion, it may be important to obtain a serum viscosity or cryoglobulin level. Ribosomal P antibody has a weak association with psychotic behavior and is found mostly in lupus patients. The finding of antibodies to nerve cells in the blood is also weakly linked with active CNS vasculitis. (These antibodies are discussed in Chapter 11.)

## Spinal Fluid Analysis

A spinal tap or lumbar puncture yields cerebrospinal fluid (CSF). If blood testing does not help make the diagnosis, analysis of spinal fluid becomes important. In CNS vasculitis spinal fluid often shows a high white cell count, elevated protein levels. If available, antineuronal antibodies may also be found. An immunologic reaction (but not necessarily acute CNS vasculitis) is suggested if oligoclonal bands or increased IgG synthesis rates are found. Patients with the antiphospholipid syndrome usually have normal spinal fluid. If large numbers of red blood cells are present in all the tubes of spinal fluid obtained, bleeding from the brain's blood vessels is suggested. Infections yield positive spinal fluid cultures for bacteria or fungi. Viruses are detected by measuring levels of viral antibodies. Elevated opening pressures with headache are found with *pseudotumor cerebri* with lupus and headaches improving from fluid removal.

## Brain Imaging

X-rays of the skull are rarely helpful. Isotopic brain scans were used from 1970 to 1985. CT scans and MRI are used to reveal strokes, tumors, bleeding, and abscesses. The MRI scans are particularly sensitive and reliable in detecting these conditions. Unfortunately, there has been a tendency to misread any scan abnormality in a patient with known lupus and call it "vasculitis." Focal lesions, or lesions limited to a specific area, suggest the antiphospholipid syndrome, whereas generalized changes are consistent with CNS vasculitis. However, many normal patients and some individuals with inactive disease have minor MRI abnormalities that are difficult to interpret and mean little.

Efforts to study cerebral dynamics, or how the brain works as opposed to the strictly anatomic information derived from CT or MRI, have led to the development of PET and SPECT. Abnormal flow can be seen with intermittent cognitive issues (lupus fog) but also can be found with vasculitis. The major use of such scans (including fMRI) is to locate the part of the brain that a seizure is coming from and to show areas of decreased blood flow (hypoperfusion), which suggest cognitive dysfunction.

A *cerebral angiogram*, whereby dye is injected into the blood vessels of the brain, is a risky procedure that is rarely positive even in the presence of vasculitis. Noninvasive magnetic resonance angiography can provide nearly as much information but is abnormal in only 10 percent of patients with CNS vasculitis, because the caliber of blood vessels involved is too small to be detected.

## Electrical Studies

*Electroencephalograms* (EEGs) have been available for decades but are of little help except to identify seizure disorders. Quantitative EEGs and brain mapping studies are more precise for localizing the part of the brain from which the seizures derive. Multiple sclerosis and lupus symptoms can be localized by using electrical studies with fancy names like *brainstem evoked potentials, visual evoked responses*, and *auditory evoked response measurements*.

*Electromyograms* (EMGs) with nerve conduction velocity testing evaluate peripheral nerve problems. They can differentiate a herniated disc from inflammatory nerve or muscle lesions, diabetic numbness, mononeuritis multiplex, and nerve compressions such as carpal tunnel syndrome.

## Behavioral Surveys

Several psychological tests have been employed to detect cognitive dysfunction, ranging from the *Minnesota Multiphasic Personality Inventory (MMPI)* to the *Luria-Nebraska test*, the *Halsted-Reitan test*, automated neuropsychiatric assessment metrics, and the *Wechsler Adult Intelligence Scale*. Most neuropsychologists have their own battery of tests customized to the nature of their practice. Specific lupus neuropsychiatric inventories are being evaluated. Although no combination of testing has been validated as being more reliable than any other, these evaluations can help physicians identify depression, psychosis, cognitive dysfunction, and neuroses, among other behavioral disorders.

## SUMMING UP

The majority of patients with systemic lupus have neurocognitive problems or active inflammation that leads to CNS problems. A wide array of possibilities may account for any given symptom, and a careful workup is necessary to avoid inappropriate therapy. The most common complaints include cognitive dysfunction, headache, and fatigue. Manifestations of vasculitis, the antiphospholipid syndrome, and altered behavior are not infrequent. Drugs, infections, and non-lupus-related disorders first have to be ruled out as a cause of the complaint or manifestation. Blood and spinal fluid testing, brain imaging, electrical studies, and neurocognitive evaluations help the physician arrive at a diagnosis. The treatment of CNS lupus can include a combination of anti-inflammatory medications, blood thinners, and emotional support.

## FURTHER READING

1. ACR Ad Hoc Committee on Neuropsychiatric Lupus Nomenclature. The American College of Rheumatology Nomenclature and Case Definitions for Neuropsychiatric lupus syndromes. *Arthritis Rheum.* 1999;42(4):599–608.
2. Ellis SG, Verity MA. Central nervous system involvement in systemic lupus erythematosus: a review of neuropathologic findings in 57 cases, 1955–1977. *Semin Arth Rheum.* 1979;8(3):212–221.
3. Kozora E, Ellison MC, West S. Reliability and validity of the proposed American College of Rheumatology neuropsychological battery for systemic lupus erythematosus. *Arthritis Rheum.* 2004;51(5):810–818.
4. Hanly JG, Su L, Farewell V, et al. Prospective study of neuropsychiatric events in systemic lupus erythematosus. *J Rheumatol.* 2009;36(7):1449–1459.

# 16

## *The Head, Neck, and Sjögren's Syndrome*

If you are a lupus patient, do you find it hard to see clearly? Do your ears ring? Do you get crops of mouth sores? Do you suck on hard candy constantly to make your mouth less dry? Have you ever lost your voice? The eyes, ears, nose, mouth, salivary glands, and larynx are occasionally affected by lupus as either a manifestation of active disease, the antiphospholipid antibody syndrome, or an adverse reaction to lupus medication. Even though they are present in only a minority of cases, pertinent head and neck symptoms and signs are too important to be overlooked. This section reviews the head and neck areas and how problems in these areas are related to lupus.

### HOW DOES LUPUS AFFECT THE OUTER EYES?

There's more to the eye than what we see. The human body's sight organ is divided into several layers, all of which can be inflamed with active systemic lupus erythematosus (SLE). *Discoid lesions* resembling the skin condition called eczema are occasionally observed around the eyelids. The eye muscles may become swollen or inflamed, which is called *orbital myositis*, or temporarily paralyzed due to a *cranial neuropathy*, because 3 of the 12 cranial nerves (peripheral nerves) control the movement of eye muscles. If diabetes and thyroid conditions are ruled out as the cause of orbital pathology, corticosteroids can relieve these conditions.

*Conjunctivitis*, or inflammation of tissues around the eyeball, is more common among lupus patients because they are more susceptible to infection. Antibiotic solutions can keep conjunctivitis in check, but the presence of conjunctivitis does not indicate more active disease. Patients with Sjögren's syndrome (see Sjögren's Syndrome section) have decreased ability to manufacture tears. When the cornea (the outer covering of the eyeball) cannot be adequately lubricated, it becomes dry and develops pits, leaving scarred areas on its surface. Artificial tears, pilocarpine, cyclosporine, eye drops, or punctal occlusion are examples of treatments usually helpful in such cases.

## DOES LUPUS AFFECT SIGHT?

### What about Cataracts, Glaucoma, or Uveitis (Iritis)?

The *uveal tract*, or middle layer of the eye, includes the iris, lens, and ciliary muscles. Lupus does not directly induce *cataracts*, or the clouding of the lens, but corticosteroids can. Similarly, these agents are associated with a greater risk of developing *glaucoma*, which is caused by elevated pressure in the eye. Cataracts can be removed surgically, and eye drops lower increased ocular pressure.

Inflammation of the iris, or *iritis* (also known as *uveitis*), is a recurrent problem in 1 to 2 percent of lupus patients. It has been observed in almost every autoimmune disease and exists as an autoimmune disorder by itself. Iritis is managed with steroid eye drops, but at times oral corticosteroids, immunosuppressives, or intraocular injections of steroids are needed.

### The Retina

Rachel woke up blind in her right eye. She had a history of mild SLE but had generally felt well. Rachel was married to a stockbroker on the West Coast who was already at work at 6 AM; she felt helpless. Michael and she had been trying to have children, and these efforts culminated in two heartbreaking miscarriages. Rachel placed a call to her internist. The internist referred her to an eye doctor. She saw him that day. He performed a fluorescein angiogram that documented a clot in her retinal artery. Rachel was admitted to the hospital, where she was anticoagulated with an oral heparin. A rheumatologist was called in to see Rachel, and her workup documented evidence for antiphospholipid antibodies. Gradually, her sight improved, and within 3 months she had only a small blind spot that did not bother her.

The back layer of the eye is known as the *retina*. It is the only part of the body in which physicians can actually see internal blood vessels in their entirety. Although antimalarial drugs or infectious agents infrequently damage the retina, 10 percent of lupus patients develop visible retinal pathology. *Retinal vasculitis*, or inflammation of the retinal vessels, can be painful and cause visual changes. Usually seen with active disease, it is treated with corticosteroids. On the other hand, sometimes areas of "infarction," or dead tissue, are noted in the retina. These *cytoid bodies*, as they are called, indicate either old, healed retinal vasculitis or signify that a clot has traveled to the eye as a complication of the antiphospholipid syndrome (Chapter 21). Steroids will not benefit these patients; blood thinning or anticoagulation is the treatment of choice.

When another cranial nerve known as the optic nerve is inflamed, *optic neuritis* results, causing varying degrees of visual impairment. This must be differentiated from blurred vision induced by corticosteroids.

## DOES LUPUS CAUSE HEARING OR EAR PROBLEMS?

In general, lupus patients have no unusual or specific hearing deficits. They may complain of *tinnitus*, or ringing in the ears, due to anti-inflammatory medications such as antimalarials or nonsteroidal anti-inflammatory drugs. This is especially common in those over the age of 60.

One lupus patient in 500 has a rare complication known as *autoimmune vestibulitis*, characterized by sudden hearing loss with or without visual changes or dizziness. Antibodies to a 68-kd inner ear protein may be associated with this. Corticosteroids reverse this deafness.

On rare occasions, the cartilage lining the outer part of the ear becomes inflamed in active SLE, producing a condition known as *chondritis*. It appears identical to another autoimmune disease called *relapsing chondritis*, where cartilage in the trachea, nose, and valves of the heart can also be inflamed. In SLE, however, chondritis is usually limited to the ear and responds to steroids.

To sum up, ear problems are very rare in SLE and, if present, usually stem from nonimmunologic sources.

## THE NOSE

Some of my patients have been wrongly accused of using cocaine when they have nasal septal perforations. The nasal septum—the cartilage membrane that divides the nose into two nostrils—can perforate, or develop holes, in 1 to 2 percent of lupus patients. *Ulcerations* may also be found on the nasal mucosa. I usually prescribe petroleum jelly (e.g., Vaseline) or a steroid preparation (e.g., Kenalog in Orabase) for these. Recurrent sinus infections that do not improve with antibiotics, decongestants, or antiallergy medications in a patient who seems to have lupus warrants a blood test for a closely related disorder known as *granulomatosis with polyangittis* (formerly Wegener's granulomatosis). A blood test for antineutrophilic cytoplasmic antibody can help differentiate these two types of vasculitis, which are treated quite differently.

## DENTAL CONSIDERATIONS

Very few patients realize the importance of good oral hygiene as an adjunct in managing SLE. Because the mouth is teeming with bacteria, some rheumatologists believe that all dental procedures should be accompanied by prophylactic antibiotics to protect patients with lupus from developing infected heart valve vegetations (Chapter 14) or other types of infections. Those who have temporomandibular joint (TMJ) involvement from SLE or oral sclerodermalike tightening of the lips with decreased opening of the jaws find chewing more difficult and may develop cavities and abscesses. They should see their dentist at least once a year for a check-up.

Sores in the mouth, or *oral ulcerations*, are seen in 20 percent of lupus patients and are discussed in Chapter 12. Sjögren's syndrome causes dryness of the mouth (see the Sjögren's Syndrome section).

## WHAT IS THE REASON FOR THE RASPY VOICE?

The voice box (vocal cords) is in the larynx. A synovially lined joint known as the cricoarytenoid joint is found in this area (Chapter 13). Lupus activity sometimes produces synovitis. When the synovium of the cricoarytenoid joint becomes inflamed as a result of active disease, a hoarse voice can develop. Ear, nose, and throat specialists see evidence of this when they perform direct laryngoscopy. Anti-inflammatory medications can relieve the problem, although sometimes the joint may be sprayed with a steroid aerosol or locally injected.

## SJÖGREN'S SYNDROME

### Do the Skin and Eyes Feel Dry?

Laura was unable to wear the contact lenses her optometrist had prescribed. A fashion model, Laura tried her best not to think about her lupus, but fortunately the condition was limited to her skin (which could be covered with hypoallergenic makeup) and symptoms of occasional aching and fatigue. The only other medicine she took was Naprosyn for intermittent joint pain. The optometrist referred her to an ophthalmologist, who diagnosed Sjögren's syndrome. She prescribed artificial tears and told Laura to drink plenty of fluids. When Laura told this to her rheumatologist, he added Plaquenil and cyclosporin eye drops (Restasis) and gave her literature from the Sjögren's Syndrome Foundation, which listed over 100 over-the-counter moisturizing agents for the ears, nose, mouth, eyes, and vagina. Laura's joint aches and fatigue improved, but she still had to use moisturizing agents.

### What Is Sjögren's Syndrome?

In 1933 Henrik Sjögren (pronounced "show-gren") described some symptoms common to a group of patients: dry eyes (*keratoconjunctivitis sicca*), dry mouth (*xerostomia*), and arthritis. In the late 1960s, doctors found that many patients with these symptoms had an autoimmune process. Sjögren's syndrome, as the disorder is now known, can be part of many autoimmune diseases or may exist by itself (termed *primary Sjögren's*) without fulfilling accepted criteria for any other process. It is estimated that 5 to 10 percent of all Sjögren's patients have SLE, although the incidence of Sjögren's in established SLE patients has not been reliably ascertained. We do know that at least 10 percent of the individuals with

**Table 16.1.** *Clinical Features of Sjögren's Syndrome*

| |
|---|
| Common |
|     Dry eyes (keratoconjunctivitis sicca) |
|     Dry mouth (xerostomia) |
|     Arthralgias (joint aching) |
| Found in 10% to 50% of patients |
|     Parotid gland enlargement |
|     Dry cough (bronchitis sicca) |
|     Vaginal dryness |
|     Atrophic gastritis |
|     Peripheral nerve disease |
|     Hypothyroidism |
| Found in <10% of patients |
|     Lymphoma |
|     Pancreatitis/biliary cirrhosis |
|     Renal tubular acidosis |
|     Interstitial lung disease |

lupus have obvious Sjögren's. However, if minimally or asymptomatic patients with lupus undergo vigorous testing for the syndrome, perhaps as many as one third would fulfill accepted Sjögren's definitions. See Table 16.1.

### How Do We Diagnose Sjögren's and Why Is It Important?

Some of the procedures used to diagnose Sjögren's include the *Schirmer's test*, which measures the amount of tearing, or *lissamine green staining* of the cornea, which looks for pitting or areas of scarring. Although simple to perform, these procedures have false-positive and false-negative results. The ultimate and most accurate diagnostic test is a *lip biopsy*, which displays a characteristic inflammatory infiltrate. Fortunately, it is rarely necessary to do this potentially uncomfortable procedure. Many Sjögren's patients have enlarged salivary glands.

Why is it important to diagnose Sjögren's? First, the syndrome is associated with disease outside the salivary glands and tear ducts. For example, a persistent, nonproductive hacking cough is a manifestation of dry lungs or *bronchitis sicca*, which predisposes one to interstitial lung disease (Chapter 14). Other related disorders include atrophic gastritis (dry stomach), hyperviscosity syndrome (thick blood), cryoglobulinemia, and subacute cutaneous lupus rashes. The anti-Ro (SSA) antibody (Chapter 11) is noted in 30 percent of those with SLE but 70 percent of those with primary Sjögren's (Table 16.2). This antibody crosses the placenta and has the capability of inducing neonatal lupus and congenital heart block (see Chapter 22). Of all rheumatic diseases, Sjögren's correlates with the highest levels of autoantibodies. It is not unusual for Sjögren's patients to have antinuclear antibody tests or rheumatoid factors with levels well over several thousand. Sjögren's is associated with the HLA-DR3 marker (Chapter 7). Also,

**Table 16.2.** *2016 American College of Rheumatology/European League Against Rheumatism Classification Criteria for Primary Sjogren's Syndrome*

| Item | Weight/Score |
| --- | --- |
| Salivary gland biopsy demonstrating Inflammation | 3 |
| Anti SSA/Ro positivity | 3 |
| Ocular staining suggestive of Sjogren's | 1 |
| Positive Schirmer's test | 1 |
| Decreased salivary flow rate | 1 |

Adapted from *Ann Rheum Dis* 2017;76:9–16. One meets criteria with a total score of 4 or greater.

Sjögren's syndrome is the only autoimmune condition that has a potential for malignant transformation. Up to 10 percent of Sjögren's patients develop a blood disorder, particularly lymphoma. I obtain from patients a serum protein electrophoresis, an inexpensive blood test, at least once a year to partially screen for this. A group of patients have dry eyes or mouth but do not fulfil criteria for Sjogren's syndrome. They have *sicca syndrome*, which unlike Sjogren's does necessarily require having an immunologic process. Sjogren's is subset of sicca syndrome, whereas the latter can derive from viruses, medications, or radiation therapy and found in very dry climates.

### How Should Sjögren's Be Managed?

Despite all that has been said, Sjögren's syndrome is usually a relatively benign process, and its treatment is symptomatic. For instance, dry eyes usually respond to artificial tears and dry mouth to everything from plugging tear ducts to sucking on hard candy (although frequently used, Lifesavers are discouraged because of their high sugar content), to drinking sparkling water with a touch of lemon, lime, orange, grapefruit, or any other citrus fruit. A humidified environment or room humidifiers can be helpful. Chicken soup moisturizes the lungs, as do several drugs that can promote humidification. Recently, some evidence has suggested that hydroxychloroquine (Plaquenil) helps to mitigate the underlying immune process of Sjögren's. Pilocarpine (Salagen) and cevimeline (Evoxac) promote increased salivary secretions. Cyclosporin or lifitigrast eye drops (Restasis, Xiidra) ameliorate dry eye symptoms and signs. Most experiences with prescribing corticosteroids for Sjögren's have been disappointing except when they are used for a short time in a rare subset of Sjögren's called *Mikulicz's syndrome*, in which the parotid or salivary glands become greatly enlarged from acute inflammation. This condition is readily identified, because patients appear to have the mumps, and the salivary glands are extremely tender to the touch.

Organ-threatening disease may benefit from the use of immune suppressive agents such as rituximab, mycophenolate mofetil, cyclophosphamide, methotrexate, or azathioprine.

## SUMMING UP

The most common cause of head and neck involvement in SLE is Sjögren's syndrome. Eye complaints are often due to medication, especially steroids, but 10 to 15 percent of patients with lupus develop complications from disease activity or the antiphospholipid antibody. Ulcers of the mouth or nose are seen in 20 percent of these patients. Involvement of the ear or larynx is rare. Patients and their physicians must carefully evaluate head and neck complaints, because failure to intervene promptly with autoimmune inflammation of the optic nerve or the ear can result in permanent blindness or deafness.

## FURTHER READING

1. Wallace DJ, ed. *The Sjogren's Book: Sjogren's Syndrome Foundation*. Oxford: Oxford University Press, 2011.
2. Heath KR, Rogers RS, Fazel N. Oral manifestations of connective tissue disease and novel therapeutic approaches. *Dermatol Online J.* 2015;21(10):pii:13030/qt7030d6gd.

# 17

## What about Hormones?

Why are women disproportionately afflicted with systemic lupus erythematosus (SLE)? Do men have milder or more severe cases than women? Are there hormonal imbalances unique to lupus? Is there any relationship between the disease and endocrine (hormonal) tissues, such as the thyroid and adrenal glands? Because it was first observed that 90 percent of lupus patients are women and 90 percent of these patients develop the disease during their childbearing years, it seemed logical to study hormonal relationships in SLE. This section reviews these approaches.

The basic science of gender immunity is reviewed in Part III, and use of hormonal interventions such as birth control pills and estrogens, among others, is discussed in Chapters 13 and 28.

### UNDERSTANDING HORMONES

A hormone is a chemical made by one organ that is transported in the blood to another organ, where it carries out its function. There is an area in the brain, known as the hypothalamus, that is responsible for manufacturing a group of chemicals known as *releasing hormones*. When these chemicals travel a short distance to another area called the anterior pituitary gland, the releasing hormones promote the production of *stimulating hormones*. These stimulating hormones are secreted into the bloodstream and travel to the peripheral endocrine glands or other body organs.

For example, the hypothalamus makes thyroid-releasing hormone, which induces pituitary production of thyroid-stimulating hormone, which, in turn, prompts the thyroid gland to make thyroid hormone. Other hormones derived by similar mechanisms include cortisol, made by the adrenal gland, and prolactin, which is made in the anterior pituitary and results in the secretion of breast milk. The female reproductive organs produce estrogen and progesterone; male hormones are called androgens, with testosterone being the most important. Figure 17.1 illustrates these hormonal pathways.

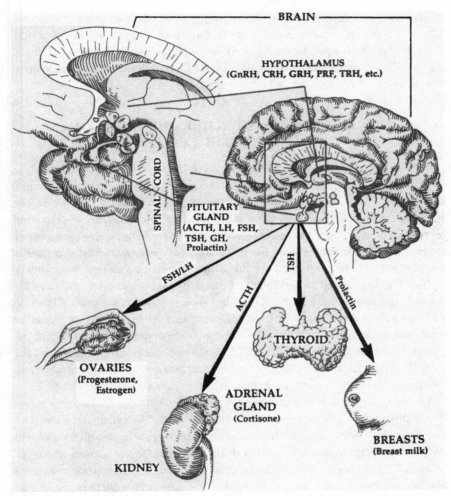

**Figure 17.1** *Hypothalamic and Pituitary Hormonal Pathways*

## HOW IS THE ENDOCRINE SYSTEM ALTERED IN SYSTEMIC LUPUS?

What happens to sex hormones in lupus patients? Sex hormones act on the immune system in three ways. First, they stimulate the central nervous system to release immunoregulatory chemicals. Second, they regulate the production of cytokines (Chapter 5). Finally, sex hormones stimulate endocrine glands to release other hormones, such as prolactin, in women.

*Estrogens* (female hormones) can promote autoimmunity, and this can indirectly increase inflammation, whereas androgens (male hormones) generally suppress autoimmunity. Estrogens increase the production of autoantibodies, inhibit natural killer cell function, and induce atrophy of the thymus gland. Further, in SLE, estrogens are metabolized differently. Due to an abnormality in a chemical pathway (called 16 alpha-hydroxylation), lupus patients have excess levels of 16 alpha-hydroxyestrone and estriol metabolites. Males with lupus have lower-than-normal levels of testosterone and other androgens.

## IS THERE A DIFFERENCE BETWEEN MEN AND WOMEN WITH SYSTEMIC LUPUS?

How do males with SLE fare? This information has been surprisingly difficult to ascertain. For instance, to study outcomes in a scientifically acceptable fashion, a large group of men with SLE must be followed closely for at least 5 and preferably 10 years. Because 90 percent of those with SLE are women, this requires studying several hundred patients. Interestingly, no studies suggest that males have a better prognosis. Published reports are evenly divided between males having a similar outcome to that of females and those suggesting that men have a poorer prognosis.

If SLE is aggravated by female hormones, why might males fare worse? This question has stumped the best and brightest rheumatologists for years. One possible answer recalls a fascinating survey performed in the 1960s that would be extremely difficult to repeat in today's research environment. In that report, the gender of fetuses from women with SLE who miscarried was tabulated, and the majority were males. This suggests that male fetuses with a lupus gene are more likely not to be born, which may explain why there are so few men with SLE.

On the other hand, a rare chromosomal disorder known as *Klinefelter's syndrome* provides investigators with contradictory clues. A normal female carries two X chromosomes (XX—both female) and a normal male one X (female) and one Y (male) chromosome (XY). Individuals with Klinefelter's are men who carry an extra X chromosome (XXY). It has been suggested that Klinefelter's patients have an increased incidence of SLE and that this is directly related to female hormone excess. Also, inactivated X chromosomes (women have XX) enriched with hypomethylation can be bound and activated by TLR7 and 9, which is associated with SLE and T cell activation.

## MENSTRUAL PROBLEMS IN SLE

One of the most frequently asked questions I encounter deals with the relationship between lupus and menstruation. *Amenorrhea,* or the absence of menstruation, is observed in 15 to 25 percent of women with SLE between the ages of 15 and 45 and can be related to prior chemotherapy or severe disease activity. Irregular periods are not uncommon. For example, nonsteroidal anti-inflammatory drugs increase bleeding, and changes in corticosteroid doses or steroid shots into joints or muscles can alter menstrual cycles. A pregnancy test should always be performed before any medical treatment directed toward amenorrhea or menstrual irregularities is initiated.

*Premenstrual syndrome* (PMS) may be more severe in SLE, and the majority of women with lupus report a mild premenstrual flare in their musculoskeletal symptoms, and they usually respond to several days of ibuprofen or naproxen (Advil, Aleve). The onset of *menopause* is associated with less SLE activity, and premature onset of it is not uncommon among lupus patients.

## THYROID DISEASE

Vanessa was feeling achy and under a lot of stress. When she visited her doctor, he decided to take an antinuclear antibody (ANA) test, which came back positive, and he told her she might have lupus. She was very edgy and couldn't focus on any task for more than 3 minutes. She increasingly became aware of palpitations and was always turning up the air conditioning. A rheumatologist was consulted, who confirmed that the ANA was positive, but it was in a low-level speckled pattern. The blood panel also included other autoantibodies, and her thyroid antibodies were markedly elevated. Blood testing showed that she had elevated thyroid function and was hyperthyroid. A diagnosis of Graves' thyroiditis was made; Vanessa did not have lupus. When antithyroid medication failed to suppress her symptoms adequately, she was given radioactive iodine to drink, which prevented the gland from making thyroid and allowed her to feel normal again. She is now maintained on a low dose of thyroid replacement.

The thyroid gland in the neck helps regulate our metabolism, and it affects how we feel by controlling the production of thyroid hormone. Thyroid-related symptoms—such as fatigue, palpitations, fevers, being too hot or too cold, and joint aches—can often be mistaken for SLE.

Autoimmune disease of the thyroid is characterized by detectable levels of antithyroid antibodies in the blood. Clinically manifested as *Graves' disease* or *Hashimoto's thyroiditis*, autoimmune thyroid disease initially appears as hyperthyroidism (overactive thyroid) and ultimately develops into hypothyroidism (underactive thyroid). Approximately 10 percent of lupus patients have thyroid antibodies, and autoimmune thyroiditis occasionally coexists with SLE. Many of these individuals also have Sjögren's syndrome. Conversely, many people like Vanessa with primary autoimmune thyroid disease have positive ANA tests without evidence of lupus.

Whether autoimmune thyroiditis is present, some 1 to 5 percent of those with SLE studied at any point are hyperthyroid, and 1 to 10 percent are hypothyroid.

In other words, thyroid abnormalities are commonly noted in lupus and are related to antithyroid antibodies about half of the time.

## DIABETES MELLITUS

The most common cause of diabetes in SLE patients is corticosteroid therapy. Steroids raise blood sugars, and the risk of developing diabetes depends on how much prednisone the patient has been taking and for how long. Diabetes sometimes disappears when steroid doses are lowered or discontinued.

The islet cells of the pancreas are endocrine tissues responsible for producing insulin. Interestingly, many individuals with juvenile diabetes (called type I) have positive ANAs even though lupus is uncommon in this group of patients.

## THE ADRENAL GLAND

*Corticotropin releasing hormone* (CRH) in the hypothalamus stimulates the production of *adrenocorticotropic hormone* (ACTH) in the pituitary, which induces the secretion of various types of cortisone (steroids) by the adrenal gland (see Figure 17.1). The adrenal gland can be affected directly and indirectly in systemic lupus.

The direct effects include an autoimmune inflammatory process known as *autoimmune adrenalitis*, whose concurrence rate with SLE has not been determined. In addition, the *antiphospholipid syndrome* (see Chapter 21) may result in clots to the adrenal gland's blood supply, which leads to infarction, or death of adrenal tissue.

The administration of oral (exogenous) corticosteroids suppresses internal (endogenous) secretions of steroids from the adrenal gland. The normal adrenal gland makes the equivalent of 7.5 milligrams of prednisone daily. Higher oral steroid doses turn off the adrenal gland. When steroid doses are decreased below 7.5 milligrams, the gland is supposed to resume steroid production. However, when one has been on corticosteroids for a prolonged time, the adrenal response is sluggish and symptoms of adrenal insufficiency, such as fatigue and aching, may become evident. When the adrenal gland does not make enough cortisone, symptoms of *adrenal insufficiency* become manifest and can mimic a lupus flare-up. See Chapter 27.

## WHAT ABOUT PROLACTIN—THE BREAST HORMONE?

*Prolactin* is a hormone that provides the stimulus needed to produce breast milk. Over the last few years several investigators have documented that a disproportionate number of lupus patients have elevated prolactin blood levels. Bromocriptine (Parlodel) and cabergoline (Dostinex) are agents that block prolactin, and they may help lupus patients.

## SEXUAL DYSFUNCTION: DO LUPUS PATIENTS
## HAVE A PROBLEM?

It's rare for women with lupus to be unable to enjoy sexual intercourse. Female sexual dysfunction because of disease activity is unusual in SLE. The two well-established exceptions are vaginal dryness from Sjögren's syndrome and vaginal ulcerations, which are rare compared to oral or nasal ulcerations. Both of these conditions can result in painful intercourse. Vaginal dryness is managed with lubricants and ulcerations, with a hydrocortisone ointment. Physiologic sexual problems unique to males with lupus have not been reported.

Sometimes women with avascular necrosis or other destructive changes in the hip have difficulty spreading their legs apart during sex. Until corrective surgery can alleviate this, lupus patients and their partners are urged to use alternatives to the missionary (man on top) position, such as the woman being on top or rear entry. (In Chapter 25, psychological and emotional aspects of lupus are discussed in more detail.)

## DO LUPUS PATIENTS HAVE ANTIBODIES TO SEX
## HORMONES?

Even though sexual problems of a physiologic nature are unusual, many lupus patients have antibodies to reproductive hormones. As many as 30 percent of women with lupus have antiestrogen and antiovarian antibodies in their blood. The presence of the antibodies does not really matter and has nothing to do with fertility, except that they are more common in patients taking birth control pills. Males with SLE have an increased prevalence of antisperm antibodies. Again, this has no known clinical relevance.

## SUMMING UP

Hormones are substances secreted by an endocrine gland in response to stimulation by the brain. They are capable of modulating immunologic reactions, but the extent to which this is clinically useful is not known except that female hormones tend to promote immune responses, whereas male hormones are more immunosuppressive. Nevertheless, male lupus is often more severe than female lupus. Patients with SLE have an increased incidence of antibodies to glandular tissue and autoantibodies to reproductive organs, but the significance of this is not known. Sexual dysfunction is uncommon except that a few women with SLE have disease-related vaginal dryness, vaginal sores, or arthritic hips.

## FURTHER READING

1. Ferrari SM, Elia G, Virili C, Centanni M, Antonelli A, Fallahi P. Systemic lupus erythematosus and thyroid autoimmunity. Front Endocrinol (Lausanne). 2017;8:138.
2. Fatnoon NN, Azarisman SM, Zainal D. Prevalence and risk factors for menstrual disorders among systemic lupus erythematosus patients. Singapore Med J. 2008;49(5):413–418.

# 18

## *The Impact of Lupus on the GI Tract and Liver*

The largest organ system in our body is the gastrointestinal (GI) tract. If it were laid out on a floor, the area from the throat to the anus would extend for 40 feet. So it should come as no surprise that such an important part of the body can be involved in lupus. Actually, it is surprising that only limited portions of the gastrointestinal system are involved in the disease. This chapter will cover the relevant information for the lupus patient.

In addition, the GI system includes closely related regions that are not part of the GI tract per se but either empty into it or have closely interrelated functions. These areas consist of the liver, pancreas, and biliary tree (bile ducts and gall bladder). To lend some order to this section, we will start at the top and work down. Figure 18.1 highlights the anatomy of the GI tract.

### TAKE A GULP!

The upper GI tract begins in the throat and ends just beyond the stomach. Starting from the top, persistent sore throats are common complaints of children with systemic lupus erythematosus (SLE), even though nothing is usually found on physical examination. (Mouth sores are discussed in Chapter 12 and dental hygiene in Chapter 16.)

The oral cavity gives way to a long tube called the esophagus, which carries food and liquid nourishment from the mouth, behind the chest cavity and heart, and finally to the stomach. Esophageal problems in SLE are of two types: those related to muscle dysfunction and symptoms related to reflux, or heartburn. The upper part of the esophagus wall contains a type of muscle called *striated* and the lower esophagus a type of muscle called *smooth*. The upper muscles are responsible for swallowing. Patients with certain other rheumatic diseases such as inflammatory myositis (dermatomyositis or polymyositis) have a high incidence of *dysphagia*, or difficulty swallowing. Interestingly, they seem to tolerate solid foods quite well, but liquids may come up through the nose and are sometimes aspirated into the lungs. Approximately 10 percent of patients with lupus have a

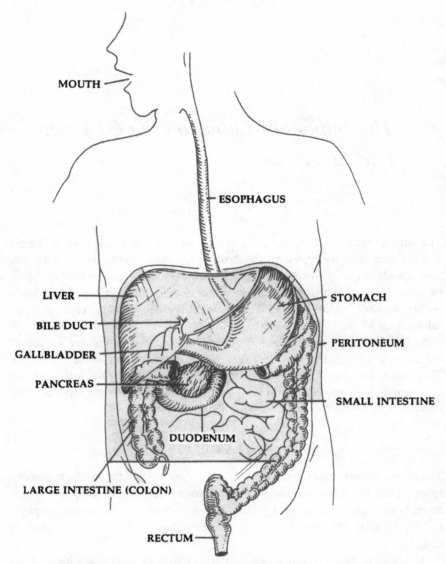

**Figure 18.1.** *Functional Anatomy of the Gastrointestinal Tract*

crossover (mixed connective tissue) disease with components of inflammatory myositis with overlapping connective tissue disorders.

Imaging or *esophageal manometry* (which measures pressure) easily identifies the syndrome. About once a year, I encounter an individual whose swallowing problem has posed such a significant threat of aspiration pneumonia or malnutrition that I have one of my colleagues in head and neck surgery perform a procedure on the muscles known as a cricopharyngectomy, which usually eliminates the problem.

## WHY DO LUPUS PATIENTS GET HEARTBURN?

Phil always had a sensitive stomach. When he started treatment for lupus, his doctor prescribed naproxen, which relieved his joint pain but gave him a mild gastritis. Phil had a long-standing history of heartburn, which worsened around the time he was diagnosed. An upper GI X-ray endoscopy was normal except for evidence of a hiatal hernia (fluid going back into the esophagus from the stomach from displacement). He tolerated the gastritis and didn't tell anybody about it. Three months later, he attended a Bruins football game. After an afternoon of fun and frolic that included eating the end-zone pizza, consuming two Bruin dogs, and drinking three beers, Phil began to feel as if he was digesting this haute cuisine again and again. He thought that if he took an extra naproxen it might help his stomach pain. The next morning he passed black, tarry stools and nearly passed out. His family took him to an emergency room. When blood was drawn, he was markedly anemic with a hemoglobin count of 6. Dr. Gordon took him to have an endoscopy (visualization of the stomach), where Phil was diagnosed as having a hiatal hernia, erosive gastritis, and a duodenal ulcer. Lucky to be alive, Phil was given a transfusion, started on Omeprazole, taken off naproxen, and given an appointment with the nutritionist.

Ten to 50 percent of lupus patients have problems with the esophagus, making them painfully aware that this organ is not lined to protect itself from acid. Though esophageal tissue is not equipped to handle acid, stomach tissue is specially lined to do so. The esophagus empties into the stomach, which makes acid. There are a couple of reasons why fluid from the stomach ends up back in the esophagus, or produces *reflux esophagitis* or *gastroesophageal reflux disorder (also known as GERD)*.

It could be the way a person is built. The stomach may be higher than usual, and the sphincter (a muscle) between the esophagus and stomach is weakened. This anatomic anomaly is a common finding in both healthy patients and particularly patients with lupus; it is called a *hiatal hernia.*

It could also be that one's lower esophageal muscles may be incompetent and fail to propel materials into one's stomach correctly. Patients with crossover or mixed connective tissue disease have components of scleroderma and/or myositis and are especially predisposed to these problems. The net result of acidic stomach fluid entering the esophagus is not only heartburn but also scarring, adhesions, and even poorer peristalsis (propulsion of the lower esophagus) from chronic "burns."

An upper GI X-ray endoscopy is usually diagnostic. On occasion, an upper GI endoscopy identifies additional problems, At this procedure the esophagus can be dilated, which may help to relieve symptoms. With heartburn, people often automatically reach for antacids, which is a natural and understandable reflex. But it's only part of the solution. Esophageal motility problems are managed by eating small, frequent meals rather than a few large ones, and patients are generally instructed not to lie down for at least 2 hours after eating. Antacids, H2 antagonists (e.g., cimetidine, ranitidine), sodium sucralfate (Carafate), and especially proton-pump inhibitors (e.g., pantaprazole, omeprazole, esomeprazole) are all effective to varying degrees.

## INTERNALS AND EXTERNALS: NAUSEA, VOMITING, BLOATING, DIARRHEA, AND CONSTIPATION

Anita experienced a change in her bowel habits. After a particularly stressful experience at work, she began having diarrhea alternating with constipation with mucousy stools. This was associated with bloating, cramping, and distension. After a complete GI workup that ruled out other possibilities, Dr. Berk diagnosed her as having functional bowel disease. Around the same time, Anita's internist told her that the muscle and joint aches she complained about in her upper back and neck areas and which were keeping her up at night were due to a closely related disorder known as fibromyalgia. Well-controlled on probiotics and a high-fiber diet, even Anita's fibromyalgia improved. Then she was diagnosed with SLE. Wondering whether lupus had affected her intestines all along, Anita requested and her doctor performed another evaluation, which showed no evidence of lupus activity in the GI tract. Dr. Berk diagnosed her as having a flare-up of functional bowel syndrome, which was resulting from generalized lupus activity.

At various times, many of my patients complain of nausea, vomiting, diarrhea, or constipation. The most common sources of these complaints are nonsteroidal anti-inflammatory drugs (NSAIDs), corticosteroids, and chemotherapy. The rest of the bowel complaints listed here are what doctors label *functional*. In other words, they represent a disorder that carries several names, including *functional bowel disease, spastic colitis*, and *irritable bowel syndrome*—all of which are related to abnormal intestinal motility or are due to malfunctioning of the autonomic nervous system. This condition correlates with the presence of fibromyalgia (see Chapter 23), which is not part of SLE. It is, however, seen in a large number of lupus patients. Occasionally, the symptoms of nausea, vomiting, diarrhea, or constipation reported by SLE patients are due to lupus or a concurrent inflammatory bowel disease such as ulcerative colitis.

## THE MICROBIOME AND BACTERIAL GUT HEALTH

It has been known for many years that in certain autoimmune conditions such as scleroderma are characterized by *small intestinal bacterial overgrowth*. This produces bloating and distension. It is more common in lupus patients who have a scleroderma overlap and responds to intermittent courses of an antibiotic known as rifaximin, as well as probiotics and other antimicrobial therapies.

Healthy individuals have large amounts of healthy bacteria in their intestine of all different types. This sum of our bacterial make-up is called the *microbiome*. Recent work has suggested that some lupus patients may have a specific types of bacterial makeup in their gut. It is unknown what this means, but it is predisposed to increased inflammation in the body. As of now, there is no specific lupus diet, but in the next few years, there may be food or food groups that make a lupus patient feel better, or others that should be avoided.

## PEPTIC ULCER DISEASE

Have you ever experienced a pain in the pit of your stomach that would not go away? Until 1975, 20 percent of patients with SLE developed an ulcer during the course of their disease. With the introduction of medications such as H2 blockers (Tagamet, Zantac, Pepcid, Axid), sodium sucralfate (Carafate), and proton-pump inhibitors such as omeprazole (Prilosec), as well as an agent known as misoprostol (Cytotec), the number of lupus patients with ulcers has decreased to less than 5 percent. Though necessary to treat the disease, NSAIDs and corticosteroids can all produce erosions in the stomach or duodenum of the small intestine, leading to ulcerations. Fortunately, selective cox-2 blocking NSAIDs (such as celecoib, or Celebrex) and nonacetylated aspirin products are much less likely to cause an ulcer than the older nonsteroidals. Gastric ulcers caused by the bacterium *Helicobacter pylori* may be more common in SLE and are treated with erythromycin-based antibiotics, ampicillin, bismuth solutions, and proton-pump inhibitors.

## IS INFLAMMATORY BOWEL DISEASE ASSOCIATED WITH SLE?

Somewhere between 1 and 4 percent of lupus patients experience severe, crampy abdominal pain with chronic diarrhea. They have developed a second autoimmune process known as *ulcerative colitis*. Characterized by inflammation of the superficial lining of the colon (large intestine), ulcerative colitis is treated with aspirin/sulfa antibiotic combinations (e.g., sulfasalazine), anti-TNF rheumatoid arthritis therapies, and, if necessary, steroids, among others. Patients with lupus may have difficulty tolerating some sulfa derivatives.

*Crohn's disease* (or *regional ileitis*) and SLE are both autoimmune diseases, but curiously, very few patients are victims of both disorders. Because both are autoimmune diseases, an increased concurrence with SLE would be anticipated. In fact, lupus and Crohn's disease have been reported together only infrequently in the world's literature. These conditions can be diagnosed by antibody testing, imaging, and colonoscopy.

## WHAT IS ASCITES?

Some lupus patients notice a swelling in their belly and feel as though they are pregnant. It has been estimated that at some point 5 to 10 percent of lupus patients demonstrate *ascites*, a collection of fluid made by peritoneal tissue. The perito-neum is a thin membrane that lines the abdominal cavity, just as the pleura and pericardium line the lung and heart. We have already shown how pleurisy and per-icarditis develop as a result of irritation of these linings (Chapter 14). Peritonitis evolves similarly. Irritation of the peritoneum results in fluid formation (ascites) throughout the abdominal area. Ascitic fluid, like pleural fluid, is either a transu-date or an exudate.

*Transudates* (clear, sterile fluids) are painless and common when pleural or pericardial effusions are also present. Nephrotic syndrome, a condition observed when the kidney leaks protein, is also associated with ascites. *Exudates* can be painful and are thicker and cloudier, producing ascites when there is an infec-tion, malignancy, pancreatitis, or serious inflammatory process in the abdomen. Usually identified at physical examination, ascites is also diagnosed by an ultra-sound or computed tomography (CT) scan.

When ascites is diagnosed, I usually arrange to have some of the fluid removed for microscopic analysis and culture to help identify its source and cause, which, in turn, suggests appropriate management. Exudative ascites can be mistaken for a "surgical abdomen," resulting in unnecessary surgery. If an infection is ruled out, ascites is treated with anti-inflammatory medication, gentle water pills (diuretics), and occasionally periodic drainage. Infections are treated with antibiotics.

## MALABSORPTION: PROTEIN-LOSING ENTEROPATHY AND CELIAC DISEASE

Have you ever felt that the food you eat isn't getting into your system? Severe diarrhea with very low serum protein (especially albumin) levels is rare in SLE, but when it does occur, it should tip off the lupus specialist that protein is being lost through the intestine as a consequence of malabsorption. Abdominal pain may also be present. Among those who suffer from malabsorption, 90 percent are children; less than 1 percent of the adults with SLE malabsorb their food. *Protein-losing enteropathy*, as this symptom complex is called, is treated with corticosteroids.

Celiac disease can be an autoimmune malabsorptive intestinal disorder found when patients are sensitive to gliadin, or wheat products. It can be diagnosed by biopsy or by ordering a celiac autoantibody panel and is treated with die-tary restriction. Half of those with gluten sensitivity don't have celiac disease but are allergic, or hypersensitive, to wheat products. Only one-third of those with gliadin associated antibodies actually have celiac disease, but those with the antibody should see if limiting gluten or wheat products helps their gastrointestinal complaints.

## LESS FREQUENT COMPLICATIONS: MESENTERIC VASCULITIS, INFARCTION, AND BOWEL HEMORRHAGE

Jackie had a severe case of lupus, being treated with 40 milligrams of prednisone a day, which her doctor wanted to raise. Jackie, however, had become diabetic and developed high blood pressure already. Because she was still getting used to having lupus, she was not ready for the increase in medication. One morning she developed a fever, severe abdominal pain, and bloody diarrhea. Her doctor hospitalized Jackie and called in a surgical consultant. The diagnosis of an acute abdomen was made, and she was taken to surgery. In surgery, her doctors discovered vasculitis along with a small perforation that resulted from steroid use. Nutrition became a major problem, and peritonitis set in that seemed resistant to all antibiotics. Her situation is critical, and her doctors are not sure she will make it. They are hopeful that aggressive, innovative approaches will help.

If cramping and abdominal pain are associated with vomiting, fever, and bloody stools, an immediate call to the doctor is in order. *Mesenteric vasculitis*, or inflammation of the blood supply to the small and large intestines, is one of the most serious complications of lupus. It calls for urgent intervention because it is life threatening. Even in the best of hands, this condition is associated with a high mortality rate. Estimates suggest that 1 to 3 percent of lupus patients may develop this complication. Patients on steroids are especially at risk because the hormone thins the lining of the bowel and makes it more susceptible to perforation.

The blood supply to the bowel can also sustain blood clots in patients with antiphospholipid antibodies (Chapter 21), which also leads to *mesenteric infarction*. This implies that not enough oxygen is getting to the bowel tissue because of an interruption in the blood supply. Both mesenteric vasculitis and antiphospholipid antibodies can induce mesenteric infarction.

Because the body cannot survive for more than a week or two with infarcted or "dead" bowel, surgical removal of this tissue is necessary. The best way for a doctor to approach mesenteric vasculitis or infarction is to be on the lookout for it. Few rheumatologists who regularly treat lupus patients see this complication more than once every 2 to 3 years. Additionally, if vasculitis is evident, corticosteroids are given; if a clot is present, the patient is given anticoagulants after surgery.

## THE BILIARY TREE

Bile is formed in the liver, stored in the gallbladder, and drained into the duodenum of the small intestine through bile ducts. Systemic lupus rarely affects this region except for the pancreas. The pancreas is a secretory and endocrine organ. It makes digestive enzymes that help the intestine break down food and empty it into the duodenum through the biliary tree. As an endocrine organ, the pancreatic islets manufacture insulin. Cirrhosis of the bile ducts is rarely noted in lupus patients who also have Sjögren's syndrome. These patients have elevated serum gamma glutamyl transpeptidase (GGT) levels and automicrochondrial or smooth-muscle autobodies. They respond to a medicine known as ursidiol.

## WHAT ABOUT THE PANCREAS?

Wendy thought she would die. Although her lupus was under reasonably good control with steroids and Imuran, she never knew back pain could be as bad as this was. It occurred suddenly after an evening of drinking beer with her college roommate, who had just broken up with Wendy's former boyfriend. At 3 AM, Wendy noticed the sudden onset of searing back pain and knew she had overdone it. Her roommate took her, screaming in pain, to the emergency room, where her serum amylase count was 2,000 and a diagnosis of acute pancreatitis was made. Dr. Dietz was not sure if the pancreatitis was from her prednisone, azathioprine (Imuran), alcohol abuse, or lupus. Her rheumatologist was asked to see Wendy. She stopped all medication except for intravenous steroids; she also ordered intravenous fluids, pain medicine, and nasogastric suction. It took a week for Wendy to start coming around, and the culprit was not active lupus but either Imuran (which was not resumed) or lifestyle habits. Wendy was told that she could not have any alcohol at any time, and she has adhered strictly to this regimen.

I hope you never experience the severe midabdominal pain radiating to your back that Wendy had, which is associated with nausea, vomiting, and fever. In lupus, several mechanisms contribute to this extremely painful form of pancreatic inflammation known as *pancreatitis.*

Certain agents used in the management of lupus have been found to provoke pancreatitis. These include corticosteroids, azathioprine (Imuran), and thiazide diuretics (e.g., hydrochlorothiazide, Dyazide). Vasculitis of the pancreatic blood supply is the second most common cause of pancreatitis in SLE. One can also develop pancreatitis for the same reasons that otherwise healthy people do—alcohol abuse, gallstones, and physical trauma to the back, where the pancreas is.

Ultrasounds or CT scans are obtained to look for gallstones or "cysts" in the pancreas (pancreatic pseudocysts), which could be perpetuating the problem. A form of autoimmune pancreatitis with elevated immunoglobin G4 subclass levels that is also associated with Sjögren's syndrome and biliary cirrhosis has also been described.

The management of pancreatitis is quite problematic. Because pancreatic vasculitis is treated with steroids and steroid-induced pancreatitis is treated with steroid withdrawal, this serious process is first approached with general measures until the cause is determined. These include giving the patient nothing by mouth, supplying intravenous hydration, putting a tube through the patient's nose that goes into the intestine to remove secretions, and administering pain medicine. If previously prescribed, thiazide diuretics and azathioprine are discontinued. If generally active lupus is evident, steroid doses can be briefly but greatly increased to treat presumed pancreatic vasculitis. Should steroids be found culpable, they are tapered but cannot be abruptly discontinued. Despite aggressive measures, recurrence is common, and the process can go on for months.

## HOW DOES LUPUS AFFECT THE LIVER?

How can one tell if one's liver is involved? Most of the time, no symptoms or signs are evident until advanced disease is present. On occasion, right-sided upper abdominal pain or distension, fevers, or a yellow appearance are clues. Lupus activity in one form or another in the liver is evident in numerous ways that are delineated in the following discussion.

Involvement of the liver in SLE is a frequently misunderstood complication of the disease. It can be affected as a result of both lupus and medications used to treat inflammation. The concept of what constitutes *autoimmune (lupoid) hepatitis* has undergone many changes since it was first described in the 1950s. This section attempts to reconcile our differing perceptions of what "lupus in the liver" really means.

*Enlargement of the liver*, or hepatomegaly, is found in 10 percent of patients with SLE. The liver is rarely tender unless the enlargement is so great that the capsule or covering of the organ is stretched. The most common causes of large livers in lupus include autoimmune hepatitis, ascites, congestive heart failure, or a complication of a large spleen, whose materials drain into the liver.

*Jaundice*, the condition we think of as turning a patient yellow, is seen in 1 to 4 percent of patients with lupus. Manifested by high serum levels of bilirubin, which are responsible for that yellow pigmentation and itching, jaundice results from autoimmune hemolytic anemia, viral hepatitis, cirrhosis, or bile duct obstruction from gallstones, tumor, or pancreatitis. Occasionally, certain medications, including NSAIDs and azathioprine, may produce jaundice.

*Hepatic vasculitis*, or inflammation of the small- and medium-sized arteries of the liver, is extremely rare and is noted in just 1 lupus patient per 1,000. It responds to corticosteroids.

*Budd-Chiari syndrome* results from a blood clot in the portal veins, which drain materials from the liver into the vena cava. Those patients with antiphospholipid antibodies appear to be uniquely at risk for developing these clots. Additionally, hepatic artery clots may occur. Untreated Budd-Chiari syndrome can lead to ascites, elevated liver pressure (called portal hypertension), and liver failure. The preferred treatment of Budd-Chiari syndrome is anticoagulation (blood thinning).

*Ascites*, already discussed, may also reflect liver failure.

## Why Are Liver Blood Tests Abnormal?

*Abnormal liver function tests* may be found in 30 to 60 percent of patients with lupus at some point and cause no symptoms. Blood enzyme evaluations included in routine blood panels such as aspartate aminotransferase (AST; also called serum glutamic oxaloacetic transaminase [SGOT]), alanine aminotransferase (ALT; also called serum glutamic pyruvic transaminase [SGPT]), alkaline phosphatase, and GGT may be elevated from a variety of mechanisms.

First, nearly all NSAIDs as well as acetaminophen (Tylenol) can elevate these enzymes, and lupus patients—for unclear reasons—appear to be particularly susceptible to this. These abnormalities are usually of little consequence and generally represent false alarms, unless they are greater than three times normal. Also, active lupus can elevate these enzymes. Most nonsteroidals can be stopped for a week or two and the enzymes rechecked. If they remain increased, the possibilities for this elevation include hepatitis, infection, biliary disease, cancer, pancreatitis, alcoholism, or active lupus.

Second, lupus patients are predisposed to a *fatty liver.* This is associated with the use of corticosteroids, nonsteroidals, and metabolic syndrome (obesity, insulin resistance and high lipid levels).

## What Is Autoimmune (Lupoid) Hepatitis?

Amanda did not feel right. She complained of vague right-sided upper abdominal discomfort for several months before seeing her doctor. Her examination demonstrated tenderness in this area, a low-grade fever, and distension. Blood tests revealed sky-high liver function studies. She was referred to a gastroenterologist, who embarked upon a workup that included a liver biopsy. It demonstrated chronic active hepatitis. Because Amanda did not have a history of viral hepatitis or alcohol abuse and because her hepatitis virus, cytomegalovirus, toxoplasmosis, and other tests were negative, autoantibodies were examined. These were consistent with autoimmune hepatitis. Amanda responded to steroids at first, but after 3 years she began developing abdominal swelling, rectal bleeding, and mental slowing. Imuran was added to her prednisone as an immunosuppressive regimen, to which Amanda responded. A special diet was strictly enforced, and mild water pills were prescribed. This prolonged matters for another year, until it was evident that Amanda was experiencing liver failure. At that point, she underwent a liver transplant and is doing fine 3 years later.

*Lupoid hepatitis* is a complicated and controversial entity. Described in 1955 and coined by Ian Mackay in 1956, lupoid hepatitis has undergone many changes in definition. The overwhelming majority of patients who were told they had lupoid hepatitis between 1955 and 1975 would not fulfill current criteria. Initially thought of as the presence of chronic active hepatitis ("hepatitis" meaning inflammation of the liver) with lupus erythematosus cells, the term *autoimmune hepatitis* seemed more appropriate, because few of these patients had typical clinical lupus. Patients with autoimmune hepatitis first notice right upper abdominal pain along with malaise, nausea, aching, and low-grade fevers. Loss of appetite, light-colored stools, and dark urine may also be present.

The development of diagnostic tests to detect hepatitis A, B, and C has changed our concepts of autoimmune hepatitis. The current working definition of autoimmune hepatitis is (i) liver disease consistent with chronic active hepatitis; (ii) absence of evidence for active hepatitis virus A, B, or C infection; and (iii) a positive antinuclear antibody test or other autoantibodies associated with the syndrome.

Even using these criteria, only 10 percent of patients at the Mayo Clinic with autoimmune hepatitis fulfilled the American College of Rheumatology criteria for lupus (Chapter 2). Many of the physical findings associated with SLE (e.g., rashes, other organ involvement) are usually absent. Because lupus patients have compromised immune systems and can develop a viral hepatitis, they take medications that can affect liver function, and some abuse alcohol just as non-lupus patients do (which can lead to a chronic active hepatitis), diagnosing autoimmune hepatitis can be tricky. About 30 to 60 percent of those with autoimmune hepatitis also have antibodies to smooth muscle or mitochondria (AMA or SMA).

## How Is Autoimmune Hepatitis Treated?

Why is it so important to split semantic terms to come up with the correct type of hepatitis? Because autoimmune hepatitis, if untreated, can be fatal within 5 years. However, it can respond to agents including steroids, 6-mercaptopurine, and azathioprine. Several of our patients have undergone successful liver transplants, and we have come a long way in our understanding of liver disease in lupus and autoimmune hepatitis. But it still takes a great deal of skill to sort out what is an autoimmune disease and what is viral and, thus, what medication is appropriate in each case.

## SUMMING UP

Difficulty in swallowing must be taken seriously. Heartburn and acid indigestion can be brought on by medication, stress, or active lupus. Nonspecific bowel symptoms are common and can be managed symptomatically unless a fever, localized tenderness, swollen abdomen, or bloody stools are present. These manifestations warrant prompt medical attention. The liver can be involved in lupus because of reactions to medication, antiphospholipid antibodies, or as a complication of infection. Vasculitis in the liver is rare, and autoimmune hepatitis should be carefully investigated and ruled out.

## FURTHER READING

1. Talotta R, Atzeni F, Ditto MC, Gerardi MC, Sarzi-Puttini P. The microbiome in connective tissue disease and vasculidites: an updated narrative review. *J Immunol Res.* 2017;2017:6836498.
2. Adiga A, Nugent K. Lupus hepatitis and autoimmune hepatitis (Lupoid hepatitis). *Am J Med Sci.* 2017;353(4):329–335.
3. Ebert EC, Hagspiel KD. Gastrointestinal and hepatic manifestations of systemic manifestations of systemic lupus erythematosus. *J Clin Gastroenterol.* 2011;45(5):436–441.

# 19
## Lupus in the Kidney and Urinary Tract

The kidneys are critical to long-term health, and medicine has come a long way in understanding how they play a central role in many diseases. Unfortunately, in up to 40 percent of lupus patients, the disease can affect how the kidneys function. Though some do not require treatment, most forms of kidney disease, termed *lupus nephritis*, warrant aggressive management. After discussing the functional anatomy of the kidney, the symptoms and signs of lupus nephritis are reviewed, followed by a classification of kidney disease and an overview of its therapy.

### HOW DOES THE KIDNEY WORK?

Think of the kidneys as the body's waste treatment plant. The body's wastes are filtered by the kidneys and then excreted in urine. The two kidneys are bean-shaped organs tucked neatly behind the abdominal cavity, level with the upper lumbar spine. Blood flows to the *nephron*, the functional unit of the kidney, and each kidney's approximately 1.2 million nephrons are divided into two parts. The first part is the *glomerulus*, a series of small, circular corpuscles through which materials are filtered and most reabsorbed back into the blood. The filtrated blood drains into the second part of the nephron, the *tubule*, which both reabsorbs and secretes electrolytes (e.g., calcium, phosphorus, bicarbonate, sodium, potassium, chloride, and magnesium), glucose, and amino acids. These tubules form into the *ureter*, which connects to the *bladder*—the collecting area of materials destined for excretion. The kidney is principally responsible for maintaining the volume and composition of body fluids, excreting metabolic waste products, detoxifying and eliminating toxins, and regulating the hormones that control blood volume and blood pressure. Additionally, it is responsible for helping control the production of red blood cells and cell growth factors.

Lupus primarily affects the glomerulus and produces a condition known as *glomerulonephritis*. The medullary *interstitium* is the tissue surrounding the loop of Henle in the renal medulla. It functions in renal water reabsorption by building up a high hypertonicity, which draws water out of the thin descending limb of the loop of Henle and the collecting duct system and can be involved in the inflammatory process.

Figure 19.1 shows the functional anatomy of the kidney.

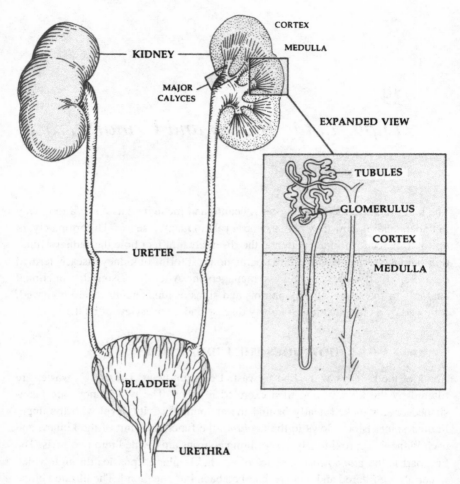

**Figure 19.1.** *The Female Kidney and Urogenital System*

## HOW CAN YOU TELL WHEN THE KIDNEY IS INVOLVED?

Lupus patients don't say, "Doc, my kidney hurts!" Pain in the kidney area would be felt if the patient had developed pleurisy, a kidney stone, or severe kidney infection or had suffered a muscular spasm of the lumbar spine. Except for pleurisy, none of these ailments have anything to do with lupus. In fact, most patients with kidney involvement have no specific complaints that can be immediately traced to the kidney. There are two circumstances that initiate awareness of a kidney problem in SLE patients: when they become *nephrotic* or *uremic*. In nephrotic syndrome, the kidney spills large amounts of protein due to a filtering defect, and serum albumin levels become very low. When serum albumin levels drop below 2.8 grams per deciliter (g/dL) or per 100 milliliters and 24-hour urine protein measurements rise above 3.5 grams, swelling is apparent in the ankles and abdomen. Lower amounts of protein loss may result in mild ankle swelling. The patient may complain of a general sense of bloating and discomfort. Pleural and pericardial effusions may be noted, and shortness of breath or chest pains are occasionally present. In uremia, a failing kidney inadequately filters wastes and toxic materials accumulate, which can damage other tissues. When a kidney is functioning at a level below 10 percent of normal, the patient will probably complain of fatigue, look pale, and emit a distinct odor. Patients suffering from advanced uremia must go on dialysis to live.

Because patients with lupus nephritis usually have few obvious symptoms, how can doctors tell whether the kidney is involved? They do it through blood and urine testing. Elevations in the serum *blood urea nitrogen* (BUN) or *creatinine* usually reflect an abnormality in kidney function and indicate renal involvement. A *urinalysis* is the most accurate assessment for the presence of lupus nephritis. Patients with SLE have cellular debris called *casts*, visible in urine when viewed under the microscope. Many different types of casts can be found, including hyaline, granular, or red cell casts. Most nephritis patients have *hematuria*, or at least small amounts of microscopic blood in their urine. The most specific correlate of lupus nephritis is *proteinuria*, or protein in the urine. The presence of protein can be determined quickly and painlessly with a urine test in the doctor's office. If proteinuria is found, most physicians attempt to quantitate it by having the patient collect the urine for 24 hours; then the amount of protein in the sample is measured. A spot urine (the urine protein/creatinine ratio) can also be used to estimate 24-hour urine excretion. Expect the 24-hour urine protein to exceed 300 milligrams when lupus is active in the kidney. Nephrotic patients have protein levels between 3,500 and 25,000 milligrams. As part of a 24-hour urine collection/ spot urine, the *creatinine clearance* can be calculated.

## WHAT ARE THE TYPES OF LUPUS GLOMERULONEPHRITIS?

When lupus affects the kidney, it makes sense for a rheumatologist to seek consultation from a kidney specialist (nephrologist) to obtain a renal biopsy. A renal biopsy is recommended if there is abnormal urine sediment (e.g., casts, hematuria) and more than 500 milligrams of protein in a 24-hour urine specimen. Renal biopsies are performed for three reasons: (i) to confirm the diagnosis of lupus nephritis as opposed to another disease; (ii) to determine if the kidney tissue is inflamed, scarred, or both; and (iii) to evaluate for potential treatments. Treating a patient with an elevated creatinine who has significant scarring but no inflammation with anti-inflammatory medication for the kidney is not advisable. There is no reason for using potentially toxic medicines without cause.

Tissue obtained at biopsy is examined by three methods. First, it is stained to look for structural abnormalities and viewed under a standard microscope. Second, the sample is evaluated for antibodies to the gamma globulins immunoglobins G,

A, and M under an immunofluorescent microscope. Finally, the tissue specimen is examined with an electron microscope to search for "electron-dense deposits," which are immune complexes that interfere with the kidney's ability to filter materials properly. Most nephrologists obtain enough material to give the pathologist an opportunity to use all three methods. Occasionally, only a small amount of tissue is available, which permits a more limited evaluation.

These methods allow kidney tissue to be classified according to the International Society of Nephrology/Renal Pathology Society system of six different patterns. In *Class I*, the light microscopy is normal and electron microscopy shows minimal abnormalities. No treatment is indicated. *Class II* disease is termed *mesangial* and reflects mild kidney involvement. Low doses of steroids are sometimes given. *Class III* is called *focal proliferative* nephritis, whereas *Class IV* is *diffuse proliferative*. Proliferative disease, both types being extensions of the same process, is a serious complication and will usually lead to *end-stage renal disease*, necessitating dialysis if it is not treated. *Class V* glomerulonephritis is known as *membranous* and is characterized by a high incidence of nephrosis with a tendency toward a slow, indolent, progressive course ending with renal failure if not treated. *Class VI* nephritis is known as *glomerulosclerosis* and represents a scarred-down, end-stage kidney with irreversible disease. However, it can also include interstitial nephritis. Historically, end-stage SLE or Sjögren's nephritis with scarring and glomerulosclerosis was labeled as Class VI nephritis. However, recent work has suggested that subtle changes in the interstitium can regulate inflammation in the kidney, and may be as the glomerulus. See Table 19.1.

A doctor usually performs a kidney biopsy in a hospital in a radiology suite with ultrasonic guidance. An ultrasound examination should confirm the location of the kidneys and that the patient has two of them. The risk of bleeding from the biopsy in experienced hands is small—1 in 100 patients needs a blood transfusion, and 1 in 1,000 will have a serious complication. Most patients are able to go home within 36 hours of the biopsy without any work or activity restrictions.

**Table 19.1.** *Kidney Biopsy Patterns Found in Systemic Lupus Erythematosus*

| ISN/RPS Class | Name | 10-Year (%) Dialysis Risk | Treatment |
|---|---|---|---|
| I | Nil disease | <1 | None |
| II | Mesangial | 10 | Low- to moderate-dose steroids |
| III | Focal proliferative | 50 | Steroids, immunosuppressives |
| IV | Diffuse proliferative | 50–75 | Steroids, immunosuppressives |
| V | Membranous | 30 | Steroids, immunosuppressives |
| VI | Glomerulosclerosis/ interstitial | High | None/not known |

ISN/RPS, International Society of Nephrology/Renal Pathology Society.

Occasionally, renal biopsies are ill advised or require special preparation. These circumstances include patients who weigh over 250 pounds (they require an open biopsy at surgery), patients who are very anemic and/or who cannot risk or refuse blood transfusions (e.g., Jehovah's Witnesses), or individuals who have unique clotting problems that predispose them to unusual bleeding risks or require continuous anticoagulation.

## HOW DO WE MONITOR KIDNEY DISEASE?

There is no one test that best assesses lupus in the kidneys. The BUN and creatinine tell doctors how well the kidney is functioning. High blood pressure signals that the kidney is under stress, and persistent elevations are associated with the development of kidney failure. Low serum albumins and urine protein measurements tell physicians how much leakage there is. Low C3 complement levels and high anti-DNAs in the blood indicate active proliferative lupus inflammation. Microscopic evaluation of a freshly voided urine specimen can roughly suggest how active the nephritis is. I follow nephritis patients by taking their weight (to measure fluid retention) and blood pressure. Blood and urine are obtained as well as a urine protein/creatinine ration or and a 24-hour urine collection is measured if indicated. These evaluations will reveal a general pattern of improvement, stabilization, or worsening and will suggest alterations of therapy if needed. In the next few years, urinary biomarkers and functional magnetic resonance imaging will teach us a lot more about inflammatory activity.

## ARE THERE OTHER FORMS OF LUPUS KIDNEY DISEASE BESIDES GLOMERULONEPHRITIS?

Although they rarely cause symptoms, many *commonly used drugs can affect renal function*, the most common of which are nonsteroidal anti-inflammatory drugs (NSAIDs). Some of them, particularly indomethacin, can raise serum creatinine as part of their action against a chemical called prostaglandin. A normal serum creatinine is up to about 1.3 mg/dL. If the creatinine is slightly above this level, nonsteroidals should probably be used only for a few days, and the blood should be carefully monitored. Circumstances in which this might arise would be an acute attack of gout or bursitis. Because creatinines are measured in terms of a logarithmic function rather than an arithmetic one, a serum creatinine of 2 indicates only 50 percent kidney function, 3 means 30 percent kidney function, and 4 signifies 20 percent kidney function. (Remember logarithms from high school? A rise in creatinine from 2 to 3 indicates a tenfold change!) Patients with a serum creatinine above 6 mg/dL usually require dialysis. The use of NSAIDs is not advised if the creatinine is above 2.

Other drugs can induce an *interstitial nephritis*, which inflames and then scars the connective tissue of the glomerulus. Certain antibiotics and anti-inflammatory drugs are included in this group. Sjögren's syndrome is associated with *tubular dysfunction* (particularly due to *renal tubular acidosis*), which leads to electrolyte abnormalities. High blood pressure also damages kidney tissue and is capable of inducing renal failure regardless of SLE activity. Patients with antiphospholipid antibodies are predisposed toward developing *renal vein thrombosis*, especially if they have membranous nephritis. This condition can result in acute renal failure, flank (side of the back) pain, and fever. It is managed with anticoagulation and steroids if the lupus is active.

## WHAT IS THE NATURAL COURSE OF LUPUS NEPHRITIS, AND HOW DO WE TREAT IT?

When Dr. Cohn told Gillian she had lupus in her kidney, it was not an easy thing to say to a promising concert pianist. At the time, her ankles were so swollen that Gillian couldn't wear any shoes other than an old pair of sneakers. Her anti-DNA levels were high and serum complement levels low. Dr. Cohn arranged for a kidney biopsy, which showed class IV (diffuse proliferative) disease with a lot of activity and little scarring. He told Gillian that she had a reversible lesion and needed chemotherapy as well as steroids. She was started on 60 mg of prednisone a day and received six monthly doses of intravenous cyclophosphamide at the hospital infusion center as an outpatient. During this time, Gillian gained 40 pounds, became moody and irritable, and could not concentrate on her practicing. After 6 months, she began to improve. Her creatinine was high normal at 1.3, and her 24-hour urine protein had decreased from 7 grams to 3. At this point, Dr. Cohn extended the cyclophosphamide treatments to every 3 months for a year and then added mycophenolate (CellCept) and tapered her prednisone to 10 mg a day. Gillian did well for a year, but her blood pressure began to go up, as did her cholesterol and blood sugars. She was started on blood pressure medicine and put on a strict low-fat, low-carbohydrate diet. Five years later her creatinine was 2.6, along with a 24-hour urine protein of 1.3 grams. Dr. Cohn arranged for a second biopsy that showed little lupus nephritis activity but a lot of damage from hypertension and scarring. Her medicine was kept the same.

Being on the road a lot, Gillian tried the best she could to keep to her diet, but it was not easy. After 10 years of nephritis, Gillian's creatinine finally crept up near 7, and she was placed on hemodialysis. Fortunately, her brother was able to donate a kidney, and she underwent a successful transplant. Fifteen years later, her creatinine is 1.0, and she is on 10 mg of prednisone a day; mycophenolate, and tacrolimus to prevent transplant rejection; a diabetes medicine; a cholesterol medicine; and a blood pressure medicine. At age 30, Gillian teaches music at a junior college.

Patients with class I and II biopsy patterns have an excellent outcome. Class V is relatively resistant to therapy, even though most rheumatologists try a course of corticosteroids with or without *immunosuppressive regimens.* Some of the drugs that fall into this category include azathioprine, cyclophosphamide, mycophenolate mofetil, or tacolimus, all of which are discussed in Chapters 27 and 28. Class VI usually leads to end-stage renal disease within months, and no specific therapy is indicated. Class III or IV proliferative nephritis is reversible some of the time with aggressive therapy. High doses of corticosteroids with or without immunosuppressives (particularly intravenous cyclophosphamide, or Cytoxan; azathioprine, or Imuran; or mycophenolate mofetil, or CellCept) can prolong kidney function and prevent the need for dialysis over a 10-year period in half the patients. (See Chapter 28.)

Is there anything you can do to prevent the effects of kidney disease? High blood pressure should be managed aggressively because it accelerates functional kidney impairment. Stress reduction helps lower blood pressure. Patients with renal disease should restrict their salt intake to no more than 3 grams a day; when renal function is 50 percent or less, normal protein intake should also be restricted. Diuretics help remove fluid in lupus patients and make them feel more comfortable, but they must be used cautiously, because they alter electrolyte balance. Potassium supplements are given to patients with normal kidney function on most diuretics. However, potassium intake is restricted in patients with markedly impaired renal function.

## HOW ARE THE URINARY TRACT AND BLADDER AFFECTED BY LUPUS?

The ureter is not involved in lupus, and the bladder is a rare target of the disease. But a condition known as *lupus cystitis* is observed in 1 to 5 percent of those with lupus. Manifested by inflammation of the lining of the bladder with blood in the urine, cystitis can be diagnosed by an office procedure known as cystoscopy. Lupus cystitis frequently correlates with gastrointestinal malabsorption. It is treated with antibiotics and anti-inflammatory lupus medications. Occasionally, pentosan polysulfate sodium (Elmiron) is prescribed, heparin or a drug called dimethylsulfoxide (DMSO) is administered directly into the bladder. Nerve stimulation is also used.

Young women are especially prone to develop urinary tract infections, and young women with lupus are particularly vulnerable to infections in general. The drugs of choice for most urinary tract infections are sulfa antibiotics, but these are often poorly tolerated by SLE patients (Chapter 9). A common problem I encounter takes place when gynecologists, urologists, or family practitioners prescribe sulfa antibiotics without realizing that lupus patients frequently develop flare-ups of SLE when they are given these drugs. Many antibiotic alternatives are available in these circumstances. Patients should always tell physicians who are treating them that they are dealing with a lupus patient.

## SUMMING UP

Lupus nephritis is very tricky to treat because it produces few symptoms or signs. Despite best efforts, patients may still evolve kidney failure. First, a doctor must confirm that it is indeed lupus that is affecting the kidney. Second, renal function and inflammation must be measured. On the basis of blood tests, urine testing, and biopsy material (if available), a careful treatment plan is formulated. Because many of the drugs used to prevent or retard this disease are quite potent in their own right, a careful balance is important.

The reader is referred to other parts of this book for details regarding dialysis and transplantation (Chapter 28); cyclophosphamide, mycophenolate mofetil, calcineurins, nitrogen mustard, azathioprine, pulse steroids, steroids, and apheresis management (Chapters 27 and 28); and pregnancy in the patient with lupus nephritis (Chapter 30).

## FURTHER READING

1. Weening JJ, D'Agati VD, Schwartz MM, et al. Classification of glomerulonephritis in systemic lupus erythematosus revisited. *Kidney Int.* 2004;659(2):521–530.
2. Yu F, Haas M, Glassock R, Zhao MH. Redefining lupus nephritis: clinical implications of pathophysiologic subtypes. *Nat Rev Nephrol.* 2017;13(8):483–495.
3. Zampeli E, Klinman DM, Gershwin ME, Moutsopoulos HM. A comprehensive evaluation for the treatment of lupus nephritis. *J Autoimmun.* 2017;78:1–10.

# 20
## The Blood and Lymphatic Systems

Before rheumatology was recognized as a subspecialty of internal medicine in 1972, lupus patients were treated primarily by another group of subspecialists— hematologists. *Hematology* is the study of diseases of the lymph glands and blood components, all of which play a key role in the well-being of individuals with systemic lupus erythematosus (SLE). This chapter looks at why many lupus patients have blood and lymphatic abnormalities. Although rheumatologists supervise the overall management of SLE, hematologists still play an important role in managing the blood abnormalities seen in lupus.

### WHAT'S WRONG WITH THE PATIENT'S BLOOD?

Whole blood is divided into three major components: red blood cells, white blood cells, and platelets. The function of each of these is reviewed in Chapter 5. In SLE, any or all of these components may be quantitatively (or numerically) high or low, or they may be malfunctioning *qualitatively*. A simple tube of blood measures quantitative values; qualitative tests also require blood samples but are more difficult to perform.

### COULD THE PROBLEM BE ANEMIA?

Are you tired? Do you feel weak? Do you look pale? If any of these answers are yes, you could be anemic. About 80 percent of SLE patients are anemic during the course of their disease. Anemia, or a low red blood cell count, is defined as a *hemoglobin* count of less than 12 grams per deciliter (g/dL) or a *hematocrit* of less than 36. The hematocrit is the percentage of red cells per 100 mL of blood and it is usually about three times the hemoglobin. A normal hemoglobin ranges from 12 g/dL to 16 g/dL and indicates the amount of a certain protein in red blood cells. Anemia in lupus is divided into two general categories: nonimmunologic and immunologic. The major symptom of anemia is fatigue, which is usually evident when the hemoglobin drops into the 10 g/dL range. Further decreases can make a person appear pale and feel weak.

## Nonimmunologic Anemias

Red blood cells are made by the bone marrow and released into the circulation. When people develop chronic inflammatory disorders, the stimulus to make red blood cells decreases. These individuals develop what is called an *anemia of chronic disease*.

A week after Sylvia had her annual gynecologic evaluation, her doctor called her to say that she was anemic. Her hemoglobin was 9.7, and it had been 13 a year before. Sylvia's lupus had been under excellent control with three aspirins four times a day, and even though she felt tired, Sylvia had only minimal aching. Her periods had always been heavy, but not unusually so. She consulted her internist, who performed a thorough evaluation. He found that Sylvia's anemia stemmed from several causes: she was iron-deficient due to her heavy periods, had an anemia of chronic disease, and was also having a problem with the aspirin. An endoscopy of her stomach showed evidence of gastritis from taking aspirin. Her doctor started her on iron and omeprazole (an ulcer medicine with the brand name Prilosec) and stopped aspirin. Her hemoglobin rose to 12 and another endoscopy showed the ulcer healing.

Lupus patients can be anemic for any of the reasons that makes otherwise healthy people become anemic. However, several of these causes are more prominent in SLE, especially when superimposed upon a pre-existing anemia or chronic disease. Among young women, a common cause is heavy menstrual bleeding and resultant *iron-deficiency anemia*. Another cause of this type of anemia is the administration of nonsteroidal anti-inflammatory drugs (NSAIDs) such as ibuprofen or aspirin, which can irritate the stomach lining, inducing secondary blood loss from an erosive gastritis. Practitioners sometime check the stools of their lupus patients for blood on a periodic basis if these patients are taking nonsteroidals. If continued NSAID administration is necessary, patients with these problems are given iron supplements and gastric agents that coat the stomach. However, doctors often discontinue the NSAIDs. Occasionally, anemias in lupus patients respond to the administration of folic acid or injections of vitamin B12. Because African Americans have an increased prevalence of SLE, sickle cell anemia and sickle cell traits should be screened for in this population. Methotrexate is an anti-inflammatory drug taken by about 10 percent of lupus patients. A folic acid–responsive anemia may develop in these patients.

A hormone made by the kidney, called *erythropoietin* (EPO), stimulates the bone marrow to make red blood cells. *Chronic renal disease* is associated with decreased EPO levels, which can lead to anemia. The availability of EPO injections has greatly improved these patients' quality of life over the last two decades. There are many other causes of anemia in lupus, but they occur in the same proportion as in the general population.

### Immunologic Anemias

Mary was a healthy college student until she suddenly became profoundly fatigued and started noticing a yellowish cast to her skin. At a victory celebration, after her team had won its Saturday football game, she passed out. Paramedics were called and took her to a hospital, where her hemoglobin level was found to be 6. An internist then undertook an anemia workup. It turned out that she had SLE with autoimmune hemolytic anemia. Even though her bone marrow was churning out red blood cells, they were being destroyed within days upon release into the circulation. A hematologist was consulted and started her on 60 milligrams of prednisone daily. Twelve weeks later, she had a hemoglobin of only 9, and she was given a course or rituximab.

Up to 10 percent of patients with lupus develop *autoimmune hemolytic anemia* (AIHA); most of these patients complain of weakness, dizziness, and fevers. They may appear jaundiced (have a yellowish complexion) as a result of the rapid destruction of red blood cells. Antibodies to the surface of red blood cells are responsible for AIHA. A red blood cell normally lives for 120 days, but in AIHA it is destroyed by antibodies much earlier. The bone marrow is then stimulated to make more red blood cells, which can sometimes compensate for this early destruction, as evidenced by an elevation in the reticulocyte count (which measures rate of formation of red blood cells). But most of the time, it is not enough.

Specialized blood testing can help to diagnose AIHA, and the deformed cells can be seen by looking at a blood smear under the microscope. Suspicions that AIHA is present can be confirmed by blood tests (such as an elevated reticulocyte count, serum LDH, decreased serum haptoglobin, or the presence of an antibody to red blood cells, which is measured using the Coombs' antibody test).

This potentially serious complication of SLE responds only temporarily to transfusions and often calls for a prolonged course of high-dose corticosteroids. Poorly responsive AIHA patients have their steroids supplemented with cyclophosphamide, azathioprine, rituximab, or mycophenolate. Sometimes a splenectomy or removal of the spleen is necessary, because this organ removes partially damaged red cells, thus contributing to anemia.

In rare cases, circulating plasma factors tell the bone marrow to turn off the production of red blood cells. The end result of this is a slowdown or shutdown of the bone marrow, termed *hypoplasia* or *aplasia*. This usually reflects active disease, and corticosteroids or cytotoxic drugs (especially cyclosporin) may be necessary (see Chapter 27). A careful drug history should be taken, because many prescription drugs (e.g., sulfa antibiotics) can occasionally cause aplasia. See Table 20.1.

**Table 20.1.** *Some Causes of Anemia in Lupus Patients*

1. Anemia of chronic disease
2. Iron deficiency
3. Folic acid or $B_{12}$ deficiency
4. Bone marrow suppression
5. Drugs (e.g., NSAIDs, immunosuppressives)
6. Sickle cell anemia
7. Kidney impairment
8. Immune anemias (e.g., hemolytic, TTP)
9. Heavy periods

NSAIDs, nonsteroidal anti-inflammatory drugs; TTP, thrombotic thrombocytopenic purpura.

### Can the Patient Have a Blood Transfusion?

Several studies have shown that lupus patients have the same blood types and distribution of blood types as the general population. However, patients with immune-mediated anemias break down transfused cells more rapidly than otherwise healthy individuals. One study suggests that up to 16 percent of lupus patients with immune anemias experience a mild allergic-type reaction when their blood is transfused. This reaction results from red cell antibodies. There is usually no problem transfusing lupus patients without immune anemias. An extra dose of corticosteroids or an antihistamine such as Benadryl can be ordered immediately prior to the transfusion to minimize any reactions. With current screening methods in the United States, the risk of HIV or other transmissible viruses is on the order of one in tens of thousands, and the use of directed donors (e.g., having friends or relatives donate blood for you) further decreases this risk. On the other hand, it is not a good idea for lupus patients to donate their blood, since it contains too many antibodies.

### HOW IMPORTANT ARE WHITE BLOOD CELLS?

Half of all lupus patients develop low white blood cell counts during the course of their disease. White blood cells, or *leukocytes*, constitute the body's defense mechanism. They are responsible for immunologic memory (lymphocytes), bacterial killing (neutrophils), and allergic reactions (eosinophils). Chapter 5 reviews the functions of the five types of white blood cells. White blood cell counts are elevated by active infections, corticosteroid therapy, and sometimes by active SLE. Low white blood cell counts derive from viral infections or active lupus or are the consequence of chemotherapy for lupus.

The usual reason for low *lymphocyte* levels is the presence of antilymphocyte antibodies, which destroy lymphocytes. *Neutrophil* counts are usually normal in SLE unless suppressed by chemotherapy. Yet though their levels are normal, there are apparently qualitative defects in neutrophil function that are manifested by a decreased ability to kill bacteria. This helps explain why lupus patients are more susceptible to infection. *Eosinophils* are elevated in 3 to 10 percent of lupus patients, and lupus patients have an increased incidence of allergies compared with the general population (Chapter 29).

## CLOTTING AND BLEEDING PROBLEMS

Platelets are the blood components responsible for clotting blood. Increased numbers of platelets reflect acute inflammation and are observed in a minority of patients with active lupus. Low platelet counts are associated with bleeding disorders. The lupus anticoagulant usually promotes clotting and can damage the body due to functional abnormalities of the platelets (see Chapter 21).

When Celeste was in the sixth grade, she noticed red spots on her legs. She told her mother, who took her to see their pediatrician. Dr. Hawkins obtained a blood count that indicated that Celeste had 20,000 platelets per cubic milliliter. Celeste was started on prednisone, after which her platelet count became normal. She was off all medication within a year. Six years later, after a bad flu, the spots reappeared and her platelet count dropped to 20,000 cubic milliliters. Her internist also found that she tested positive for antinuclear antibodies and anti-double stranded DNA. Even though she denied any of the signs or symptoms of lupus and enjoyed being out in the sun, Celeste was told she had lupus with idiopathic thrombocytopenic purpura. She was started on prednisone and her platelet counts normalized within a few weeks. Celeste now feels fine and is off all medication.

Decreased platelet counts along with the presence of platelet antibodies is called *idiopathic thrombocytopenic purpura* (ITP). It is usually seen in children and young women, most of whom have no symptoms other than that they bruise easily. Approximately 20 percent of patients with ITP also have a positive antinuclear antibody test, and 20 percent of these patients ultimately develop lupus. A normal platelet count is between 130,000 and 400,000 per cubic millimeter. One sixth of all lupus patients run platelet counts below 100,000 during the course of their disease. Easy bruising is noted when the counts drop below 50,000, and counts less than 20,000 can be life threatening in the sense that these individuals can suffer spontaneous internal bleeding. Anyone who notices numerous black-and-blue marks, excessive bleeding from the gums, very heavy periods, or little red spots (*petechiae*) on the skin should obtain a platelet count. Many ITP patients lack other signs and symptoms of SLE, and many are not even sun sensitive.

I often add steroid treatment for patients with a platelet count between 60,000 and 100,000 per cubic millimeter only if lupus is active outside the platelet system or the counts drop further. This condition is usually fairly responsive to steroids, but occasionally I add azathioprine, vincristine, rituximab, mycophenolate mofetil, or cyclophosphamide (Chapter 27). Intravenous gamma globulin and platelet transfusions temporarily raise platelet counts, as does plasmapheresis. Removal of the spleen, the organ that traps platelets coated with antibodies, is usually curative. Most patients with ITP and lupus also have antiphospholipid antibodies (Chapter 21); some also have AIHA (Evans' syndrome).

A rare and frightening complication of SLE is *thrombotic thrombocytopenic purpura* (TTP). Called a "pentad" because of its five signal markers of fever, hemolytic anemia, neurologic impairment, kidney failure, and low platelet counts, TTP can lead to multiple organ failure when disseminated clots form throughout the body. The disease generally results from antibodies that activate the immune system to inhibit the ADAMTS13 enzyme.

It can be brought on by a viral infection or other forms of sepsis, and it was fatal until recently. The critical life-saving element is the treating doctor's awareness of this rare disorder as a possibility and the ability to diagnose it promptly. Plasmapheresis can cure the condition, which rarely comes back once it has been successfully treated, and rituximab is often helpful. Recently, an agent that blocks the activation of complement, *eculizumab*, has been used.

Some lupus patients also have *qualitative platelet defects*. Aspirin, platelet antibodies, and chronic renal failure can all alter functional blood clotting, even when platelet counts are in the normal range. Steroids and NSAIDs disrupt platelets and induce *purpura*, those black-and-blue marks on the skin that result partially from damage to fragile capillaries. This benign but annoying condition causes no symptoms and need not cause alarm if platelet counts are in the normal range. No treatment is necessary.

## DOES LUPUS CAUSE SWOLLEN GLANDS?

When the disease is active, the increased numbers of inflammatory cells and immune complexes can cause lymph glands (or nodes) to enlarge. Lymph glands, loosely arrayed in chains throughout the body, drain and filter particulate materials. Whereas arteries supply blood and nutrients to the body, veins return blood and nutrients to the heart and are helped along by lymph glands. Half of all lupus patients have enlarged lymph nodes that can be felt on a physical examination at some point during the course of the disease. On occasion, the nodes can be up to 1.5 inches in diameter. This prominence has been called *Kikuchi's syndrome*. Infections also enlarge lymph glands, as can malignancies; before active lupus is treated, these possibilities must be ruled out. *Lymphadenopathy* (another name for swollen lymph glands) from SLE is treated with anti-inflammatory medication.

## HOW IS THE SPLEEN INVOLVED IN LUPUS?

In the left upper part of the abdomen lies a large, vascular lymphatic organ called the *spleen*. The spleen filters the blood and destroys and removes damaged red blood cells, white blood cells, and platelets. This process is part of what rheumatologists and immunologists call the *reticuloendothelial system* (RES). The spleen can become larger when a greater number of cells than usual require removal.

Circulating immune complexes are also cleared by the spleen, and in SLE their clearance can be impaired. Impaired RES clearance increases the deposition of immune complexes in tissue, which, in turn, causes damage or inflammation. About 10 percent of lupus patients have enlarged spleens on physical examination. Abdominal computed tomography or ultrasound easily shows an enlarged spleen. The spleen rarely produces pain unless it is very large and the capsule is stretched. *The most common cause of left upper abdominal pain in SLE is pleurisy, because the lung and ribs overlie the spleen.*

On occasion, the spleen is removed to treat AIHA or ITP. Even though a person can have a normal life expectancy without a spleen, some individuals become vulnerable to numerous infectious agents, especially a form of bacterium that leads to pneumococcal pneumonia. Every patient who has had the spleen removed (splenectomy) should be vaccinated against this bacterium and watched closely for infection.

### WHAT IS MGUS?

Approximately 5 percent of lupus patients have an "extra protein" found when doctors order a serum protein electrophoresis (Chapter 11). Our proteins consist of albumin and globulins. Within the gamma globulin fraction, small proteins made by the bone marrow can found. Seen in 1 percent of healthy individuals, these *monoclonal gammopathies of uncertain significance, or MGUS*, can become a myeloma or lymphoma in 10 to 12 percent over a 20-year period of observation. I usually send lupus patients with MGUS to a hematologist for a baseline evaluation. MGUS patients have no symptoms.

### WHAT DOES THE THYMUS DO?

The thymus is a lymph organ at the base of the neck; it is responsible for establishing a system of immune surveillance. In adult life, the gland atrophies and is barely recognizable. The thymus in lupus patients does not look any different than it does in a healthy person. Removing the gland, with a *thymectomy*, usually has no effect upon the disease.

### SUMMING UP

Anemia, the most common blood abnormality in lupus patients, can cause fatigue and pallor. The anemia can result from a nonimmunological cause—iron deficiency or chronic disease—or it can result directly from immunological conditions caused by lupus. Immune-mediated anemias are serious and potentially life threatening. They often mandate high doses of steroids and other immunosuppressive therapies.

Low white blood cell counts are also commonly observed and result from antilymphocyte antibodies. White blood cells (called neutrophils) do not kill bacteria as well as they should in SLE, and this increases the risk of infection.

Antibodies to platelets lower platelet counts, especially in patients with the lupus anticoagulant. Very low platelet counts can result in serious internal bleeding and must be managed with steroids and other immunosuppressive therapies.

Lymph glands swell with active lupus, but this can be treated. The spleen also enlarges when its filtering capacities are overwhelmed, but treatment can resolve this problem as well.

## FURTHER READING

1. Velo-García A, Castro SG, Isenberg DA. The diagnosis and management of the haematologic manifestations of lupus. J Autoimmun. 2016;74:139–160.
2. Habets KL, Huizinga TW, Toes RE. Platelets and autoimmunity. Eur J Clin Invest. 2013;43(7):746–757.
3. Newman K, Owlia MB, El-Hemaidi I, Akhtari M. Management of immune cytopenias in patients with systemic lupus erythematosu—old and new. Autoimmun Rev. 2013;12(7):784–791.

# 21
## *Why Do Blood Clots Develop?*

As many as one third of all deaths due to complications from lupus arise from blood-clotting abnormalities. The saga of how the medical world came to see that patients with SLE were especially susceptible to blood clots is one of the more interesting and convoluted tales in rheumatology. After 40 years of struggling with the problem, rheumatologists finally realized that the solution lay in tying the knot right under our noses. Fortunately, rapid developments in this area over the last decade should greatly decrease complication and mortality rates in this group at risk.

### LUPUS AND FALSE-POSITIVE SYPHILIS TESTS

In 1940 Dr. Harry Keil and his colleagues at Johns Hopkins linked 10 women together with a very peculiar finding. They all had lupus and they all tested positive for syphilis, but they did not have the venereal disease. Many of these tests were performed as part of routine premarital exams. I still remember several patients relating to me that in the 1940s and 1950s they were told they had syphilis, even though they were virgins. Engagements were broken, and misunderstandings abounded. Further studies showed that up to 20 percent of all lupus patients had a false-positive "Wassermann" test, as the syphilis test was called in those days. However, these patients with lupus had no unique or specific clinical features that differentiated them from others with the disease.

The Wassermann test relied upon *reagin*, an antibody found in syphilis patients. Further work showed that the antigen to which this antibody reacted was *cardiolipin*, a phosphorus-fat component of cell membranes called *phospholipid*.

### WHAT IS THE LUPUS ANTICOAGULANT?

In 1948 another Johns Hopkins team led by Dr. C. Lockard Conley and his colleagues reported that an antibody found in the blood of lupus patients prolonged phospholipid-dependent clotting tests. In time, it was called the *lupus anticoagulant*. This term has turned out to be a misnomer because—except in unusual circumstances—it is associated with the formation of blood clots rather than increased bleeding. For years no investigator linked patients with false-positive syphilis tests to those who had the lupus anticoagulant. It did not seem important, because these findings were considered laboratory curiosities, and lupus patients were strange in any case. Little, if any, clinical relevance was attached to these oddities for some 35 years.

## ANTIPHOSPHOLIPID ANTIBODIES COME OF AGE

In the early 1980s a team of English investigators headed by Graham Hughes began looking in earnest at antibodies to the troublesome phospholipid antigens. Using newly available immunologic techniques, they identified several antiphospholipid antibodies that had important clinical implications. One of these antibodies, the *anticardiolipin antibody*, was first correlated with an increased risk of *thromboses*, or blood clots. As the testing process was further refined, a myriad of clinical associations were confirmed. *Approximately one third of all lupus patients possess antiphospholipid antibodies, and one third of these patients have complications as a result of this antibody.* Because several antiphospholipid antibodies are associated with blood clots, what was originally called the anticardiolipin syndrome is now termed the *antiphospholipid syndrome*.

## WHAT IS THE ANTIPHOSPHOLIPID SYNDROME?

As previously mentioned, many patients have antiphospholipid antibodies but only a small proportion of these individuals have problems resulting from them. For example, 10 to 30 percent of all patients with rheumatoid arthritis, scleroderma, and other forms of vasculitis have antiphospholipid antibodies, even though clotting complications are extremely unusual. Further, many infectious diseases, particularly AIDS, are associated with these antibodies and never cause clotting problems. The reasons for this are twofold. First, lupus patients are uniquely susceptible to the antiphospholipid syndrome because they have an additional protein cofactor known as anti-beta$_2$ glycoprotein-1 that makes antiphospholipid antibodies that promote clotting. Also, antiphospholipid antibodies are directed against different *isotypes*, or types of immunoglobulins (Chapter 11). Immunoglobin G (IgG) anti-cardiolipin antibody, for example, is much more likely to lead to blood clots than immunoglobin M (IgM) or A (IgA) anticardiolipin antibody. Higher amounts of antibody also increase the risk of clots.

The term *antiphospholipid syndrome* is applied to a group of clinical complications that result from antiphospholipid antibodies. The overwhelming majority of patients with this syndrome have lupus, but a very small percentage of otherwise healthy people have the antiphospholipid syndrome. The criteria for antiphospholipid antibodies are delineated in Table 21.1.

**Table 21.1.** *Criteria for the Classification of the Antiphospholipid Syndrome*

---

**Clinical criteria**

Vascular thrombosis: one or more episodes within 5 years

Pregnancy morbidity: one or more unexplained deaths of a morphologically normal fetus after at least 10 weeks of gestation; *or* before the 34th week of gestation due to pre-eclampsia, eclampsia, or placental insufficiency; *or* 3 or more unexplained spontaneous abortions before the 10th week of gestation

**Laboratory criteria**

IgG or IgM isotype anticardiolipin antibodies on two occasions at least 3 months apart

Lupus anticoagulant on two occasions at least 6 weeks apart

Antibodies to beta$_2$ glycoprotein (IgG or IgM isotypes) on two occasions 12 weeks apart

One clinical plus one laboratory criteria must be present

---

S Miyakis et al., *J Thromb Haemost,* 2006. IgG, immunoglobin G; IgM, immunoglobin M.

## WHAT IS THE IMPORTANCE OF ANTIPHOSPHOLIPID ANTIBODIES?

Quite simply, antiphospholipid antibodies and the lupus anticoagulant can cause blood clots, and blood clots are potentially serious. These clots can form anywhere in the body, especially in arteries or veins. If they appear in the brain, they can produce a stroke (Chapter 18). In Libman-Sacks endocarditis, the heart valves can become a source for infection and can produce emboli (traveling blood clots) to the brain, which lead to strokes (Chapter 14). In the body's vascular system, phlebitis (inflammation of a vein) from a clot is not uncommon, especially in the calves of the legs. Sometimes leg clots can travel to the lungs and produce pulmonary emboli (Chapter 14). Multiple pulmonary emboli may lead to pulmonary hypertension.

In our blood, antibodies to platelets or red blood cells can be closely associated with antiphospholipid antibodies. Several serious conditions are associated with these antibodies, including autoimmune hemolytic anemia and thrombocytopenia. Pregnant women with antiphospholipid antibodies can miscarry and must be closely monitored (Chapter 30). Other conditions are also found in this syndrome, such as livedo reticularis of the skin (Chapter 12).

The risks of clotting are not necessarily related to disease activity and can become troublesome when lupus is in remission. Table 21.2 summarizes these findings and shows how antiphospholipid antibodies can be complicating factors in lupus that relate to many different parts of the body.

## WHY DOES ABNORMAL CLOTTING DEVELOP?

We still don't know why antiphospholipid antibodies predispose patients to blood clots. Several theories that are difficult to test have been put forward. Current thinking suggests that these antibodies bind to platelets and activate them. This

**Table 21.2.** *Complications Caused by Antiphospholipid Antibodies in Lupus*

| |
|---|
| Obstetric |
|   Fetal loss/miscarriages |
| Hematologic |
|   Arterial and venous clots (thromboses) |
|   Low platelet counts (autoimmune thrombocytopenia) |
|   Anemia (autoimmune hemolytic anemia) |
| Neurologic |
|   Strokes |
|   Migraines |
|   Transient ischemic attacks (stroke warnings) |
| Cardiologic |
|   Libman-Sacks endocarditis |
| Pulmonary |
|   Pulmonary emboli |
|   Pulmonary hypertension |
| Dermatologic |
|   Livedo reticularis |
|   Ulcers and gangrene |

combination increases the risk of forming clots. Or possibly antiphospholipid antibodies could bind to *endothelial cells*, the cells that line blood vessels, or inhibit the release of certain chemicals that dilate blood vessels. Patients with lupus are prone to develop an acquired deficiency of several proteins important in clotting. These include protein C, protein S, annexin V, Factor V Leiden mutation, the MTHFR gene mutation, and antithrombin 3. A lack of any of these proteins induces what physicians call a *hypercoagulable state*, or a milieu in which clotting risks are high.

A small percentage of patients with antiphospholipid antibodies are more likely to experience bleeding than clotting. This group either has very low platelet counts—less than 30,000 per cubic millimeter ($mm^3$); normal is more than 150,000/$mm^3$—or lacks a blood clotting factor called factor II (also known as prothrombin).

## WHAT IS THE RELATIONSHIP BETWEEN ANTIPHOSPHOLIPID ANTIBODIES, THE LUPUS ANTICOAGULANT, AND FALSE-POSITIVE TESTS FOR SYPHILIS?

Because many patients with antiphospholipid antibodies feel well until they develop a clot, it is frequently difficult to convey the complicated interactions between clotting factors and antibodies in a meaningful way. Figure 21.1 is designed to help the reader visualize these interrelationships.

The majority of patients with the lupus anticoagulant also have positive tests for antiphospholipid antibodies, and vice versa. As previously noted, many of

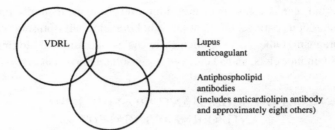

**Figure 21.1.** *Relationships between Various Methods for Detecting Antiphospholipid Antibodies*

these individuals also have a false-positive syphilis test. The prevalence of the lupus anticoagulant depends on how the testing is performed. A *partial thromboplastin time* (PTT) measures how long it takes to activate the body's intrinsic clotting cascade. Most lupus patients have normal PTTs when tested by conventional methods. However, the PTT can be modified by a variety of methods that reduce the amount of phospholipid in the test clotting mixture. This brings out evidence of an antibody to the *prothrombin activator complex*, or clotting factors X and V (10 and 5, respectively), which is an antiphospholipid antibody. It is probably not the anticardiolipin antibody, but it is closely related. That's why some patients with a positive anticardiolipin antibody can have a negative modified PTT and others with a positive lupus anticoagulant test have negative anti-cardiolipin antibody testing.

Some of the names for lupus anticoagulant tests include the Russell viper venom test, the RBNP, and the kaolin PTT. Ten percent of patients with SLE have an abnormal conventional PTT and 30 percent, a prolonged modified PTT. Another 20 percent of lupus patients have a false-positive VDRL, a test for syphilis that detects antiphospholipid antibodies that are not usually associated with clotting problems.

## WHAT TESTING SHOULD BE DONE TO SCREEN FOR CLOTTING RISKS?

Most of my new lupus patients are screened for the lupus anticoagulant and anticardiolipin antibody and have a syphilis serologic test performed. The cost of doing these three tests relatively inexpensive and can be life-saving. If these tests are negative or only borderline positive in patients with an abnormal clotting history, I measure protein C, protein S, anti-beta$_2$ glycoprotein-1, Factor V Leiden mutation, and antithrombin 3 levels and look for the presence of other antiphospholipid antibodies for which testing is now commercially available. Anticardiolipin antibodies can appear and disappear as the disease waxes and wanes. Steroids can decrease anticardiolipin levels or make them disappear alto-gether. Some lupus patients have antiphospholipid antibodies present only when they are pregnant. Other less common deficiencies of additional clotting factors occasionally induce clots, and a hematology consultant may wish to test for these.

## HOW SHOULD ANTIPHOSPHOLIPID ANTIBODIES BE TREATED?

Management of the antiphospholipid syndrome is controversial. Its therapy is not without side effects, and only one third of the patients with antiphospholipid antibodies ever experience a clinical problem. Over the years, my practice has evolved guidelines that I have found useful.

My patients with a positive test for the lupus anticoagulant, IgG isotype (>25), IgM isotype (>50), or anticardiolipin antibody are told to take one baby aspirin a day. There is some preliminary evidence that this decreases the risk of thromboses. If a patient cannot tolerate even low-dose aspirin, all three antimalarial drugs used to treat SLE can prevent clots, so I prescribe one of them (Chapter 27). Aspirin can be combined with antimalarial therapy. However, many patients who have had a thromboembolic event—especially while taking aspirin or antimalarials—require lifelong anticoagulation with warfarin (Coumadin) or heparin. For many years, heparin was only available as an injection that worked for 8 hours and had to be constantly monitored. Since the early 2000s, a low molecular weight hep-arin has been available in both injectable (Enoxaparin-Lovenox) and oral forms such as rivaroxaban (Xarelto) and apixaban (Eliquis). At first, they saw little use because they were prohibitively expensive and not covered by insurance, but ac-cessibility and pricing has greatly improved. Also, experience has shown that they are as reliable as warfarin and that Lovenox might also have anti-inflammatory properties as well.

The treatment of certain thromboembolic events requires hospitalization = to use heparin (or occasionally streptokinase), which dissolves the clots, followed by oral warfarin. The antiphospholipid syndrome demands a higher dose of war-farin than that used in other diseases because the treatment is trying to achieve an international normalization ratio (INR), or blood-thinning level, of 2.5 to 3.5 as opposed to the usual 2.0 to 2.5. If the clots are arterial, the addition of a platelet antagonist such as dipyridamole (Persantine) or clopidogrel (Plavix) may be helpful. Even though corticosteroids decrease levels of antiphospholipid antibodies or eliminate them from the blood, they promote clotting and do not necessarily decrease the risk of thromboemboli.

A few patients have what has been termed *catastrophic primary antiphospholipid syndrome*. In other words, they experience repeated thromboembolic insults de-spite platelet antagonist therapy with aspirin, antimalarials or other agents, or therapeutic warfarin. This rare subset of patients has an inflammatory component present and can be difficult to treat, but giving them chronic heparin intravenously or subcutaneously, along with immunosuppression and rituximab, is helpful.

## SUMMING UP

Approximately one third of lupus patients have an antibody to phospholipids, which in the presence of certain predisposing factors unique to lupus, causes abnormal clotting. Individuals at risk are identified by performing antibody tests of phospholipids (especially to anticardiolipin antibodies), by using studies that check for prolonged clotting times, or by testing for syphilis and obtaining a false-positive result. Between 10 and 15 percent of those with SLE have clinical evidence of abnormal clotting, which can result in strokes, recurrent miscarriages, pulmonary emboli, and low red cell or platelet counts. There are few or no symptoms or warning signs. Few dietary or activity restrictions can aid prevention. Clotting complications can be prevented or minimized with platelet antagonist therapy (e.g., aspirin, antimalarials). Patients with thromboembolic events on platelet antagonists should be given warfarin, and a small subset of patients need chronic heparin.

## FURTHER READING

1. Schreiber K, Sciascia S, de Groot PG, et al. Antiphospholipid syndrome. *Nat Rev Dis Primers.* 2018;4:17103.
2. Sciascia S, Coloma-Bazán E, Radin M, et al. Can we withdraw anticoagulation in patients with antiphospholipid syndrome after seroconversion. *Autoimmun Rev.* 2017;16(11):1109–1114.
3. Chaturvedi S, McCrae KR. Diagnosis and management of the antiphospholipid syndrome. *Blood Rev.* 2017;31(6):406–417.

# 22

## *Lupus through the Ages: Lupus in Children and the Elderly*

Lupus comes in many sizes, shapes, and varieties unique to the age of onset, the presence of a specific autoantibody, and the appearance of certain clinical features. Most systemic lupus erythematosus (SLE)—some 85 percent—occurs in individuals between the ages of 20 and 60. Does the disease manifest itself differently in youth and a more advanced age? The answer is yes. Four distinct types of SLE have been described that represent the remaining 15 percent of patients with the disease: neonatal lupus, lupus in childhood, lupus in adolescence, and older-age-onset SLE.

### NEONATAL LUPUS

At first, the concept that one can be born with lupus seems frightening. When a report appeared in 1954 that an infant was diagnosed with discoid lupus and its mother developed lupus shortly thereafter, the rheumatology community was concerned about the presence of such a chronic disease in infancy. However, between 1954 and the present, only a few thousand such cases have been described in the world's literature. Neonatal lupus is certainly quite rare.

If the neonatal period is defined as within 30 days of birth, how can one develop lupus during this period? In the 1950s lupus erythematosus (LE) cells were shown to cross the placenta and produce positive LE cell results in healthy infants of lupus mothers for several weeks. It turns out the immunoglobin G (IgG) but not immunoglobin M or A autoantibodies cross the placenta. Three IgG-containing autoantibodies that cross the placenta can damage fetal tissue: anti-Ro (SSA), anti-La (SSB), and anti-RNP (Chapter 11). Fortunately, all of these autoantibodies disappear by the eighth month after birth, because the baby is not able to make them. A review of the literature suggests that the prevalence of these autoantibodies in children with neonatal lupus is anti-Ro, 90 percent; anti-La, 53 percent; and anti-RNP, 2 percent.

## How Does a Physician Detect Neonatal Lupus?

The autoantibodies responsible for neonatal lupus settle in different tissues, especially the skin and heart. A review of published cases suggests that 54 percent of infants with neonatal lupus have varying degrees of myocardial dysfunction or congenital heart block, 37 percent have cutaneous lupus lesions, and 7 percent have both. Additionally, less than 8 percent have liver, gastrointestinal, blood, neurologic, or lung manifestations of lupus. Two-thirds of all reported patients are female.

*Congenital heart block* is the most serious complication of neonatal lupus. Anti-Ro and anti-La are attracted to fetal heart pacing tissue and can interfere with its development. Congenital heart block is defined by a slow fetal heart rate, evidence of heart block on an electrocardiogram at birth, or abnormalities on a fetal heart echocardiogram (ultrasound). The death rate is 20 percent, but many babies can be saved by implanting a pacemaker. The incidence of congenital heart block in the general population is 1 in 20,000 births. Overall, the risk for mothers with SLE of having a child with congenital heart block is estimated at 1 to 2 percent. If they carry anti-SSA, anti-SSB, or anti-RNP antibodies, the risk is about 5 percent; if they do not, it is about zero. Minor pacing abnormalities with myocardial dysfunction may respond to corticosteroids.

*Cutaneous neonatal lupus* is manifested by the development of discoid or subacute cutaneous-type lesions during the neonatal period. The rashes, which disappear spontaneously after several months, respond to sun avoidance and steroid creams. Approximately 1 case of cutaneous neonatal lupus is found for every 14 mothers with SLE who carry the anti-Ro or anti-La antibody.

## What Kind of Disease Is Found in the Mothers?

Surprisingly, many women who have children with neonatal lupus feel perfectly healthy and do not have lupus. In a summary of the world's literature where maternal health has been ascertained, 40 percent had SLE, 38 percent had no disease, 13 percent had a diagnosis of Sjögren's syndrome, and 9 percent had other autoimmune diagnoses. It should be remembered that 70 percent of all Sjögren's patients have anti-Ro. Why do healthy women have babies with neonatal lupus? Simply because 1 healthy women per 1,000 carries the anti-Ro or anti-La antibody. Many women are family members of patients with autoimmune diseases. Moreover, some healthy women develop clinically evident lupus or Sjögren's within several years of giving birth to a child with neonatal lupus, but most remain in good health.

## What Is the Outcome of Children with Neonatal Lupus?

With or without treatment, cutaneous lupus disappears within a few months. As previously mentioned, the mortality rate of congenital heart block is 20 percent.

Those who survive generally do quite well. Unfortunately, occasional reports have shown that some of the children born with neonatal manifestations of lupus develop SLE 10 to 15 years later. It is therefore strongly advised that all children with neonatal lupus be screened for SLE during their adolescent years.

## What Should Mothers with SLE Know about Neonatal Lupus?

Mothers with SLE who lack the anti-Ro, anti-La, or anti-RNP antibody are not at risk for delivering children with neonatal lupus. The 30 to 40 percent with lupus who carry these autoantibodies should be told that the risk of congenital heart disease or block in their child is about 5 percent and of neonatal cutaneous lupus, 2 percent. Because cutaneous lupus is benign, the only precaution I take is to perform weekly fetal echocardiograms between the 16th and 24th week of gestation to make sure that the fetal heart rate is not too slow. Fetal pacemakers can be implanted into the womb if necessary. Studies using different forms of steroids (e.g., betamethasone, dexamethasone), apheresis, or other anti-inflammatory regimens have not shown impressive efficacy. I have never recommended that women with these potentially risky autoantibodies terminate a pregnancy, because a neonatal lupus risk of 1 in 14 is small, and these children usually lead normal lives.

## LUPUS IN CHILDREN

Somewhere between 5,000 and 10,000 children in the United States have lupus. Even though it looks like adult lupus under the microscope and is treated with the same medications, there are important conceptual and treatment considerations that enter into the overall equation.

First, lupus proportionately occurs more often in boys than men. Adult males make up 5 to 15 percent of the lupus population, but boys represent 20 to 40 percent of those with childhood lupus. Lupus is more severe at early ages and milder in older age groups. Whereas half of those with adult SLE develop organ-threatening disease (e.g., heart, lung, kidney, or liver involvement), 80 percent of those with childhood-onset SLE develop organ-threatening conditions. In some centers, up to 70 percent of children with lupus can have kidney disease, as opposed to 30 to 40 percent of adults. As a result, children with SLE require more aggressive monitoring and management. This becomes especially apparent because they are less likely to complain or to understand the seriousness of the inflammatory process. Fortunately, lupus is usually fairly easy to diagnose in children. The average lupus patient in the third decade has symptoms for 1 to 2 years before being diagnosed; in children, a diagnosis is usually made within 3 months.

The outcome of adult diseases is often discussed in medical journals and textbooks in terms of 5- or 10-year survival; in children, we are trying to achieve a 50-year survival. Because many of those with childhood SLE live a normal life course, anything a doctor does has long-term implications. For example, corticosteroids may stunt growth and influence a child's stature for a lifetime. Chemotherapies may render a patient sterile and rarely cause cancer many years later, which naturally has an impact on dating, career, and lifestyle choices. Certain medications used to treat lupus—such as the nonsteroidal anti-inflammatory indomethacin—are specifically ill advised in young children. Other medications are not available as liquids or in strengths that can easily and safely be used by children.

There are only a few hundred pediatric rheumatologists in the United States. All parents of children with SLE should have their pediatrician or healthcare provider network seek out one of these practitioners for counsel and advice.

## LUPUS IN ADOLESCENTS

Pubertal teenagers with SLE have the same clinical manifestations as young adults with the disease. However, several psychosocial considerations are unique to adolescents.

Adolescents are notorious for not complying with prescriptions and medication. They find out very quickly what steroids do to their appearance and mood. Many would rather not take a medication that promotes fluid retention, acne, facial hair, easy bruising, and a puffy face. A fair percentage pretend to take their steroids but don't. Fragile social relationships with friends can be altered by sun avoidance, a skin rash, hair loss, swollen joints, and fatigue. They often have special concerns when confronted with issues of dating, marriage, or childbearing. All too often, physicians treat adolescents as adults and fail to address these issues. This mistake can be deadly. The importance of compliance with medication, regular blood monitoring, and being honest with the physician must be specifically spelled out and frequently reinforced. See Chapter 25 for a more detailed discussion.

## LUPUS AMONG THE ELDERLY

Two groups of individuals with SLE are found among patients over the age of 60: those who have had lupus for years and those who are developing it for the first time. For those with a history of long-term SLE, the golden years are usually just that. Lupus tends to burn itself out after many years and rarely progresses after menopause. Patients still need to be careful in the sun and may have joint inflammation, but newly evolved organ-threatening disease is extremely rare.

The onset of lupus past the age of 60 is often very subtle. Studies have suggested that it takes an average of 3 years of symptoms before nondrug-induced SLE is diagnosed. Drug-induced lupus makes up some of the new lupus cases in older age groups, so a careful drug history should be taken. This topic is discussed in detail in Chapter 9. Several other diseases mimic SLE, and differentiation can be difficult. In individuals over the age of 60, rheumatoid arthritis, polymyalgia rheumatica, and primary Sjögren's syndrome can all produce positive antinuclear antibody tests, inflammatory arthritis, stiffness, aching, and elevated sedimentation rates. A rheumatology consultation is often helpful in arriving at the correct diagnosis.

Late-onset SLE includes more males among its victims and is clinically manifested by aching, stiffness, dry eyes, dry mouth, and pleuritic pain. Organ-threatening disease is quite rare and found in less than 20 percent of patients. Rashes, fevers, swollen glands, Raynaud's phenomenon, and neuropsychiatric lupus are also much less common than in young adults. Low-dose steroids, methotrexate, and antimalarials along with nonsteroidal anti-inflammatory drugs are frequently employed as treatment.

Less than 2 percent of all SLE onset occurs after the age of 70. Lupus in the elderly has a favorable outcome and deaths from the disease are extremely unusual.

## SUMMING UP

Lupus in newborns is very rare. Cutaneous neonatal lupus disappears spontaneously. Sometimes the presence of congenital heart block may require permanent treatment with a pacemaker or medication that controls the heart's rhythm, but this condition usually has a favorable outcome. Recent reports suggest that a minority of neonatal lupus patients may develop lupus during adolescence. Childhood lupus is frequently serious and organ threatening. Aggressive management increases the chances for a good quality of life during adulthood. The teen years are fraught with compliance problems and psychosocial complications that require special attention. For those who develop symptoms of SLE after age 60, drug-induced lupus and other forms of inflammatory arthritis must be ruled out first as possible culprits. Senior citizens with lupus usually have mild, nonprogressive disease.

## FURTHER READING

1. Brucato A, Cimaz R, Caporali R, Ramoni V, Buyon J. Pregnancy outcomes in patients with autoimmune diseases and anti-ro/SSA. *Clin Rev Allergy Immunol.* 2011;40(1):27–41.
2. Macdermott EJ, Adams A, Lehman TJ. Systemic lupus erythematosus in children: current and emerging therapies. *Lupus.* 2007;16(8):677–683.
3. Arnaud L, Mathian A, Boddaert J, Amoura Z. Late-onset systemic lupus erythematosus: epidemiology, diagnosis and treatment. *Drugs Aging.* 2012;29(3):181–189.

# 23

## *Is It Really Lupus?*

### DIFFERENTIAL DIAGNOSIS AND DISEASE ASSOCIATIONS

Of adult males in the United States, 13.7 percent have a positive antinuclear antibodies (ANA) test, but probably less than 400,000 have lupus. Many people fulfill one, two, or three American College of Rheumatology (ACR) criteria for systemic lupus erythematosus (SLE) but lack the requisite four criteria reviewed in Chapter 2. What do they have? Are other autoimmune diseases present? And while we're on the subject, are there any other disorders that lupus patients tend to get or are spared from? When a physician considers the presence of other similar diseases, this decision process is called *differential diagnosis*. This chapter will put these issues into a practical, logical perspective.

### HOW CAN WE TELL IF IT'S LUPUS?

If a person's rheumatic complaints do not fulfill the criteria for systemic lupus or any other rheumatic disease, what is the problem and how can the doctor tell for sure? First, cutaneous (discoid) lupus and drug-induced lupus have definitions separate from those for SLE, which are reviewed in Chapter 2. A host of patients with various forms of lupus do not always fulfill the ACR criteria even when the diagnosis is self-evident. For example, evidence from biopsies of the kidney will provide clear-cut proof of lupus if the kidney is affected by the disease.

The average person with symptoms of lupus can take 1 or 2 years to be diagnosed, because the full-blown disease is not present. We call this evolution by its Latin term, *forme fruste lupus*. Similarly, a small percentage of patients with *palindromic rheumatism* develop SLE over a 5- to 10-year period. A palindrome is a word or phrase that is the same spelled forward or backward, such as "Madam, I'm Adam" or "Dad." Patients with palindromic rheumatism can be fine one day and have rashes or swollen knees the next. Three days later they are fine, with no hint of there ever having been a problem. These flare-ups are cyclical, and blood tests are often negative. Half of these patients go on to develop rheumatoid arthritis (RA), but some become lupus patients.

What if lupuslike symptoms have appeared for years? Many patients have nonspecific complaints of fatigue or aching along with a positive ANA. Most immunology laboratories have ANA panels that can be performed. As discussed in Chapter 11, certain autoantibodies are simply not seen in healthy people. If any patient seeks my consultation and has any of the following abnormal tests with the previously noted complaints, I know that a real immunologic disorder is likely: anti-DNA, anti-Sm, anti-RNP, C3 complement, C4 complement, high Westergren sedimentation rate, positive rheumatoid factor, anti-CCP, high creatine phosphokinase (CPK), false-positive syphilis test, anticardiolipin antibody, antineuronal antibody, anti-histone antibody, antiribosomal P antibody, anti-Ro (SSA), anti-La (SSB), or a broad gamma globulin band on serum protein electrophoresis. *In questionable situations, the presence of these antibodies can't be confirmed by a second, independent laboratory*. Some of the tests are difficult to perform, and occasionally false-positive results are obtained.

What can a doctor do to confirm the disease in a suspected lupus candidate who has a positive ANA, lupuslike symptoms, and negative tests for other antibodies? If joint or muscle complaints are prominent, lupus can be distinguished from fibromyalgia (see the section What Is the Relationship between Lupus and Fibromyalgia?) by a *bone scan* or a hand magnetic resonance imaging. Lupus can inflame the joints; fibromyalgia does not. In lupus, a bone scan may pick up increased blood flow to the joints as well as bone and muscle inflammation, whereas fibromyalgia will produce a normal bone scan. An ultrasound can demonstrate inflammation of the hands (synovitis). Inflammatory that would respond to a group of medications different from those used in noninflammatory fibromyalgia arthralgias. Another useful procedure is the *lupus band test*. Its applications are reviewed in detail in Chapter 12, but in essence the presence of a specific combination of immune reactants at the junction of the dermis and epidermis under the skin is seen only in SLE even if there is no rash. Finally, half of all first-degree relatives (parents, siblings, or children) of SLE patients demonstrate a positive ANA on blood testing even though only 25 percent will ever develop an autoimmune disease and less than 10 percent will become lupus patients. Nonspecific symptoms in these individuals should be followed closely.

The biggest mistake a doctor can make is to classify a patient as having SLE when he or she doesn't have the disease. Occasionally, I come across what I can only call a "lupus wannabee." These individuals are convinced they have the disease on the basis of reading and talking to their friends. It is very difficult to convince them that they don't have it. Some want to be diagnosed as having lupus perhaps for psychological reasons: they want loved ones to pay more attention to them or feel sorry for them, or they want to prove to family members that they are not "crazy." Some may eventually find a doctor who will agree with their self-diagnosis and treat them. But this is not the sort of illness that can be placated with innocuous and harmless treatments. The therapy for SLE involves toxic, expensive, and time-consuming treatment. Disease-modifying therapies (anything other than a nonsteroidal anti-inflammatory drug [NSAID]) should never be given unless a firm diagnosis has been made or an organ-threatening complication is clinically evident. Labeling a patient with SLE who does not have the disease can make it difficult for him or her to obtain gainful employment, health insurance, or life insurance, and it can mean lifelong stigmatization.

## WHAT IS ANA-NEGATIVE LUPUS?

Heidi was sure she had lupus even though six different doctors had obtained six different negative ANAs in six different labs. She had a butterfly rash on her cheeks, was tired and achy, and had a checkerboard mottling (called livedo reticularis) on her legs. Finally, the third rheumatologist she saw was sympathetic to her predicament. Even though her blood chemistry profiles, chest X-ray, electrocardiogram, sedimentation rate, CPK, anti-DNA, and complement levels were negative or normal, Dr. Schwartz obtained additional blood for testing. Heidi had a positive anticardiolipin antibody and a false-positive syphilis serology. These antibodies are seen in 20 percent of discoid lupus patients and are associated with livedo reticularis. Dr. Schwartz also referred Heidi to a dermatologist, who did a lupus band test on her cheek rash; it came back positive. A bone scan showed increased blood flow to her hands and feet, suggesting an inflammatory arthritis. Dr. Schwartz diagnosed Heidi as having ANA-negative lupus because she fulfilled the criteria by having arthritis, sun sensitivity, discoid rashes, and a false-positive syphilis serology. Three years later, Heidi's ANA blood test became positive.

Until 1985, 10 percent of all lupus patients had a negative ANA test. The introduction of improved testing material for performing the ANA test has decreased this 3 percent. Between 1980 and 1989, my office treated 464 patients who fulfilled the ACR criteria for lupus; 17 of them were ANA negative. In analyzing this group, we found that patients fell into four basic categories. One third had antiphospholipid antibodies and one third had biopsy-documented kidney lupus. Of the remaining third, half ultimately became ANA positive. The last group had advanced disease; prolonged treatment with steroids and chemotherapy made their ANA disappear. A variety of rarer causes of ANA-negative lupus exist, such as the presence of anti-Ro (SSA) antibody without ANA. Nevertheless, if a patient does not fall into any of these four categories, some of the lupus-related or lupus-mimicking disorders discussed in this chapter might be the culprit.

## WHAT IS AN UNDIFFERENTIATED CONNECTIVE TISSUE DISEASE?

Many patients feel ill, have a positive ANA, and have a couple of swollen joints but do not fulfill the ACR criteria for SLE. Their doctor says, "You don't have lupus; you have a collagen disorder of some kind." Over the last few years, rheumatologists have examined this group of patients and followed them over a

**Table 23.1.** *Undifferentiated Connective Tissue Disease*

1. Defined as autoimmune features in patients who do not fulfill the American College of Rheumatology criteria for lupus or any other autoimmune disorder. It is 5 to 10 times more common than lupus.
2. Mandatory symptoms or signs are at least two swollen joints, Raynaud's, or documented dry eyes not due to medication or infection.
3. Mandatory laboratory abnormalities are positive antinuclear antibody, rheumatoid factor, or anticyclic citrullinated peptide.
4. Three of the following eight features must be present: myalgias, autoimmune rash, pleurisy or pericarditis, persistent fever (above 99.6°F) without infection, swollen glands, elevated sedimentation rate or C-reactive protein, and antiphospholipid antibody.

period of years. The insights garnered from these observations allow us to finally clarify what to call patients who have an "almost lupus" condition. Several years ago, the University of Utah enlisted the cooperation of 10 academic centers to identify patients who had autoimmune features, had early disease, and did not fulfill criteria for lupus, RA, scleroderma, or any other disorder. The 410 patients labeled as having undifferentiated connective tissue disease (UCTD) were enrolled. The outcomes after 5 years among the group were no disease (18 percent), lupus (14 percent), scleroderma (5 percent), RA (4 percent), primary Raynaud's (18 percent), polymyositis (1 percent), mixed connective tissue disease (MCTD; 4 percent), and UCTD (36 percent). (See Table 23.1.)

In other words, although many patients evolve another rheumatic disease, there are probably a million Americans with UCTD. Its features include rashes, swollen joints, fatigue, fevers, swollen glands, Raynaud's, pleurisy, high sedimentation rates, and a positive ANA. Rarely organ threatening and less serious than SLE, most UCTD patients are managed with NSAIDs (e.g., ibuprofen), hydroxychloroquine (Plaquenil), and occasionally low doses of steroids or methotrexate. It's important to remember that these classifications are used by doctors and insurance companies for categorization purposes, as estimates of disease prevalence, and as criteria for enrollment in research studies. Your doctor needs to treat you as a unique individual with a specific set of symptoms, signs, and laboratory findings whose management is tailored to best improve the way you feel and decrease potential risks.

## WHAT NONRHEUMATIC DISORDERS MIMIC LUPUS?

Many diseases mimic SLE; they fall into several broad general categories. For example, almost every disorder of *hormonal imbalance*—from thyroid abnormalities or pregnancy to evolving menopause to diabetes—can appear with symptoms such as fatigue, aching, and feeling feverish that may lead the doctor to order lupus blood tests. *Blood or tissue malignancies* ranging from lymphoma to breast cancer can give positive ANAs and induce constitutional complaints. *Infectious processes*, especially from viruses, are associated with positive ANAs as well as lupuslike symptoms. All these possibilities should be ruled out before a diagnosis of lupus is made. Neurologic disorders, such as multiple sclerosis or myasthenia gravis, can coexist with or be difficult to differentiate from SLE. Finally, the presence of *substance abuse, malnutrition, primary psychiatric disorders*, or *allergies* needs to be considered.

## HOW CAN WE DIFFERENTIATE LUPUS FROM OTHER AUTOIMMUNE DISEASES?

Especially during the first year of symptoms, RA, scleroderma, MCTD, inflammatory myositis, and other forms of systemic vasculitis can be very difficult to differentiate from each other. It is not usually critical to make the diagnosis at first, because steroids and immunosuppressive therapy can be used to treat critical complications of any of these disorders.

RA, which afflicts 4 million Americans, is ten times more common than SLE in the United States. In its initial presentation, RA can be difficult to tell from lupus, but within several months, the diagnosis usually becomes obvious. Twenty-five percent of patients with lupus have a positive rheumatoid factor, and 25 percent with RA have a positive ANA. Antibody to cyclic citrullinated peptide, if present, is quite specific for RA. The hallmark of RA is an autoimmune reaction in the synovium, the tissue lining the joint. It is uncommonly complicated by systemic organ involvement, and deforming rheumatoid joint disease causes erosions (actual bone destruction) that resemble a mouse bite on X-rays. Lupus induces joint deformities less than 10 percent of the time, and erosions are almost never seen. An occasional patient has distinct features that fulfill the ACR criteria for both RA and SLE. Called *rhupus*, this rare disorder is managed with drugs useful for both diseases, such as nonsteroidals, steroids, methotrexate, and antimalarials.

Most patients with *scleroderma*, an autoimmune disease characterized by inflammation that heals with tightening of the skin and scarring of the tissues, also have a positive ANA. The 200,000 Americans with scleroderma-related disorders (e.g., progressive systemic sclerosis, CREST syndrome [or, *calcinosis, Raynaud's, esophagitis, sclerodactyly, telangiectasia*], autoimmune Raynaud's, MCTD) are frequently misdiagnosed as having SLE. A few lupus patients fulfill criteria for both diseases (called *lupoderma*), and in most cases the condition eventually evolves into a pure scleroderma. In reality, a process known as MCTD probably makes up the majority of these cases. By definition, as well as being ANA positive, MCTD patients must have a positive anti-RNP. Their condition resembles lupus, but they tend to have puffy hands, complain of heartburn and swallowing problems, are at an increased risk for developing pulmonary hypertension, and have interstitial scarring of the lungs on chest X-ray. Raynaud's phenomenon is almost universally seen in MCTD. Our survey of 464 patients with SLE shows that 25 of them, or 5 percent, also met the definition for MCTD.

*Inflammatory myositis,* as in dermatomyositis or polymyositis, is a feature of lupus in 10 to 15 percent of patients. However, the very high CPKs seen in dermato- or polymyositis, its distinct skin papules, and its association with malignancy and heliotropelike rashes are not observed in SLE. In other words, lupus is occasionally characterized by a mild, bland, frequently asymptomatic muscle inflammatory process.

RA, lupus, scleroderma, inflammatory myositis, and MCTD all involve inflammation of the small- and medium-sized arteries and arterioles. *Polyarteritis nodosa* and *microscopic polyangiitis* are primary vasculitides of those caliber vessels. They can mimic lupus, and most patients have a positive ANA. The diagnosis of polyarteritis or microscopic polyangiitis is confirmed by blood testing (known as ANCA, or antinuclear cytoplasmic antigens) with myeloperoxidase (MPO) staining that is fairly specific for systemic vasculitis, along with evidence of inflammation of the vessels documented by an angiogram or biopsy.

A group of patients have features of two to six of the disorders previously mentioned, but they do not seem to fit perfectly into any one of them. They are said to have a *crossover syndrome.* Many individuals initially exhibit a crossover syndrome that evolves into a distinct, definable disorder over time. Occasionally, rare forms of vasculitis affect medium- and small-sized vessels, which heal with scars known as granulomas; these are difficult to differentiate from lupus at first. *Granulomatosis with polyangiitis,* or *Wegener's granulomatosis,* and *eosinophilic granulomatous with polyangiitis,* or *Churg-Strauss,* are ultimately diagnosed by the pathologic finding of granulomas or a positive c-ANCA staining with PR3 blood test in Wegener's. An unusual form of vasculitis called *Behcet's* is rarely diagnosed as ANA-negative lupus. Its features of mouth ulcers, eye inflammation, and central nervous system involvement resemble SLE, but the lack of a positive ANA usually leads physicians to a correct diagnosis. Finally, as mentioned in Chapter 22, older people can develop an aching in the hips and shoulders with severe stiffness and a high sedimentation rate. Some of these individuals, who are ultimately diagnosed with *polymyalgia rheumatica,* have positive ANAs as a function of age, and lupus must be ruled out. Fever, fatigue, aching, and even mouth sores can be seen in other autoimmune disorders. These include inflammatory bowel disease (e.g., *ulcerative colitis, Crohn's disease*), *celiac disease,* and *Hashimoto's thyroiditis.* There is an increased prevalence of lupus-associated features in neurologic autoimmune syndromes such as *multiple sclerosis* and *myasthenia gravis.*

Several features of autoimmune disease can also appear by themselves without fulfilling criteria for any of the disorders above mentioned. These include Raynaud's phenomenon, idiopathic thrombocytopenic purpura, and Sjögren's syndrome.

# DOES HAVING LUPUS DECREASE THE RISK OF GETTING OTHER DISEASES?

For reasons that are not clear, several disorders have a "negative" association with lupus—in other words, having lupus decreases your chances of getting certain diseases. These include *amyloidosis, sarcoidosis, ankylosing spondylitis*, and HIV infection.

# WHAT IS THE RELATIONSHIP BETWEEN LUPUS AND FIBROMYALGIA?

Fibromyalgia, or fibrositis, has repeatedly been mentioned throughout this book. It is not a disease but a central sensitization syndrome in which sensory-afferent signals overwhelm the body's ability to filter them (see Table 23.2).

## What Is Fibromyalgia?

Fibromyalgia is a syndrome that afflicts 6 million Americans. About 90 percent of them are women, and most develop it between the ages of 20 and 50. It is a pain-amplification syndrome characterized by chronic neuromuscular pain, widespread stiffness, and aching of at least 3 months' duration. To fulfill the ACR criteria for fibromyalgia, one must have tender points (defined as wincing or withdrawing in pain when 4 kilograms, or 9 pounds, of pressure is applied) in at least 11 of 18 designated points in all four quadrants of the body (right side, left side, above the waist, and below the waist, as shown in Figure 23.1). If tender points are found in fewer than four quadrants, the patient has not fibromyalgia but a *regional myofascial syndrome*. Most of the tender points are in the upper back and neck area, buttocks, and chest.

**Table 23.2.** *Central Sensitization Syndromes*

---

*Central sensitization syndromes* are defined as the bombardment of sensory-afferent impulses into the dorsal root ganglion of the spinal cord from the periphery that overwhelm the body's ability to dampen them. This is associated with the following conditions:
Fibromyalgia (seen in up to 30% with lupus)
Functional bowel syndrome (irritable colon, spastic colitis)
Tension headache
Irritable bladder (female urethral syndrome)
Chronic fatigue syndrome (myalgia encephalomyelitis)
Chronic pelvic pain, endometriosis; dysmenorrhea
Localized syndromes: temporomandibular jaw dysfunction syndrome, myofascial pain syndrome, repetitive strain syndrome, whiplash, pseudo-carpal tunnel syndrome
Autonomic nervous system dysfunction (e.g., mitral valve prolapse, hypervigilance syndromes)

---

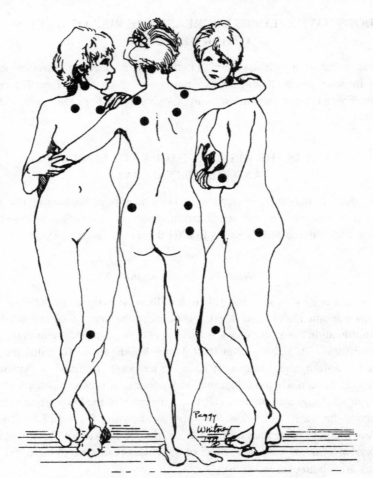

**Figure 23.1.** *Tender Point Locations in Fibromyalgia*

In addition to musculoskeletal symptoms, patients with fibromyalgia may complain of nonrestorative sleep (waking up in the morning after lying down for 8 hours but not feeling refreshed); functional bowel symptoms such as abdominal cramping, bloating, and distension; a sensation of swelling, with numbness and tingling; profound fatigue; and occasionally cognitive dysfunction. These symptoms are similar to those discussed in Chapter 15.

The cause of fibromyalgia is unknown, but pain amplification probably results from a dysfunctional interaction of neurotransmitters (such as epinephrine, dopamine, or serotonin), the autonomic nervous system, hormones, and cytokines (Chapter 5) when exposed to repetitive noxious stimuli. Fibromyalgia can be brought on by trauma, infection, or an inflammatory disorder, among other causes, and it is aggravated by psychosocial stressors.

## How Many Lupus Patients Have Fibromyalgia?

Several surveys have suggested that about 20 percent of all lupus patients also ful-fill the ACR criteria for fibromyalgia (there are several other similar definitions). The most common causes of fibromyalgia in SLE are a reaction to active mus-culoskeletal lupus, transient symptoms after a viral infection or trauma, poor coping mechanisms, and a steroid withdrawal syndrome. The latter occurs, for example, when your doctor sees how well things are going and decreases predni-sone doses from 20 milligrams to 15 milligrams a day. Decreased steroid doses can result in a flare-up of muscle and joint aching without a worsening in lab-oratory testing, objective synovitis, or swelling indicating a lupus flare. These symptoms often lead patients to call their doctors, who then raise the prednisone back to 20 milligrams daily. This may be a mistake. These complaints represent withdrawal symptoms and will disappear spontaneously over a 1- to 3-week pe-riod. Not only do alterations in steroid doses aggravate fibromyalgia, but the skin of all patients on corticosteroids develops an increased sensitivity to pressure that imitates fibromyalgia.

## How Can We Tell Lupus from Fibromyalgia?

Differentiating active lupus from fibromyalgia is critical. This is often made dif-ficult by two confounding factors: lupus patients can have concurrent fibromy-algia and 20 percent of fibromyalgia patients have a positive ANA. In patients with SLE, complaints of fatigue, muscle aching, and stiffness can represent active lupus or fibromyalgia. If a recent infection, trauma, adrenal insufficiency, or ste-roid tapering is ruled out, active lupus is usually detected by the presence of a rash or swollen joints on physical examination or is evident in tests for anemia, elevated sedimentation rate, a high anti-DNA, or low complement levels. A common mis-take among internists and even rheumatologists is to take a patient's symptoms at face value and treat them with toxic medication even though no laboratory param-eter validates that a lupus flare-up is present. Fibromyalgia flare-ups respond only temporarily to rises in corticosteroids, and the patient may actually feel worse within several weeks.

## How Do Doctors Treat Fibromyalgia?

Fibromyalgia is managed in several ways. First, doctors reassure patients that even though it's a real syndrome, it is neither life threatening nor crippling. Rheumatologists usually provide brochures from the Arthritis Foundation or fibro-myalgia support organizations that document its nonprogressive nature. Second, physicians encourage patients with fibromyalgia to adjust their lifestyles in a way that will ensure restful sleep, pacing of time, and improved coping mechanisms. Counseling may be recommended. Also, physical measures such as moist heat, gentle massage, biofeedback, and coolant sprays followed by muscle stretching (called "spray and stretch") are also employed. An occasional injection of a local anesthetic (with or without a local steroid) can be used at the trigger point of pain. A patient's work station and job description are analyzed in an effort to minimize alterations in body mechanics that could irritate muscles and stress joints. Electronic acupuncture (e.g., acuscope, neuroprobe, TENS units) may also be helpful.

Several families of medication, used alone or in combination, are useful for fibromyalgia, especially when employed with complementary approaches that enhance mind–body connection by promoting relaxation and anxiety reduction. These include tricyclic antidepressants (e.g., cyclobenzaprine, amitriptyline) to relax muscles and promote sleep; specific serotonin reuptake inhibitors (e.g., citalopram, fluoxetine) to reduce anxiety and help fatigue; serotonin norepinephrine reuptake inhibitors (e.g., duloxetine [Cymbalta], milnacipran [Savella]) to combine the previous effects; dopamine 3 receptor antagonists (e.g., pramipexole [Mirapex]), which help restless legs syndrome interfering with sleep; benzodiazepines, which relax muscles, promote sleep, and diminish anxiety (e.g., alprazolam, clonazepam); anticonvulsants for burning or numbness (e.g., gabapentin, pregabalin [Lyrica]); nonnarcotic analgesics (e.g., tramadol); nonsteroidal anti-inflammatory agents for analgesia (e.g., ibuprofen, naproxen); and tizanidine to lower substance P levels. Most of these agents are generic and have not been well studied for fibromyalgia. Savella, Cymbalta, and Lyrica are approved by the Food and Drug Administration for the syndrome and improve symptoms in 30 percent of those who take any of them by an average of 30 percent.

## SUMMING UP

Lupus is often difficult to diagnose. If established criteria are not fulfilled, additional blood tests, bone scanning, or a lupus skin biopsy band test can assist in making the diagnosis. ANA-negative lupus is rare, and a physician confronted with this diagnosis should embark on a workup to exclude other diseases that mimic lupus, such as scleroderma, RA, vasculitis, polymyalgia rheumatica, fibromyalgia, UCTD, or Behcet's syndrome. Low-titer positive ANAs are found in patients with malignancies and infections, which must be ruled out before the diagnosis of lupus becomes established. Most autoimmune disorders have overlapping features with SLE and must be considered, because their management may substantially differ. Finally, lupus patients are at an increased risk for having concurrent fibromyalgia, which is also managed differently from SLE. Sorting out lupus from fibromyalgia flare-ups presents a major challenge for patients and their healers.

## FURTHER READING

1. Wallace DJ, Wallace JB. *Making Sense of Fibromyalgia.* 2nd ed. Oxford: Oxford University Press, 2014.
2. García-González M, Rodríguez-Lozano B, Bustabad S, Ferraz-Amaro I. Undifferentiated connective tissue disease: predictors of evolution into definite disease. *Clin Exp Rheumatol.* 2017;35(5):739–745.
3. Rooney R. Systemic lupus erythematosus: unmasking a great imitator. *Nursing.* 2005;35(11):54–60.

# Part V
# THE MANAGEMENT OF LUPUS ERYTHEMATOSUS

Having read about the various symptoms, signs, and laboratory features of lupus, we must now consider ways to treat the disorder. I've taken a therapeutic approach that will help patients feel better by working with their physicians and healthcare team, by showing them how to maximize coping skills, and by promoting an understanding of the rationale behind specific treatment plans.

The treatment of lupus erythematosus is divided into four categories: physical measures, medication, surgery, and counseling. All four are closely interrelated, although surgery plays a minor role in the management of SLE. Simply stated, "the head bone is connected to the lupus bone." A doctor might prescribe all the correct medications, but if emotional stress overcomes the patient's will to recover, it could all be for naught. We review these areas in this section. Feel free to skip around or consult the index for any specific treatment feature that might interest you, but remember: the treatment of lupus is multifaceted and will be unsuccessful unless all four categories are given careful attention.

# 24

## *How to Treat Lupus with Physical Measures*

Let's look at physical measures first. We have a fair amount of control over these management techniques, and, to some extent, controlling the environment represents a common-sense approach. The physical or environmental factors we are going to discuss include the effect of sunlight, diet, exercise, heat, rest in the treatment of fatigue, and the impact of weather. The Lupus Foundation of America Web site (http://www.lupus.org) continuously updates patient and consumer information.

### DO LUPUS PATIENTS REALLY NEED TO AVOID THE SUN?

The sun emits ultraviolet radiation in three bands known as A, B, and C. Only the first two, ultraviolet A (UVA or "tanning") and ultraviolet B (UVB or "burning"), are harmful to lupus patients. (The mechanisms by which sun damages the skin and aggravates lupus are discussed in Chapters 8 and 12.) On the one hand, many of my lupus patients say the sun does not bother them and ask if they really need to avoid it. On the other hand, another group of my patients are so sun sensitive that they develop a rash along with fatigue and aching even when they are exposed to open, uncovered fluorescent lights.

The truth about sun exposure lies somewhere in between. When rheumatologists sent lupus patients questionnaires about how they feel in the sun, 60 to 70 percent replied that they avoid the sun because it gives them a rash or makes them feel tired, achy, or feverish. However, when dermatologists administered ultraviolet light to a small, defined area of skin and later biopsied it to look for inflammation or irritation, they found that only 30 percent of their patients with systemic lupus erythematosus (SLE) had reproducible light sensitivity. The reason for this discrepancy is that ultraviolet light damages the skin in a time- and dose-related fashion. I have patients who tell me that they can tolerate 15 minutes of sun exposure but begin to feel sick after 20 minutes. Ultraviolet light is present even on a cloudy day: UVA is constant throughout the day, but UVB (which is more harmful in lupus) is strongest between the hours of 10 AM and 3 PM (standard time). Ultraviolet light is more powerful at higher altitudes, and it can also be reflected on certain surfaces, such as sand and snow. I advise my sun-sensitive patients to perform their necessary outdoor activities in the early morning or late afternoon, so they can avoid the peak UVB period. Medications that increase one's sensitivity to the sun include most sulfa-containing antibiotics and certain tetracyclines.

Do sunscreens help? In most cases they can be useful, but an understanding of how they work is important. Most of the commercially available sunscreens are rated on a scale known as SPF (sun protection factor). An SPF of 15, for example, means that one is 15 times more protected than with no protection. SPFs below 15 are of little value in lupus, and those over 30 may cause the skin to dry, burn, sting, or itch. These ratings apply only to UVB light; some commercially available preparations also block UVA. One of my colleagues, Rick Sontheimer, MD, at the University of Utah, has put together a listing of useful sunscreens, which is reproduced in Table 24.1. Sunscreens are over-the-counter preparations, which means that a prescription is not necessary. If one is going to be out in the sun for 5 minutes or less, protection usually is unnecessary. For longer periods of sun exposure, a sunscreen can be applied every 2 to 3 hours to any uncovered

**Table 24.1.** *Sun Protection and Sunscreens in Lupus Patients: Important Principles*

**Safe Sun Habits**

*Schedule outdoor activities before 10* AM *and after 4* PM. so that you avoid being exposed to the most intense and damaging ultraviolet (UV) rays in sunlight. Even on cloudy days as much as 80% of UV rays still penetrate the cloud cover. You must *protect your skin on cloudy days just as on sunny days. Limit exposure to reflected UV rays* from surfaces such as water, concrete, sand, snow, tile, and reflective window glass in buildings.

The window glass in homes blocks some UV rays, especially the sunburning UV rays (UVB). However, considerable amounts of *long-wavelength UV rays (UVA) may still pass through such glass. Special UV-blocking plastic films* that can easily be applied to home window glass are available (Llumar UV Shield Window Film, 1-800-255-8627, http://www.llumar.com; North Solar Screen, 1-866-230-4700, http://www.northsolarscreen.com).

Clothing can be an excellent form of sun protection. Cover up *with loose-fitting and lightweight clothing* (long pants and long-sleeved shirt when possible), *sunglasses, and 4-inch wide-brimmed hats.* Tightly woven fabric blocks UV rays best. UV protection drops significantly when the fabric becomes wet. Dark colors protect better than light colors. The average white t-shirt provides an SPF (sun protection factor) of only 6 to 8. Sun-protective clothing lines with a rating of SPF 30 or greater are available: Solumbra/Sun Precautions, 1-800-882-7860, http://www.sunprecautions.com; Sun Protective Clothing, 1-800-353-8778, http://www. sunprotectiveclothing.com; Coolibar, 1-800-926-6509, http://www.coolibar.com.

**Sunscreens**

*Sunscreen products (also called "sunblocks") should be applied 15 to 30 minutes prior to sun exposure to be most protective.* Sunscreen should be reapplied after prolonged swimming or vigorous activity. *Water-resistant* sunscreens protect skin for 40 minutes of water exposure, and *waterproof* sunscreens protect for 80 minutes.

**Table 24.1.** (continued)

---

*Sunscreen needs to be applied liberally.* As much as 1 ounce. may be needed to cover the entire body. Particular attention needs to be paid to the back of the neck, the ears, and the areas of the scalp with thin hair.

*Use sunscreens with at least a 30 SPF.* Select a broad-spectrum sunscreen that contains ingredients that effectively block both UVB and UVA rays. Such ingredients include *avobenzone (Parsol 1789), titanium dioxide,* and *zinc oxide.* Sunscreen gels work well on oily skin or when sweating. Sunscreen lotions help dry skin, and sunscreen sprays work best on the body. Sticktype sunscreens can be used on the lips or around the eyes to avoid eye irritation or for maximum protection of the ears.

The sunscreens listed below are only suggestions for special needs. You may use a sunscreen of your choosing as long as it fulfills these criteria: (i) it has an SPF rating of 30 or higher and (ii) it is truly broad spectrum by virtue of containing at least one of the following most effective UVA-blocking ingredients: *avobenzone (Parsol 1789), titanium dioxide,* or *zinc oxide.*

**Broad-spectrum UVA/UVB**
- Neutrogena UltraSheer Dry Touch Sunblock SPF 55 (with Helioplex)[a]
- Coppertone Spectra3 Triple Protection 50
- Coppertone Shade Sunblock SPF 30
- SolBar Zinc Cream SPF 32
- Total Block Clear Sunblock 65
- Skinceuticals Physical or Ultimate UV Defense SPF 30

**Oil-free sunscreens for those prone to acne**
- Coppertone Spectra3 Triple Protection 50
- Neutrogena Oil Free Sunblock 45
- SolBar Zinc Cream SPF 32
- Total Block Clear Sunblock SPF 65
- Coppertone Oil Free Sunblock Lotion for Faces SPF 30

**Sunscreens for very sensitive skin (generally contain titanium dioxide or zinc oxide)**
- Elta Block SPF 30/32
- Estee Lauder Sunblock SPF 30
- Vanicream SPF 35

**Waterproof/sweat-resistant sunscreens**
- Elta Block Super Waterproof or Sport SPF 30
- SolBar Cream SPF 50

**Moisturizer/sunscreen combinations**
- Elta Facial Moisturizer and Block SPF 30/32

---

Mexoryl-based sunscreens are now available in Europe but not yet in the United States. L'Oreal makes Ombrelle, and Anthelios is made by La Roche Posay. These can be purchased online. Some data suggest that Mexoryls are superior sunscreens.

[a]Helioplex is a Neutrogena patented technology that preserves the efficacy of avobenzone to block UV even after prolonged exposure to the sun.

Adapted with permission of Dr. Richard Sontheimer, University of Utah School of Medicine.

area, especially the face. Protective clothing and wide-brimmed hats are also useful.

A small subset of my patients (less than 5 percent) are extremely sensitive to ultraviolet light. Most of them carry the anti-SSA (Ro) antibody (Chapter 11). Sun-sensitizing chemicals are found in certain perfumes, mercury vapor lamps, xenon arc lamps, halogen or tungsten iodide light sources, and photocopy machines; excessive exposure should be avoided. Fluorescent lighting rarely presents a problem if the fixtures have a covering. Sleeves that block UV emanation without reducing illumination from fluorescent lighting are available. Tinting car windows and wearing special protective sunglasses may be advisable. Even lupus patients who are not sun sensitive must be aware of the potential damage of UV light and should take precautions.

Despite these precautions, the lupus patient who exercises prudence and caution need not become an "environmental cripple." Lupus patients should approach the issue of ultraviolet light with common sense and not become obsessive or panic.

## IS THERE A DIET FOR LUPUS?

Individuals with SLE should eat a well-balanced, healthy, nutritious diet. Diet books for arthritis are a multimillion-dollar industry, and one of the questions most commonly asked of rheumatologists deals with the role of diet in lupus. It might seem surprising, but few nutritional modifications apply to SLE. Things that do affect lupus can be divided into two categories: factors that are lupus related and those that are medication related.

For starters, fish oil has anti-inflammatory properties. This has been documented in patients with rheumatoid arthritis and in animal models of SLE. Eating several fish meals a week is equivalent to taking several extra aspirins. It will never cure the disease, but it might bring about a modest improvement in well-being. Fish oil capsules are appropriate substitutes, but they can irritate the stomach, and it takes several capsules a day to substitute for one fish meal.

One food supplement to stay clear of is alfalfa sprouts. They contain an amino acid known as L-canavanine, which increases inflammation in patients with autoimmune disease. All members of the legume family contain L-canavanine, but it is highly concentrated in alfalfa sprouts. Well-documented flare-ups of lupus disease have been associated with increased consumption of alfalfa sprouts and have disappeared when sprouts are avoided. Alfalfa is an ingredient in many food products, and some aggressively marketed "natural" vitamin remedies contain alfalfa. Such products (e.g., Km) should probably be avoided by patients with SLE. I advise my patients to bring me copies of the labels on health-food products they purchase to make sure the items don't contain any ingredients that might be harmful in SLE.

Numerous medications are used to treat SLE, but only one has any dietary implications. Corticosteroids can raise blood sugar, serum cholesterol, and triglyceride levels and increase blood pressure. Therefore, steroid-dependent patients who require a dose of more than 10 milligrams of prednisone a day should decrease their sugar, salt, and fat intake.

See Chapter 18 for a review of the *microbiome* and bacterial overgrowth in SLE and the potential implications of this for future dietary recommendations.

## WHAT ABOUT VITAMINS OR HERBS?

No specific vitamin is recommended for lupus, but under special circumstances certain vitamins may be useful. For example, vitamin B12 and folic acid treat some of the anemias seen in SLE patients, vitamin B6 has a mild diuretic effect, and vitamin D derivatives play a role in managing specific types of osteoporosis (thinning of the bones) that are observed in the disease (Chapter 13).

No herbs or homeopathic remedies have been specifically evaluated for SLE, but controlled studies suggest that St. John's wort has mild serotonin boosting properties that might aid fatigue and depression, whereas gingko biloba may improve cognitive dysfunction. One of my rheumatologist mentors, Dan Furst, MD, and his wife, Elaine Furst, RN, at the University of California, Los Angeles, have put together a useful "Herb Chart" that I have adapted and reproduced it in Table 24.2 for informational purposes. It appears that some herbs can be helpful, others harmful, and still others have no effect.

**Table 24.2.** *Herb Chart (for Antiarthritics, Skin Treatments, and Gastrointestinal Treatments)*

| Herb | Claimed Uses | Active Ingredients | Potential Side Effects |
|---|---|---|---|
| Alfalfa | Antiarthritic | Nonprotein amino acid (L canavanine) and some saponins | In large quantities, could produce pancytopenia (decreased white blood cell count, anemia); could reactivate systematic lupus erythematosus |
| Arnica | Analgesic, anti-inflammatory (external application) | Sesquiterpenoid lactones (helenalin, dihydrohelenalin) | May cause contact dermatitis; cannot be taken internally; causes toxic effects on the heart and increases blood pressure Information on toxicity is lacking; could cause uterine bleeding |
| Black cohosh | Antirheumatic, sore throat, uterine difficulties | Substances that bind to estrogen receptors of rat uteri; also acetin, which causes some peripheral vasodilation | |
| Burdock | Treatment of skin conditions | Polyacetaline compounds that have bacteriostatic and fungicidal properties | Side effects may result from addition with belladonna |
| Butcher's broom | Improve venous circulation, anti-inflammatory | Steroidal saponins (not corticosteroids) | Unknown; self-medication for circulatory problems is dangerous |
| Calamus | Digestive aid, antispasmodic for dyspepsia | Unknown | Use only Type 1 (North American) calamus, which is free of carcinogenic ISO A Sarone (may promote cancers) |
| Calendula (marigold) | Facilitate healing of wounds (lacerations) | Unknown | Unknown |
| Capsicum | Counterirritant used to treat chronic pain (herpes zoster, facial neuralgia, or surgical trauma) | Capsaicin (proven analgesic in osteoarthritis, used externally) | Use caution in application; avoid getting into eyes or other mucous membranes; remove from hands with vinegar |

*(continued)*

**Table 24.2.** (continued)

| Herb | Claimed Uses | Active Ingredients | Potential Side Effects |
|---|---|---|---|
| Catnip | Digestive, sleep aid | *Cis-trans*-nepetalactone (attractive only to cats) | Unknown; does not mimic marijuana when smoked |
| Chamomiles, yarrow | Aids digestion, anti-inflammatory, antispasmodic, anti-infective | Complex mixture of flavonoids, coumarins, *d*-bisabolol motricin, and bisabololoxides A+B | Infrequent contact dermatitis and hypersensitivity reactions in susceptible people |
| Chickweed | Treatment of skin disorders, stomach and bowel problems | Vitamin C, various plant esters, acids, and alcohols | Unknown |
| Comfrey | General healing agent, stomach ulcer treatment | Alantoin, tannin, and mucilage, some vitamin $B_{12}$ | Hepatoxicity (liver); can lead to liver failure, especially when the root is eaten; also causes atropine poisoning due to mislabeling |
| Cranberry | Treatment of bladder infections | Antiadhesion factors (fructose and unknown polymeric compounds) prevents adhesion of bacteria to lining of bladder | Increased calories if used in large doses (12 to 32 oz. per day) as treatment rather than as preventative (3 oz. per day) |
| Curcumin (turmeric) | Anti-inflammatory | Ginger plant | A lot of recent interest |
| Dandelion | Digestive, laxative, diuretic | Taraxacin (digestive), vitamin A | Free of toxicity except for contact dermatitis in people allergic to it |
| Devil's claw | Antirheumatic | Har pagoside | None |
| DongQuai | Antispasmodic | Coumarin derivatives | Large amounts may cause photosensitivity and lead to dermatitis, possible bleeding |
| Echinacea | Wound healing (external), immune stimulant (internal) | Polysaccharides, cichoric acid, and components of the alkamide fraction | None reported, but allergies are possible; be sure product is pure and not adulterated with prairie dock (can cause nausea, vomiting); may flare lupus |
| Evening primrose | Treatment of atopic eczema, breast tenderness, arthritis | *Cis*-gamma-linoleic acid (GLA) (some suggestive data) | No data; borage seed oil (20% as GLA) may be a substitute and does have toxic side effects (liver toxicity, carcinogen) |
| Fennel Fenugreek | Calms stomach, promotes burping Calms stomach, demulcent | *Trans*-anethole, fenchone, estragole, camphene, L-pinene Unknown | Do not use the volatile oil—causes skin reactions, vomiting, seizures, and respiratory problems; no side effects with use of seeds. None |

**Table 24.2.** (continued)

| Herb | Claimed Uses | Active Ingredients | Potential Side Effects |
|---|---|---|---|
| Garlic | GI ailments, reduces blood clot pressure, prevents clots | Allin (sulphur-containing amino acid derivative), ajoene | Large doses are needed (uncooked, up to 4 grams of fresh garlic a day), which may result in GI upsets; can "thin" the blood (anticoagulant) |
| Gentian | Appetite stimulant | Glycosides and alkaloids; increases bile secretion | May not be well tolerated by expectant mothers or people with high blood pressure (possibly increasing pressure) |
| Gingko biloba | Helps dementia | Antioxidant | Well tolerated |
| Ginseng | Adaptogen, cure-all, antistress agent | Triterpenoid saponins | Be sure the product is pure; some insomnia, diarrhea, and skin eruptions have been reported; possible immune stimulant (antagonizes other medications) |
| Goldenseal | Digestive aid, treatment of genito-urinary disorders | Alkaloids (hydrastine and berberine) | In *huge* doses, may cause uterine cramps |
| Honey | Sore throat, antiseptic, anti-infective, antiarthritic, sedative | Fructose, glucose, sucrose, tannin | Do not give to children under 1 year of age; may cause botulism in infants |
| Lovage | Diuretic, promotes burping | Lactone derivatives (pH thalides) | Some photosensitivity with volatile oil of lovage |
| L-Tryptophan | Sleep aid, antidepressant | Essential amino acid that increases chemical serotonin, leading to some sleepiness | Be sure product is pure; contaminants may cause a serious blood disorder and a scleroderma-like illness |
| Mistletoe | Stimulates smooth muscle (American), antispasmodic and calmative (European) | Phoratoxin and viscotoxin (depending on the plant species) | Berries are highly toxic, and the leaves may also cause cell death; in animals lowers blood pressure, weakens, constricts blood vessels |
| Nettle | Antirheumatic, antiasthmatic, diuretic, against BPH | Histamine, acetylcholine, 5-hydroxytryptamine | Skin irritation from the active ingredients |
| New Zealand green-lipped mussel | Antiarthritic | Amino acids, mucopolysaccharides | No toxicity or side effects except in those allergic to seafood |
| Passion flowers | Calmative, sedative | Unknown or disputed | None |

(*continued*)

**Table 24.2.**  (continued)

| Herb | Claimed Uses | Active Ingredients | Potential Side Effects |
|---|---|---|---|
| Peppermint | Calms stomach, promotes burping, antispasmodic | Free menthol and esters of menthol | Do not give to infants and young children, who may choke from the menthol |
| Pokeroot | Rheumatism, cure-all | Saponin mixture (phytolaccatoxin), mitogen, pokeweed mitogen (PWM) | Vomiting, blood cell abnormalities, hypotension, decreased respiration, gastritis |
| Rosemary | Antirheumatic, digestive, stimulant | Camphor, borneol, cineole, diosmin (a flavonoid pigment) | Large quantities of the volatile oil taken internally cause stomach, intestinal, and kidney irritation |
| Rue | Antispasmodic, calmative | Quinoline alkaloids, coumarin derivatives | Skin blisters and photosensitivity following contact; gastric upsets when taken internally; may be an effective antispasmodic but is too toxic to be used |
| St. John's wort (Hypericum) | Antidepressant, anti-inflammatory, wound healing | 10% tannin, xanthones, and flavonoids that act as monoamine oxidase inhibitors (antidepressants) | Photosensitivity dermatitis in those who take the herb for extended periods; Prozac-like; increases serotonin |
| Sairei-to | Antiarthritic | 12 herbs in combination | Diarrhea, abdominal pain, rash |
| Sassafras | Antispasmodic, antirheumatic | Safrole | Active ingredient is carcinogenic in rats and mice |
| Senna | Cathartic | Dianthrone glycosides (sennosides A+B) | Diarrhea, gastric and intestinal irritation with large and/or habitual doses |
| Tea tree oil | Antiseptic (external application only) | Terpene hydrocarbons, oxygenated terpenes (terpinen-4-ol) | No side effects except skin irritation in sensitive individuals |
| Valerian (garden heliotrope) | Tranquilizer, calmative | Unknown | None noted |
| Yucca | Antiarthritic | Saporins | None noted |

*Source:* Compiled by Elaine E. Furst, R.N., and Daniel E. Furst, M.D. Modified from Taylor VE, *The Honest Herbalist.* 3rd ed. Binghamton, NY: Haworth Press; 1993: 336–351.

## CAN LUPUS PATIENTS EXERCISE?

Judicious exercise is a very important part of managing lupus. It can strengthen muscles, improve flexibility, and promote a sense of well-being. Inactivity can promote osteoporosis, muscle weakness, and wasting. Patients who are not fit are less able to respond to various stresses in the environment.

The optimal conditioning program involves engaging in activities that strengthen muscle tone and improve endurance without putting too much stress on a single joint. Isometric exercises, stretching exercises, Tai Chi, yoga, and Pilates involve strengthening muscles without moving the involved joint. These are good ways to start. Later on, walking, swimming, and bicycling are excellent activities. To start, one can take a 5-minute walk twice a day and build up to an hour-long walk three to five times a week. Limits of endurance are highly variable among individuals. The "talk test" asks: Can you talk comfortably while exercising? If not, it's best to slow down or stop. Also, one should *never* exercise beyond the point of minimal discomfort.

When a joint or muscle is painful, local heat can be applied. Moist heat (e.g., shower, bath, hot tub, jacuzzi, thermophore) is superior to dry heat. If an area is acutely injured, the application of ice will minimize swelling during the first 36 hours. Inflamed joints must not be exercised. This can be harmful. For example, engaging in such activities as tennis, bowling, golf, weight lifting, or rowing with an inflamed or swollen hand, wrist, or shoulder can aggravate the disease (isotonic exercises). But the injured area should not be ignored completely. An inflamed joint should be put through its full range of motion several times a day. This helps prevent contractures and muscle atrophy.

## WOULD A REHABILITATION PROGRAM HELP?

As discussed in Chapter 13, the inflammatory arthritis of lupus causes visible swelling of the joints in 20 to 30 percent of patients with the disease and deformities in less than 10 percent. Patients with inflammatory arthritis often benefit from a formal rehabilitation program.

*Physical therapists* are licensed allied health professionals (look for RPT—registered physical therapist—after the name). They help improve conditioning, instruct you on how to move inflamed joints without damaging them, and introduce you to muscle-strengthening regimens. They can also apply hot packs, administer ultrasound, give gentle massages, and employ spray-and-stretch techniques (using a coolant spray followed by gentle tissue stretching) for tender fibrositic tissues. An RPT will be glad to suggest a conditioning program to your doctor.

*Occupational therapists* often work with physical therapists. They are also licensed allied health professionals and provide valuable, underutilized expertise (look for OTR—registered occupational therapist—after the name). They will perform an "Activities of Daily Living" (ADL) evaluation. After examining what an individual does in the course of a day at work and at home, the therapist can advise on methods of energy conservation and joint protection. In other words, they can suggest a way to cook a meal or get on or off a toilet seat with the least amount of stress on an inflamed or damaged joint, which can also minimize discomfort. An OTR is expert in recommending assistive devices such as splints or braces and practical modifications in the workplace or home (e.g., special spoons, toothbrushes, shoehorns) that make life easier. Consider this example of how an OTR works.

> Kim is a paralegal for a large law firm. Her employers provided her with a work station that enabled her to do word processing, answer telephones, and acting as a receptionist. But she soon began complaining of neck and upper back pain as well as numbness and tingling in her hands. Although she has had SLE for 4 years, she never had any musculoskeletal problems other than occasional aching until she took this job. Her doctor ordered an occupational therapy consultation, which carefully evaluated her work station. The OTR recommended a higher chair with a firmer back and a swivel screen for the computer. She instructed Kim to type for no more than 20 minutes at a time. After implementing the changes, Kim began to feel better. The OTR showed Kim how to squat rather than stoop when picking up a file weighing more than 10 pounds and how to lift files to equalize the weight on both sides of her body. Her doctor suspected that she might have carpal tunnel syndrome, which would cause numbness and tingling in her hand. He injected the carpal tunnel with cortisone, and she wore wrist splints provided by the OTR at night for several weeks. Kim is now pain-free.

*Vocational rehabilitation* counselors provide job training for patients who are unable to continue working at their current jobs. Their services are usually obtained through worker's compensation and disability insurance programs. Some examples of vocational rehabilitation candidates are sun-sensitive farmers or fishermen or office employees with hand deformities who are unable to type.

*Psychologists* as well as physical and occupational therapists assist lupus patients in learning relaxation techniques that promote improved sleep habits and reduce stress. Some of these techniques include biofeedback, yoga, gentle massage, and hypnosis. (Chapter 25 discusses stress and coping mechanisms, along with some of these techniques, in greater detail.)

## WHY ARE LUPUS PATIENTS ALWAYS TIRED?

One of the most common complaints I hear from my patients is that they are always tired. There are many reasons for this. Lupus is associated with anemia and active inflammation, both of which promote fatigue. Some of the medicines that doctors prescribe for high blood pressure and inflammation, for example, can make one drowsy. Alternatively, the stresses of dealing with a serious disease and its associated depression are also exhausting. Many of my lupus patients whose blood tests show no active disease deny that they are depressed but still complain of fatigue. A partial explanation is on the horizon. Some evidence shows that a group of proteins known as *cytokines* are associated with fatigue (Chapter 5), and cytokine dysfunction is an established feature of lupus.

The best way for a lupus patient to manage fatigue is to follow this course of action:

1. *Determine the cause of fatigue.* Ask your doctor to undertake an evaluation for reversible causes of fatigue such as anemia, hypothyroidism (low thyroid levels), elevated blood sugars, or a lupus flare. If one of these is the cause, it can be treated. Consider additional causes of fatigue and rule them out: malnutrition, substance abuse, pain medicine, depression, bipolar disease.
2. *Pace yourself.* Keeping active prevents the cytokines from getting the better of you. Staying in bed all day only increases fatigue. Commit yourself to an hour or two of activities followed by a rest period of 15 to 20 minutes. Repeat this several times a day. Most lupus patients can perform 8 to 10 hours of productive work a day if they alternate periods of activity with periods of rest. Working 6 hours straight can be traumatic; it promotes a feeling of exhaustion that may call for several days of recovery.
3. *Take appropriate medication.* Many lupus medications decrease fatigue, in particular corticosteroids and antimalarials. Your physician may wish to prescribe certain other medications to treat fatigue. Depending on the circumstances, some of these include iron, thyroid, psychoactive stimulants, specific serotonin reuptake inhibiting antidepressants, and tricyclic antidepressants, or combinations.
4. *Get a restful night's sleep.* Many lupus patients have a secondary fibromyalgia that is associated with sleep disturbance. Not getting a restful night's sleep saps your energy and promotes fatigue. Tricyclic antidepressants relax the muscles and help induce restful sleep without being habit forming or dangerous.
5. *Walk.* A conditioning program with aerobic exercise such as walking gets more oxygen into the tissues, strengthens muscles, and will give you a sense of well-being while also reducing fatigue.

## CAN WE BLAME IT ON THE WEATHER?

It has been jokingly suggested that patients with rheumatic disease make excellent meteorologists. Changes in barometric pressure frequently lead to symptoms of increased stiffness and aching in the joints. In other words, when the temperature goes from hot to cold or the humidity from dry to wet, lupus patients complain of a feeling of stiffness. But patients with lupus needn't worry about their weather-predicting abilities. Fewer symptoms are observed in patients who live in desert climates, where the temperature and humidity are consistent. Those who live in the midwestern United States, in contrast, might be a little more achy or stiff on certain days. When traveling to different parts of the country, they may find that it takes a day or two to acclimate to their new environment.

## HOW DOES SMOKING AFFECT LUPUS?

Smoking is bad for those who don't have lupus, but it makes lupus even worse. Tobacco smoke contains hydrazines, which are reviewed in Chapter 8. Patients with lupus who smoke have more active cutaneous disease and, according to the Harvard's nurses, more lupus in general. In addition, nicotine frequently aggravates Raynaud's phenomenon, accelerates vascular disease, worsens high blood pressure, makes antimalarials less effective, and increases the greater risk of stroke, which is already a worry of patients with SLE. There are simply no good reasons to smoke.

## SUMMING UP

A good deal of lupus treatment involves things in the environment that can be controlled. A lot can be accomplished by avoiding the sun, eating a healthy, well-balanced diet, engaging in a moderate amount of general strengthening and conditioning exercise, pacing oneself, and avoiding frequent changes in barometric pressure. Now let's continue with things patients can do for themselves. The next chapter teaches you how to cope better. See Table 24.3.

**Table 24.3.** *Summary of Physical and Adjunctive Measures for Lupus Patients*

1. Ultraviolet light is harmful in SLE except perhaps for a band of UVA-1 light. Two-thirds of lupus patients report sun sensitivity. Sun exposure is greatest at higher altitudes and mid-afternoon.
2. Other than a well-balanced, healthy diet, there are no specific recommendations for lupus patients. Those on steroids should watch salt, sugar, and carbohydrate intake.
3. The only vitamins or supplements specifically beneficial for systemic lupus erythematosus is vitamin D. The others are harmless, but alfalfa sprouts, those that contain sulfa or ephedrine should be avoided.
4. Isometric exercises, specifically those that strengthen and stretch are helpful in lupus. Specifically, Tai' Chi, yoga and Pilates are beneficial. Isotonic activities (e.g., jogging, tennis, bowling) are advised only if one's joints are not inflamed.
5. Nearly all lupus patients have varying degrees of fatigue. The most common causes include medication, depression, anemia and inflammation. Fatigue is managed with pacing oneself, or having periods of activity alternating with periods of rest.
6. Smoking can flare lupus and decrease the effectiveness of antimalarials.
7. Changes in the barometer, such as weather that goes from hot to cold or wet to dry (and vice versa) is associated with more stiffness and aching until the body acclimates to these perturbations.

**FURTHER READING**

1. Ting WW, Sontheimer RD. Local therapy for cutaneous and systemic lupus erythematosus: practical and theoretical considerations. *Lupus.* 2001;10(3):171–184.
2. Barbhaiya M, Tedeschi SK, Lu B, et al. Cigarette smoking and the risk of systemic lupus erythematosu, overall and by double-stranded DNA antibody subtype, in the Nurses' Health Study cohorts. *Ann Rheum Dis.* 2018;77(2):196–202.
3. O'Riordan R, Doran M, Connolly D. Fatigue and activity management education for individuals with systemic lupus erythematosus. *Occup Ther Int.* 2017;2017:4530104.

# 25

## *You Can Help Conquer Lupus*

When confronted with a diagnosis of lupus, most patients are initially frightened about the prognosis. Often, their first reaction is to ask what they did wrong. Coping with the diagnosis of lupus can be a difficult proposition. So many aspects of the disease must be dealt with that can at times seem overwhelming. Studies have shown that over half of lupus patients express a broad range of feelings, including stress, anger, depression, fear, guilt, and pain.

This chapter offers an overview of the principal psychosocial problems that lupus patients encounter and formulates meaningful, constructive approaches for dealing with them. Active lupus and medications given to treat the disease may also be associated with mood and behavior alterations, cognitive dysfunction, fatigue, and fibromyalgia. The reader is referred to Chapters 15, 24, and 26 for a review of these concerns.

### WHY COPING IS DIFFICULT

This section lays out some of the most common problems and offers a discussion of constructive approaches that can be taken to alleviate some of them. Coping with lupus calls for dealing with many different types of problems at once.

### But You Don't Look Sick!

Jane is a high-powered attorney with a prestigious big-city law firm. She usually works 50 hours a week at the office and frequently takes work home on weekends. When she began having joint aches and muscle weakness along with fatigue, her doctor diagnosed her as having systemic lupus and started her on low-dose steroids and Plaquenil. To keep up at work, she stopped dating and going out with friends. No one at work suspected she was ill, and no one was told. On weekends, Jane would stay in bed, barely able to move, so that she could make it to work the next week. Dr. Jones told Jane that the drugs would take months to make any substantial difference in how she felt and that she needed to get extra rest and take care of herself.

Jane, however, was afraid of losing her position and did not have time to be sick. Jane surprised herself when she finally broke down and confided in friends, who were supportive and told her to follow her doctor's advice.

For better or worse, most newly diagnosed lupus patients look perfectly healthy. Only 10 percent of patients with systemic lupus erythematosus (SLE) develop a deforming arthritis, and most rashes (and paleness) can be hidden with make-up. Steroids take many weeks to puff up the face or alter one's appearance. These delays are fine if you don't want anyone to know what's going on, but it discourages the support and empathy that people who care about you might provide. Ignoring the disease can lead to a subconscious withdrawal from your vocational and social interests, mask your need for rest (as it did in Jane's case), and set the stage for disaster later on.

## My Doctor Is Not Listening

In the beginning, most patients experience some relief after being diagnosed with SLE. Some have exclaimed, "I'm not crazy after all!" A honeymoon period takes place in which the diagnosing doctor can do no wrong, followed by a period of questioning when the patient does not feel better immediately. I schedule a counseling session with my patients when they are first diagnosed, explain all the pitfalls of the disease, and outline a treatment plan. Failing to do this will cause problems with patients later on.

Often doctors become too judgmental and difficult to approach. Sometimes we unintentionally intimidate our patients, who are afraid to tell us of serious problems they are having that may affect treatment. Patients should not be afraid and must stick up for their rights. I always respect patients who tell me, "I need 15 minutes of your time without interruption" and give an organized, well-thought-out presentation of their problems. Also, they should not be afraid to ask for a second opinion. A good doctor will never object to this. Mutual honesty and respect, a sense of understanding of lifestyles and limitations on both sides, and open lines of communication are vital. A patient's relationship with his or her doctor is akin to a complex commitment; the doctor is half of the ticket to good health, and both sides have to put up with each other's idiosyncrasies.

Relatedly, patients should not antagonize their doctors. Several years ago, a group practice of four rheumatologists rated their combined 25 active lupus patients in terms of how much they liked or disliked them, and the same 5 patients were rated as "most disliked" by all four physicians. A psychiatrist was brought in and found that the 5 disliked patients displayed more hostility, anxiety, depression, immaturity, and uncooperative behavior patterns than the other 20 lupus patients. This group also had a tendency to doctor shop; in other words, they did not stop with a second opinion—they got 10 opinions in all specialties. Anxiety, depression, and even anger are normal reactive emotions to an illness like lupus. But there are times when the doctor should be trusted; mutual trust and cooperation are vital.

## Fear and Anxiety

JoAnn was told she had lupus by her doctor, who seemed at the time very busy and distracted with other things. She had many questions to ask, blurted a few out, and did not want to bother him further. She knew that sun exposure was bad for her but did not know how much sun she could have at any one time, so she made up her own treatment. JoAnn rarely went outside. She bought a sunscreen that was the wrong strength and did not know how or when to apply it. Whenever friends invited her out during the daytime, she declined. She became fearful about keeping up her front lawn and for the first time hired a gardener. When she turned them down for a third time, JoAnn's friends stopped asking her to the lunchtime bridge games she had enjoyed so much in the past. Becoming more fearful and anxious, she tried to explain this to her doctor, who did not seem to have time to hear her out. Family members noticed that JoAnn was jumpy and agitated. When they asked her what was wrong, she said "nothing" because she did not want to impose. Family members started decreasing contact with her. Finally, she took a self-help course that was sponsored by the local Lupus Foundation and sought counseling, which started to turn things around. She is no longer afraid to confront her doctor.

Lupus patients have many justifiable fears: "Will I be able to work?" "Can I take care of myself?" They express fear of pain, fear of disease flare-ups, fear of death or disfigurement, fear of drugs and their side effects. This, in turn, creates anxieties that are capable of inhibiting normal social functioning and serve to promote further isolation. "What if nobody believes me?" "Am I over- or underdoing it?" If a patient is not open and honest with friends, overanxious behavior will turn them off. Recognizing these fears and concerns and learning to deal with them is important for all lupus patients, who should express their concerns to trusting friends, family, or healthcare professionals or take a self-help course, as JoAnn did.

## Anger

After Linda was accepted to medical school, she was diagnosed with lupus nephritis. She was told that she would need high-dose steroids for months and that these would alter her mood and behavior as well as her ability to concentrate. She also had to take chemotherapy, which would make her quite sick every month. She decided to defer schooling for a year, only to learn that the school would have rejected her if it had known about her lupus. Linda became angry. It was difficult to control her emotions on 60 milligrams of prednisone a day. She was cruel to her mother, who had taken an extra job to help support her through college and no longer found time to help her younger brother with his science homework. While shopping at a super-market, Linda, after waiting for 10 minutes on a checkout line, got into a confrontation with the store manager. When her brother got an F in science, she realized that her anger was misplaced and, with the support of her doctor, began to channel her energies constructively toward beating the disease and pushing it into remission within a year. Linda is now a second-year medical student and is thinking of going into rheumatology.

If you have lupus, you have every right to be angry. There are several levels of anger. Rage is a violent, uncontrollable anger. Hostility, resentment, and indigna-tion are somewhat less intense. Yes, it's annoying if you have to give up enjoyable activities, especially outdoors. It is also frustrating and upsetting if the treatment that will make you better won't work for several months, if you have to have sur-gery, or if you can no longer think about having children. It is hard for others to see how much you hurt. But don't let anger bottle up inside you. Stress has been known to cause flare-ups of fibromyalgia and can possibly aggravate your lupus. Anger takes up a lot of precious energy and pushes away others who care about you. Try to channel your energy into productive work. Ask yourself why you are angry. How can you detect it? Can you ignore it? Step into your friend's or employer's shoes. How do they feel about what is going on? Think of how you can prevent yourself from getting angry and how to relieve anger when it builds.

### Guilt

Her mother had lupus, and Nancy always knew there was a chance she would get it. But when it happened, the diagnosis seemed to drop out of the clouds. Since she had been laid off, Nancy was now convinced that the loss of her job was due to her poor performance and not the economy, even though she had had good job performance ratings. Convinced that a higher authority was punishing her for being lazy, Nancy would sulk around the house and blame herself for everything that could possibly go wrong. Her mother made this worse by overcompensating and saying that because she, the mother, carried lupus genes, it was all *her* fault. Nothing constructive was accomplished in the household for months until Nancy's husband told her that he would leave if she didn't get some counseling that would help her develop a more positive attitude. She went for the counseling. Her lupus is now in remission, and she has a new job.

Guilt is the sense that you did something wrong or that you blame yourself for something over which you had no control. Many patients inflict guilt upon themselves. "What have I done to my children, who now have a chance of getting lupus?" or "Does not feeling well enough to participate in the garden club mean that I am in a weakened position so that others can manipulate me?" Don't say, "I should have done this instead." Block that emotion as best you can. Guilt is self-defeating, and guilt can be a "self-fulfilling prophecy." Have a positive attitude and be ready to modify your thoughts and behaviors. Counseling, such as Nancy had, can help you acquire the tools to maintain positive attitudes.

## Pain

Pain should be viewed as a sensation that is natural, inevitable, and tolerable but one that must be controlled. Most lupus patients have physical pain, but it is usually relatively mild. Only a small percentage end up attending pain centers or taking narcotic analgesics. Fear of pain, however, is a major problem. Most joint and muscle pain is inflammatory in nature and managed with anti-inflammatory medicines, not pain pills. Inappropriate reactions to pain, particularly fear of exercise and mobilization, can waste or atrophy the muscles and make joints immobile. This further promotes social isolation.

Patients can help themselves deal with pain. For example, biofeedback helps to control the heart rate, blood pressure, skin temperature, and muscle tone. It can alleviate pain from headaches, spasm, and Raynaud's phenomenon. Guided imagery and meditation promote relaxation and decrease muscle spasms. Acupuncture, especially electronic acupuncture (acupressure), numbs nerve fibers and decreases noninflammatory pain.

## Stress and Trauma

Stress is a force to which the body responds. There are good forms of stress—those that energize the body—as well as types of stress that alter the immune system. Can stress cause lupus? Several years ago, members of lupus associations were asked to fill out questionnaires that included queries about how they thought their lupus had started. Between 10 percent and 15 percent replied that they thought that emotional stress or physical trauma had brought on their disease. However, when we looked at it the other way around—examining doctors' records to see whether patients actually *were* under unusual stress (defined on a "Life Events Inventory" as a death of a loved one, divorce, or loss of a job) or had a serious injury shortly before being diagnosed—this percentage fell into the 1 to 3 percent range, which is not statistically significant. In other words, *it is unlikely that stress or trauma by itself causes lupus* There are no evidence-based studies in the literature documenting this, but a single well-controlled study from the Harvard Nurses Study over a 40-year period has suggested an "association" between post-traumatic stress disorder and those who develop years later.

Can stress aggravate lupus? It is very clear that stress and trauma can cause a pre-existing lupus to flare-up. A large body of evidence has shown that certain animals with autoimmune disease have a defective corticotrophin-releasing hormone (CRH; which is made in the brain's hypothalamus) neuron, which accelerates inflammation under stressful circumstances. Numerous studies have shown that this is brought about via interactions between the hypothalamic–pituitary–adrenal axis, autonomic nervous system, and cytokines. Not all stressed lupus patients experience flare-ups, and many patients have flare-ups when they are not stressed. Nevertheless, I have had several patients with chronic, stable, mild lupus whose disease spread to other organs or who had severe inflammatory joint reactions after a motor vehicle accident or severe emotional trauma.

Issues of stress and trauma, particularly when problems arise after an accident, can become subject to legal as well as medical definitions. For medicolegal purposes, these reactions should occur within 60 days of the incident. Documentation of a flare should be evidenced by (i) worsening of inflammatory indices (e.g., sedimentation rate, C-reactive protein [CRP], anti-DNA), (ii) increased lupus activity noted on physical examination, (iii) additional lupus medicine being prescribed or an increase in dosing of ongoing medications, (iv) more visits to the doctor, or (v) referral to a mental health professional or new psychotropic medicine prescribed to deal with stress noted in the medical record. In state workers' compensation laws, we find the term "continuous trauma," which refers to ongoing, persistent stress or harassment that causes increased disease activity. Also included in this terminology is the tendency of a traumatic incident or continuous trauma to light up, accelerate, or aggravate lupus. There have been several cases in which patients with early nondiagnosed but symptomatic (and medically documented) pre-lupus who had their disease "turned on." Emotional stress can alter the immune system. Studies performed on healthy individuals who lose loved ones show that their immune functioning is altered during the bereavement period. Our "head bone" is connected to our T cells, which, in turn, affect lupus.

## Depression

Even though Judith was told her lupus was mild, things didn't seem right. Always a perfectionist who planned each activity and goal carefully, she felt that something else had to be wrong. After all, Judith could not sleep at night; she tossed and turned even though she had a new bed. She was no longer asked out on dates. She seemed distracted and always complained of headaches and cramping, and she was sure that her pulse was too fast. She no longer enjoyed watching a good movie and forgot how to tell jokes or laugh. Judith was convinced that a serious medical illness was eluding her doctors, so she went to the Mayo Clinic and the Cleveland Clinic only to be told that her local physician was correct in her diagnosis. After joining a patient support group sponsored by the lupus society, Judith met other people with lupus who proved very insightful and pointed out each other's problems. After the third session, the group unanimously told her that she was depressed and that her symptoms were part of this reaction. The group leader, a psychologist, recommended a psychiatrist, who started her on an antidepressant. Within 4 months, she was off all medication and leading a normal life.

Depression is the most common coping problem in lupus. Lupus itself and some of the medications used to treat the disease can induce a clinical chemical depression. Additionally, lupus patients can develop a reactive depression: they are upset that they have the disease. In the simplest terms, *depression* is a feeling of helplessness and hopelessness. It is characterized by spells of crying, loss of appetite (or increased appetite), nonrestful sleep, loss of self-esteem, inability to concentrate, decreased social interests, indecision, and loss of interest in the outside world. Physiologic signs and symptoms such as headache, palpitations, loss of sexual drive, indigestion, and cramping may go along with depression. Depression affects one's body, mood, relationships, and physical activities.

Some suggestions of ways to cope with depression are detailed in the next section. First, your doctor should verify that the depression is not due to central nervous system lupus or medications you are taking. For example, steroids both induce and help depression. Chemical or biological depression is treated differently from reactive or psychological depression.

## HOW TO COPE BETTER

Depression, fear, and anxiety are the most common reactions noted in SLE patients. How should they deal with these emotions? How can they cope better? Adequate coping requires taking action, and several good approaches are available.

### Goals and Attitudes

If you are a lupus patient, your first step is to define and try to assess what is bothering you. Professional help may be needed to do this. Then you deal with these concerns by listing realistic goals and expectations. Develop a method for problem solving: problems can be eliminated, circumvented, modified, or worked out. Use all your available resources: financial, personal, and intellectual. Be willing to reassess if you cannot meet your goals or expectations. Don't try to change others; try to change yourself. Set realistic goals to improve your quality of life. Pace yourself and allow for periods of activity that alternate with periods of rest. Ask yourself what hopes you have and—if they are unrealistic—try to replace them with other hopes. Try to balance a loss with a gain. How can you improve your spiritual well-being? Learn to relax, rest, and exercise. If you don't have a sense of humor or if it is suppressed, discover laughter. Laughter is an excellent tonic for the body. Give affection to others, and you'll receive it back. Learn to share yourself. Don't worry about tomorrow—focus on what you can do today. What kinds of things do you like to do, and how can you do them? Exchange negative thoughts for positive thoughts and reinforce them. Socialize. All these things will help to make you feel better about yourself and to conquer depression.

### Marriage, Family, and Sexuality

Darleen and George were happily married for 5 years when Darleen was diagnosed with SLE. George had grown up with learning difficulties and had had limited educational opportunities. Darleen tried to tell him what lupus was, but he didn't seem to pay attention. When Darleen was put on steroids and gained 20 pounds, George made fun of her appearance. One night her joints were so swollen that she couldn't even get into the car to go to George's friends' house for dinner. George said that her joints looked okay to him and started yelling at her. Over the next few months, George started drinking heavily and lost interest in sex. Darleen was scared to talk to him, and one day he just didn't come home.

Unfortunately, some reports suggest that within 5 years of the diagnosis of lupus of married women, nearly half of them are divorced. This results from many of the emotional changes previously discussed and a coping problem on the spouse's part. ("What do you mean you can't go out with me tonight? You look fine!") When women complain of difficulty in keeping up with household chores, or workplace demands, or responsibilities to their children, relationships become precarious. After they have been diagnosed, I ask lupus patients to bring their boyfriends or husbands to a counseling session. They shouldn't feel that they are "out of the loop" or that the doctor may be hiding things from them. If possible, spouses should be included in any decisions.

Spouses should know that steroids can alter appearance, mood, and behavior and that family responsibilities might have to be shifted for a time. Parents may ignore problems, smother the patient, or act somewhere in between and be appropriately supportive. It is up to the patient to decide what role they should be assigned, if any, as part of the recovery plan.

Surprisingly, very few of the reasons for divorce among patients with lupus have anything to do with sexuality. A detailed survey showed that only 4 percent of women with SLE had major problems with physical aspects of sexuality. Most of these cases dealt with a dry vagina from Sjögren's syndrome (also causing dry eyes, dry mouth, and arthritis) that is difficult to lubricate and can cause painful intercourse. Other cases involved women who understandably complained of emotional issues such as being too tired to participate in sex. Destructive hip changes from arthritis or avascular necrosis also make sex difficult, but they are easily resolved with creative sexual positions and/or corrective surgery. Divorce or separation arises from not being frank with a loved one, from altered expectations, from lack of knowledge about lupus and how it can affect mood and behavior, and from husbands' reactions to learning that their wives cannot bear children—which does not apply to all women with lupus. (See Chapter 30, "Can a Woman with Lupus Have a Baby?") It's important for lupus patients to keep all communication channels and support systems open.

### Support Groups, Self-Help, Social Media, and Counseling

The Arthritis Foundation and lupus support and advocacy organizations provide self-help groups supervised by trained professionals like psychologists or social workers. They provide intrinsic support, disease education, emotional warmth, means for friendly communication, and closeness with others. Working together, they can help a patient reverse a negative self-image and self-defeating attitudes through a supportive atmosphere. This can lead to more hope, improved self-esteem, a redirection of energy, and a sense that one is not alone. Over the last 20 years, social media has mobilized lupus patients on the internet via blogs, Twitter, Facebook and other patient support groups. The most reliable and responsible sites are supported by respected organizations such as the Lupus Foundation of America, Arthritis Foundation, and Lupus Research Alliance where professional facilitators monitor their content and provide additional content through their websites.

Sometimes, one-on-one psychological counseling is advisable. On occasion, medication is required, and this may be prescribed by a psychiatrist. Psychiatrists are medical doctors, all of whom are taught about lupus and autoimmunity in medical school. Psychotherapists and rheumatologists should work together as teams. Tricyclic antidepressants promote restful sleep, raise pain thresholds, relax muscles, and improve mood. Specific serotonin reuptake inhibitors may be used with or without tricyclics. Taken in the morning, they often increase energy levels, promote weight reduction, relieve depression, and diminish obsessive-compulsive tendencies. Combination tricyclic/serotonin and/or norepinephrine boosters such as Effexor are also effective. Additional goals of psychological intervention are to increase self-control, patience, tolerance, flexibility, and creativity.

### Cognitive Therapy, Biofeedback, and Stress-Reduction Strategies

*Cognitive-behavioral therapy* is a useful approach for patients with lupus who have difficulty learning, retaining knowledge, processing, recalling, finding words, focusing, concentrating, planning, or organizing. Cognitive dysfunction or impairment is usually intermittent and in part reflects spasms of blood vessels that supply oxygen to the brain and that are part of a dysfunctioning autonomic nervous system (reviewed in Chapter 15). Cognitive therapists are usually psychologists, occupational therapists, or speech therapists. They urge their clients to use memory aids, such as placing project lists and Post-Its around the house, decreasing distractions, forming mental pictures to assist with associations, and not getting frustrated when trying to find words. Therapists show patients how to use cues, designate one spot at home as the repository for all reminder notes, and write things down so they will not forget. Having regular daily routines, using timers or alarm clocks, and having a regular filing system are also helpful.

There has been a lot of interest in the role of *mindfulness* in lupus. This is a psychological process that brings one's attention to experiences occurring in the present moment which can be developed through the practice of meditation and other training. Utilized to develop self-knowledge as enlightenment or complete freedom from suffering that emanated from a Buddhist-like tradition. Mindfulness-based interventions are effective in reducing *rumination* (dwelling on a specific subject) and worry. Another tool that works well with mindfulness is *virtual reality*. Virtual reality is a computer-generated scenario that simulates a realistic experience.

Relaxation exercises can decrease sympathetic nervous system activity, slow the heart rate, and improve oxygen delivery to the muscles and brain. *Biofeedback* teaches patients to control their body responses to minimize anxiety, provide relaxation, and promote pain relief by making normally unconscious bodily actions conscious. Deep-breathing exercises, relaxation tapes, and visualizing pleasant environments (called "guided imagery") decrease muscle tension, pain, and stress. Biofeedback is particularly helpful in patients with Raynaud's phenomenon. In *EEG biofeedback,* helpful beta brain waves are encouraged while disruptive alpha waves are suppressed. *Yoga* combines deep breathing, meditation, and specific postures that integrate mental, physical, and spiritual energies to enhance well-being. *Transcendental meditation* enables patients to focus on a single thought or object to create an inner calm that banishes stress. *T'ai chi* adds passive movements to achieve this result. Also, never underestimate the power of *prayer* along with quiet contemplation.

## Children and Adolescents

Children with lupus need to be treated like any other children. Although there are restrictions on sun-related and certain other activities, *they should not suffer because of their parents' guilt, and they should not be overprotected.* Many children instinctively deny their lupus; this is okay if they take their medicine and follow the usual precautions. Be matter of fact with them in discussing the disease. The advent of social media, texting, and other methods of instant communication have further complicated treating adolescents due to increased pressures inflicted by immature acquaintances with hurtful impulses.

Alternatively, children of mothers with SLE are often unusually astute and aware of their mothers' problems. Most of my female patients with young children have been asked at least once, "Mommy, are you going to die?" Be honest with your children and don't hide important things from them. They are bound to find out. Couch whatever you tell them in hopeful and positive terms. They can be a source of pride and joy and deserve to be part of your support system.

*Teenagers with lupus present special problems.* They are concerned with hair loss, rashes, and fatigue, which prevent them from participating in social activities, especially those with sun exposure (Chapter 24). They want to know about pregnancy. Adolescents need a certain degree of independence and responsibility; they need friends and often try to be away from parents, whom they perceive as embarrassing to them. Steroids alter appearance, hair growth, mood, and behavior, and this affects dating, jobs, and school life. Compliance is a major problem, and the consequences of not taking the prescribed medication or less of it should be emphasized.

Joelle is a 16-year-old girl with multisystem active lupus. It had been under good control until she fell in with a new crowd that went to the beach every day and stayed out very late at night. It was summertime, and her rashes started getting worse. This flared her joints and started causing low-grade fevers.

Because she put on a partially adequate sunscreen, Joelle did not think that sunbathing was wrong and told her mother she was going out with friends. Instead of taking the 20 milligrams of prednisone prescribed, she took only 10 milligrams because she did not want her face to look puffy or to develop facial hair. Ultimately, her doctor noticed that her anemia was so severe that she was on the verge of needing a transfusion. She was therefore hospitalized. A few days of intravenous high-dose steroids stabilized her, and the medical interns and residents on the case spent extra time with Joelle giving her emotional support. Her family was called to Joelle's bedside, and the doctors discussed with them the importance of compliance, sun avoidance, and the dangers of not adequately treating the disease. A support system was devised to prevent further problems.

Approaching an adolescent with lupus requires unique solutions. First, talk to school personnel and see whether they will work with the child. See whether there is any way concerned classmates and educators can be informed about the disease and the special considerations that may apply. Also, determine whether there are important people in the teenager's life who are role models, such as trainers, coaches, teachers, clergy, or extracurricular activity instructors who can be brought into the loop. Finally, try to direct the teen's energies into constructive hobbies or interests or safe projects.

### Avoid Unproven Remedies

There are times when lupus patients can feel desperate, and medical quackery is a multibillion-dollar-a-year industry whose claims seem tempting at certain moments. Any promotion that offers a cure for lupus should be suspect. Don't believe testimonials if the article has not appeared in the peer-reviewed medical literature. Be careful of treatments that are very expensive, such as chelation therapy, fetal animal hormone extracts, or monthly gamma globulin infusions. Some "natural vitamin and mineral" products contain alfalfa sprouts or other suspect chemicals that can aggravate lupus: L-tryptophan was an over-the-counter "natural" supplement whose metabolites induced scleroderma in 2,000 people and killed 50 of them before it was removed from the market in 1989. Mexican border clinics that promise cures treat lupus with steroids combined with a dangerous nonsteroidal anti-inflammatory drug called phenylbutazone, which is no longer available in the United States because it can cause leukemia and bone marrow shutdown. Some Chinese herbal remedies contain sulfa derivatives and other substances that trigger allergic reactions in most lupus patients. Some lupus patients flare when using the herbal cold medicine echinacea. Consult a physician before using any nonprescription drugs or potions.

*Evidence-based medicine* is when studies show that a specific therapeutic approach is beneficial using statistics and the scientific method. One of the first things I learned in medical school was "Do the patient no harm." And *you* should remember "Caveat emptor!" Ask for the evidence-based medicine that demonstrates the effectiveness of a specific therapeutic approach.

### SUMMING UP

If you have lupus, you have at least several hundred thousand Americans for company. Take hold of yourself and don't become overly upset. If there's no organ-threatening disease, you have a normal life expectancy; even if there *is* such disease, you will still live a long, long time. The disease will not go away. Although its course waxes and wanes, it is a permanent, chronic condition. It's okay to be angry, frightened, guilty, anxious, and depressed at first, but these emotions can be overcome. The sooner you develop adequate coping mechanisms, build up a good support system among family and friends, and start to work on a positive and realistic lifestyle, the better you will feel physically and mentally. Be empowered and learn how to use social media to your advantage. Who knows, all of these strategies may even make the lupus better!

## FURTHER READING

1. Bricou O, Taïeb O, Baubet T, Gal B, Guillevin L, Moro MR. Stress and coping strategies in systemic lupus erythematosus: a review. Neuroimmunomodulation. 2006;13(5–6):283–293.
2. Roberts AL, Malspeis S, Kubzansky LD, et al. Association of trauma and posttraumatic stress disorder with incident systemic lupus erythematosus in a longitudinal cohort of women. Arthritis Rheumatol. 2017;69(11):2162–2169.
3. Thomas DE. The lupus encyclopedia: a comprehensive guide for patients and families. Baltimore: Johns Hopkins Press, 2014.

# 26

# Taming Inflammation:
# Anti-Inflammatory Therapies

Even though most patients with systemic lupus erythematosus (SLE) don't like it, more than 90 percent take medication. Among the most prescribed and accepted of the many drug therapies for lupus are what doctors call "the anti-inflammatories." These remedies include *aspirin products* and other *nonsteroidal anti-inflammatory drugs*, or NSAIDs. A survey has documented that at any given time, 80 percent of all SLE patients are taking one of these agents on a regular or intermittent basis.

This chapter will endeavor to help lupus patients negotiate the tricky ins and outs of NSAIDs in an effort to maximize potential benefits while minimizing toxicity.

## ASPIRIN AND ITS FIRST COUSINS ONCE REMOVED

The fever-lowering property of willow bark (*Salix alba*) was known to the ancients and used by Hippocrates, Galen, and Pliny. The active salicylate ingredient was isolated in France in 1827, and acetylsalicylic acid (aspirin) specifically identified in 1899 in Germany. When Dr. Marian Ropes founded the first lupus clinic in Boston in 1932, aspirin was the only real medication at her disposal. For reasons that are still unclear, only one well-designed study has ever assessed the efficacy of aspirin in SLE. Fortunately, it was a definitive one. In 1980, the National Institutes of Health proved beyond the shadow of a doubt that aspirin was helpful in SLE.

### What Does Aspirin Do and Not Do in SLE?

The salicylate class of medicines, of which aspirin is the most important, ameliorates lupus by lowering fevers, treating headaches, diminishing joint or muscle aches and inflammation, and decreasing both serositis (pleurisy, pericarditis, peritonitis) and malaise. It has no effect on skin, heart, lung, kidney, liver, central nervous system, or blood involvement of the disease. Salicylates do not modify the disease; that is, they do not put lupus into remission, and they do little about the underlying immune process. Aspirin relieves lupus through the inhibition of prostaglandin, a chemical that promotes inflammation and pain in arthritic disorders.

Low-dose aspirin (baby aspirin, 81 milligrams) may be prophylactic in lupus patients with antiphospholipid antibodies (Chapter 21). Why is this so of low-dose and not regular aspirin? Low-dose salicylates inhibit a chemical that promotes clotting; regular aspirin also inhibits this chemical but additionally inhibits a second chemical that counteracts this. Taking 1 grain (81 milligrams) of aspirin daily may decrease the risk of strokes or miscarriages due to the lupus anticoagulant.

## WHAT ARE NSAIDS AND WHY ARE THEY USED IN LUPUS?

Pharmaceutical companies began their search for a better aspirin in the 1940s, and in 1952 they came up with *butazolidin* (Phenylbutazone). However, this dangerous drug is no longer marketed in the United States. It was followed by *indomethacin* (Indocin) in 1965, *ibuprofen* (Motrin) in 1974 and *naproxen* (Naproxen, Aleve). Since then, numerous additional preparations have been introduced. They are listed in Table 26.1 and discussed in this chapter. All of these preparations are more potent than aspirin, so that fewer pills are required to achieve the same effect.

All the NSAIDs, including aspirin, function similarly; their most important effect is inhibiting prostaglandin. But very few drug trials using these agents in SLE have been published. In fact, no NSAID is approved by the Food and Drug Administration for use in SLE. Despite this, as noted, 80 percent of all lupus patients take NSAIDs on a regular or intermittent basis. Some patients take NSAIDs on a daily, regular basis whereas others only use them when they have pain or inflammation. The reasons for this are that the NSAIDs are effective in relieving fevers, headaches, muscle aches, malaise, arthritis, and serositis associated with SLE. All NSAIDs have widely varying pain-relieving properties.

### Which NSAID Should Be Used?

The ideal NSAID is inexpensive, safe, and effective; however, none of them fits this billing exactly. Ibuprofen (Advil, Motrin) and naproxen (Aleve, Naprosyn) are available in over-the-counter and prescription strengths. I prefer that my patients use the Advil or Aleve liquigels, because they take effect within 18 minutes and tend to be gentler on the stomach. Naproxen is stronger than ibuprofen and lasts twice as long (8 to 12 hours), and it is my agent of choice in doses up to 1,500 mg daily. Ibuprofen can be given in doses up to 3,200 mg daily. There is also some evidence that naproxen has a superior cardiovascular

**Table 26.1.** *Major Nonsteroidal Anti-inflammatory Drugs (NSAIDs)*

Salicylates
  Aspirin
  Sodium salicylates (Trilisate, Salsalate, Disalcid)
  Diflusinal (Dolobid)
  Magnesium salicylate (Magan's, Doan's)
Proprionic acid derivatives
  Oxaprozin (Daypro)
  Naproxen (Naprosyn, Anaprox, Aleve)
  Flurbiprofen (Ansaid)
  Ibuprofen (Motrin, Advil)
  Ketoprofen (Orudis, Oruvail)
  Fenoprofen (Nalfon)
Acetic acid derivatives
  Sulindac (Clinoril)
  Diclofenac (Voltaren, Cataflam)
  Tolmetin (Tolectin)
  Indomethacin (Indocin)
Selectic cox-2 antagonists
  Celecoxib (Celebrex)
Oxicam derivatives
  Piroxicam (Feldene)
  Meloxicam (Mobic)
Others
  Etodolac (Lodine)
  Ketrolac (Toradol)
  Nabumetone (Relafen)
  Meclofenamates (Meclomen, Ponstel)

safety profile to other NSAIDs. A variety of other agents may be best for certain patients. Indomethacin and ketorolac are the strongest and most toxic and should not be used for more than a few days for acute swelling or pain. Celecoxib (Celebrex) is a selective inhibitor of cycloxygenase-2. It is much more expensive, but it may be appropriate in patients on blood thinners and in those who have had a gastrointestinal bleed.

## Why Must We Be Careful When Using NSAIDs?

NSAIDs can be extremely effective. Their use can mark the difference between holding a job and being on disability. They can greatly improve one's quality of life. However, numerous caveats apply when using these drugs. First, *all patients taking NSAIDs on a daily basis should have complete blood counts as well as liver and kidney blood chemistries every 3 to 4 months.* An increase in liver enzymes to greater than 2.5 times normal mandates discontinuation of the NSAID so as to protect the body from liver failure. Similarly, patients with lupus nephritis probably should not take NSAIDs unless they are for a specific circumstance and are administered under close medical supervision for a limited period (e.g., to treat acute gout or bursitis) and renal function is carefully monitored. All NSAIDs have the capacity to induce kidney impairment (99 percent of the time its transient). In patients with normal liver and kidney function, the risk of developing altered function ranges from 0.1 percent to 10 percent, depending on the agent employed. Fortunately, most patients have no symptoms, and these abnormalities are almost always reversed when they stop taking the drug.

Most important, all NSAIDs commonly induce erosions in the stomach, and this may lead to bleeding ulcers. Nationwide, 3 percent of all patients taking NSAIDs on a regular basis develop bleeding ulcers. A low hemoglobin or hematocrit (part of the complete blood count), black stool, or a positive Hemoccult test (stool smear for blood) is often the first sign of trouble. Tobacco, steroid use, and alcohol abuse increase the risk of ulcers. The use of H2 blockers (Zantac, Pepcid, Axid, Tagamet), antacids, or sucralfate (Carafate) relieves dyspepsia and heartburn associated with NSAIDs (seen in 20 to 30 percent of those taking them) but does *not* prevent the development of ulcers. I advise patients who need to be on NSAIDs and have had gastric erosions or ulcers to add proton-pump inhibitors (lansoprazole/Prevacid, omeprazole/Prilosec, Nexium, Aciphex, or Protonix) or misoprostol (Cytotec) to their regimen. These drugs *do* prevent ulcers from developing, but long-term continuous use can produce low magnesium, kidney dysfunction, and osteoporosis in a very small percentage.

Other adverse reactions can result from NSAIDs. These include bloating and fluid retention, easy bruisability, diarrhea, ringing in the ears, headaches, provocation of allergy or asthma attacks, and rashes. Because NSAIDs prolong bleeding times, they should be discontinued at least a week before any surgery so as to minimize bleeding risks. Doctors may try as many as 10 agents before they find one that works and has no side effects. The choice of NSAID preparations is a highly individual one, and what works for one person may not work for another.

### Do Topical NSAIDs and Salicylates Work?

In the United States, compounding pharmacists are allowed to make generic NSAIDs (especially ketoprofen, or physicians can prescribe diclofenac [Flector Patch, Voltaren Gel]) as topical therapies. Rubbed into painful joints every 6 hours, they relieve local symptoms and only very rarely produce systemic complaints. Topical NSAIDs have an excellent safety record—topical diclofenac is only 6 percent systemically absorbed. Some compounders have added to their gels cyclobenzaprine, lidocaine, gabapentin, or carbamazepine and other chemicals that relax muscles and decrease nerve irritation, with varying degrees of success. Except for diclofenac, the production of these preparations is not standardized, and some are quite expensive. Topical salicylates are widely available over the counter. They often are combined with soothing agents such as camphor or menthol or analgesics (e.g., Salon Pas, Ben Gay).

## WHAT ABOUT ACETAMINOPHEN (TYLENOL)?

Acetaminophen is an analgesic medication that modestly decreases pain (e.g., headache) and lowers fevers. It has mild anti-inflammatory effects, so it is usually not recommended in lupus cases. Rheumatologists occasionally come across patients who cannot take any NSAIDs; for them, doctors may advise acetaminophen. It is also used to relieve pain for a week prior to surgery—when NSAIDs should not be used (because they prolong bleeding times)—and when a pregnant woman has other non-lupus illnesses causing pain or discomfort such as headaches, fevers, or back strain. Acetaminophen preparations may be combined with tramadol or codeine or analgesic opiates. Chronic, daily use warrants kidney, liver, and hematologic testing at 3-month intervals.

## SUMMING UP

Salicylates have been used for more than 100 years, and other nonsteroidals have been used for more than 40 years. They are effective in treating fevers, headaches, arthritis, arthralgia, muscle aches, and serositis. None of these agents have any disease-modifying properties in lupus and have no place in treating serious SLE without disease-modifying drugs. The choice of a particular drug depends on the medical history; several agents are usually tried before one is found that is effective and safe. Call your doctor if you encounter any problems with these drugs. All the preparations listed in this section require regular blood testing and a rectal examination with a stool smear for blood at least once a year. With appropriate monitoring, NSAIDs can be given concurrently with other anti-lupus medications. See Table 26.2.

**Table 26.2.** *Use of NSAIDs and Salicylates for SLE*

---

1. None of the NSAIDs or aspirin products are approved for use in lupus. Over 80% of patients take them on at least an intermittent basis alone or in combination with other lupus therapies.
2. When used to treat fevers, pleurisy, headaches, menstrual flares, swollen glands, or joint pain, they can be quite effective but do not modify the course of lupus.
3. Continuous daily use warrants blood monitoring at regular intervals.
4. The safest form of NSAIDs or salicylates are topical forms, as they are only about 6% absorbed systemically.
5. Indomethacin or ketorolac should only be used for a few days. Naproxen is the most effective and safest NSAID from a cardiovascular standpoint. H2 antagonists relieve gastrointestinal discomfort and proton pump inhibitors decrease ulcer formation.

---

NSAID, nonsteroidal anti-inflammatory drugs.

## FURTHER READING

1. Horizon AA, Wallace DJ. Risk:benefit ratio of nonsteroidal antinflammatory drugs in systemic lupus erythematosus. *Expert Opin Drug Saf.* 2004;3(4):273–278.
2. Karsh J, Kimberly RP, Stahl NI, Plotz PH, Decker JL. Comparative effects of aspirin and ibuprofen in the management of systemic lupus erythematosus. *Arthritis Rheum.* 1980;23(12):1401–1404.

## 27

# Big Guns and Magic Bullets: Disease-Modifying Drugs

Up to this point, we've covered nonmedical aspects of therapy as well as the over-the-counter basics and prescriptions—nonsteroidal anti-inflammatory drugs (NSAIDs)—that help control symptoms and pain. Now we move on to other prescription drugs. Over 90 percent of all lupus patients will be given one of these agents at some time in the course of their disease. These drugs are termed "disease-modifying" because they can actually alter the course of lupus. Rheumatologists have nicknames for them such as DMARDs (disease-modifying anti-rheumatic drugs), among others. The DMARDs for lupus fall into three general categories: antimalarials, steroids, and immunosuppressives.

### WHAT DOES LUPUS HAVE TO DO WITH MALARIA?

When a rheumatologist mentions to a patient that she might benefit from antimalarial therapy, the usual response is one of confusion. The relationship was discovered by accident. The first use of antimalarials dates back to 1630, when the Countess Anna del Chinchon, wife of the viceroy of Peru, fell seriously ill with a high fever. In desperation, the family allowed local Native Americans to treat her with bark extracts from a "fever tree," and she made a miraculous recovery. The cinchona tree was named after the grateful countess, who proceeded to corner the market and arrange for its exportation to Spain. Years later, quinine was found to be the active ingredient of cinchona bark. In addition to its ability to diminish fever, it was noted to have anti-inflammatory and anti-infectious properties, including beneficial activity against malaria.

When Japan conquered Java during World War II, they effectively prevented the Allies from obtaining natural quinine. Faced with a serious threat of malaria among their troops in the southwestern Pacific theater, the Allies bootlegged an artificial quinine recipe from the notorious German I. G. Farbenindustrie combine (which made the gas chambers used in the concentration camps) and called it Atabrine (quinacrine). In 1943 the US Surgeon General declared Atabrine to be the drug of choice to prevent malaria, and 4 million American, Canadian,

Australian, New Zealand, and British soldiers took it daily for 3 years. There were anecdotal reports that soldiers with rheumatoid arthritis or lupus experienced improvement in rashes and joint symptoms when they took quinacrine; this led the British to conduct a study on its efficacy in lupus. The findings were published in the English journal *Lancet* in 1951. Antimalarials have been prescribed by rheumatologists ever since. Efforts to improve upon quinacrine led to the introduction of chloroquine (Aralen) in 1953 and hydroxychloroquine (HCQ, known by the brand name Plaquenil) in 1955. The production of Atabrine was discontinued in 1992; it is now available from compounding pharmacists as generic quinacrine.

## How Do Antimalarials Work?

Antimalarials have remarkably different and often divergent actions. They block ultraviolet light from damaging skin; have an anti-inflammatory effect similar to that of NSAIDs; lower cholesterol levels by 15 to 20 percent; inhibit clotting; block certain pro-inflammatory cytokines; and, most important, alters the acid–base balance of the cells, which limits their ability to process antigens. If antigens are allowed to be processed, this leads to the promotion of inflammation. Unlike steroids and chemotherapies, antimalarials do not lower blood counts or make patients more susceptible to infection. They are mild by nature, and altering the acid–base balance of cells takes time before a significant effect is noted. They also influence innate immunity by blocking activation of certain toll receptors. HCQ, for example, has an onset of action of 3 to 6 months, but its efficacy does not peak for several more months. Most patients are unaware of its benefits for 3 to 6 months.

## What Symptoms and Signs of Lupus Respond Best to Antimalarials?

In patients with non-organ-threatening systemic lupus erythematosus (SLE), antimalarials benefit several systems. The skin is helped by the interruption of ultraviolet light and anti-inflammatory actions. Discoid lesions, redness, mouth ulcers, and hair loss improve in 90 percent of these patients. Joint manifestations also diminish as swelling and aching decrease. Over time, inflammation of the pleura and pericardium lessens, as do constitutional symptoms of fatigue and cognitive dysfunction. Antimalarials are mild cortical stimulants in the sense that they can give patients energy. This is particularly true with quinacrine and, to a lesser extent, chloroquine or HCQ. Antimalarials are probably useful in patients with Sjögren's syndrome (dry eyes, dry mouth, and arthritis) or steroid-induced high cholesterol, and in patients with antiphospholipid antibodies that pose a risk for blood clots.

In 1991 a group of Canadian rheumatologists studied 47 patients whose mild, non-organ-threatening lupus was under good control with HCQ. Published in the prestigious *New England Journal of Medicine*, half of the patients were randomized to receive a placebo (sugar pill), and half continued their HCQ. This was a double-blind study—that is, neither the patients nor the researchers had any idea which drug was being given to whom. The HCQ group had many fewer disease flare-ups and organ-threatening complications over a 6-month period. This study confirmed previous suggestions that the institution of antimalarial therapy early in the disease course decreases the risk that lupus will spread to critical organs.

### What Antimalarial Should Be Taken and in What Dose?

The only antimalarial currently approved by the Food and Drug Administration (FDA) is HCQ. Rheumatologists vary widely in their use of this drug. I have my newly diagnosed lupus patients without critical organ disease take HCQ for at least 2 years. After 2 weeks of 200 mg a day as a test dose, the usual maintenance dose is 400 milligrams (two tablets) once daily (dosing is usually set at about 5 mg/kg per day). During the third year of therapy, I may reduce the dose to 200 milligrams a day (one tablet). Most of my patients are 80 to 90 percent better after 2 to 3 years. Sometimes acute flare-ups necessitate higher doses of the drug; the FDA allows up to 800 milligrams of HCQ to be given daily for short periods of time.

Some lupus patients might require longer or different HCQ regimens. These include patients with Sjögren's syndrome. It may be 1 to 3 years of therapy before dry eyes and dry mouth show clinical improvement. Patients with critical organ disease or serious joint inflammation who require steroid therapy might benefit from the concurrent use of HCQ as long as they are on corticosteroids, because the antimalarial is steroid sparing (it allows lower doses of steroids to be given), lowers cholesterol raised by steroids, and may decrease the tendency of steroids to promote clots.

What about the patient who has only a partial response to HCQ? After 6 months of treatment, many patients tell me that they are 50 percent better but still have rashes or joint swelling. In these cases, I first make sure they have had an adequate trial of all appropriate NSAIDs that can be given along with antimalarials. If this is the case, we can add methotrexate (see Immune Suppressives), lefluomide, azathioprine, low doses of oral steroids (see Why Are There So Many Different Kinds of Steroids?), or another antimalarial. Studies have suggested that the long-term administration of HCQ is associated with fewer flare rates and less damage accrual. As a result, many rheumatologists are using HCQ indefinitely for many years.

### WHAT ABOUT OTHER ANTIMALARIALS?

What other antimalarials are appropriate for lupus? *Chloroquine* (Aralen) was FDA approved for lupus and rheumatoid arthritis and is still widely used outside the United States for these indications. It is no longer FDA approved for lupus because HCQ is much safer. Nevertheless, chloroquine is a much more potent drug. It is particularly effective for skin rashes and joint inflammation, and therapeutic benefits are noticeable in a month. I prescribe chloroquine when patients with severe skin or joint lupus cannot wait 6 months for HCQ to work, but I switch them over to HCQ within 3 to 4 months to minimize serious eye toxicity. Quinacrine is still available through 2,000 compounding pharmacists in the United States. These old-time pharmacists make the drug from scratch by grinding up quinacrine powder. Quinacrine is indicated for lupus patients who cannot risk any potential damage to their eyes, those who cannot tolerate HCQ (it is chemically different), and those whose main complaint is profound fatigue. Quinacrine is synergistic with HCQ or chloroquine: the drugs mix well together, and their combined benefits are greater than those of both agents separately. The usual dose for quinacrine is 100 milligrams daily, although as little as 25 milligrams a day can be effective. Quinacrine works within a month, and after 2 years it can be tapered to 5 days a week, then 3 days a week, and finally once a week.

For those who remember my late friend Ray Walston standing and dancing on a box labeled Atabrine during the soldiers' variety show in the movie *South Pacific*, it has been half-jokingly suggested that this mild cortical stimulant played a role in the Allies' victory in World War II.

### General Adverse Reactions and How to Handle Them

HCQ is generally very well tolerated. A surveillance study showed that only 8 percent of lupus patients given the drug discontinued it during the first 12 months. Approximately 10 to 15 percent of patients develop generalized complaints of aching, nervousness, headache, queasiness, or nausea. When a patient relates these problems to me, I stop HCQ for 72 hours and then restart it at 200 milligrams daily. The body adjusts to the drug, and within a few months the dose can be increased to 300 to 400 milligrams. Doses as low as 200 milligrams a day can be effective in lupus; they just take longer to work. Another 5 percent of patients develop a rash on HCQ.

Chloroquine has the same side effects as HCQ, but they occur more often. In addition, the drug may sometimes (less than 1 percent of the time) cause hair to gray, damage muscle cells, and lower blood counts. These reactions are almost unheard of with HCQ. Long-term use of both drugs can cause black or blue skin pigment deposits. Quinacrine produces mild abdominal cramps and diarrhea in up to 30 percent of patients. Also, there may be a reversible yellowing of the skin in 40 percent of patients taking at least 100 milligrams daily (lower doses rarely cause skin changes). As a mild "upper," quinacrine is capable of inducing a toxic psychosis with manic behavior in 1 of 500 patients, but that disappears with its discontinuation. Blood counts should be monitored, although the risk of problems in the absence of an allergic rash is 1 per 30,000. If an allergic rash breaks out, therapy should cease immediately.

## What about the Eyes?

My pet peeve is that too many lupus patients have been frightened away from antimalarials by doctors who warn them about potential eye toxicity. First, quinacrine does not affect the eyes in currently used doses. Second, eye toxicity caused by HCQ is extremely unusual. Melanin (normal skin pigment) deposits at the back of the eye, or retina, can be promoted by antimalarials, causing blind spots (called scotomas), because humans cannot see through melanin. Patients tell me all the time that after a month on the drug, they have blurred vision. They are not making it up. Many patients started on HCQ are also on steroids, and steroids can not only cause blurred vision but also can lead to cataracts and glaucoma. If a lupus patient sees a retina specialist every 6 months, the deposits will be noticed before they cause any symptoms, and if the drug is stopped, the deposits will disappear in weeks. A newer imaging of the retina, known as ocular coherence tomography, appears to me more reliable for evaluating HCQ retinotoxicity. Using this procedure, *the risk of permanent eye damage from HCQ with normal kidney function in any patient who has had eye examinations every 6 months and who has taken the drug in doses of less than 5 mg/kg per day for less than 10 years is zero at 5 years and about 3 percent after 10 years.*

In contrast, chloroquine can cause permanent eye damage and must be used very carefully. The risk of eye toxicity with chloroquine is 10 percent after 10 years, and the changes it causes are not necessarily reversible. All patients on chloroquine should be examined every 3 months. Additionally, cloudy vision caused by swelling of the front of the eye (called *corneal edema*) is common with chloroquine and rare with HCQ. It is usually so mild that most patients continue to take the drug, and it goes away once these agents are stopped. With increasingly sophisticated technologies, ophthalmologists are coming up with newer methods to evaluate retinal function. The American Academy of Ophthalmology recommends that unless unusual circumstances (e.g., liver or kidney impairment) are present, HCQ patients should have a baseline exam at treatment initiation, 5 years later, and annually thereafter.

## IS CORTISONE REALLY NEEDED?

Steroids are the most effective and most misunderstood treatment for lupus. They are also the most used and abused therapeutic interventions for the disease. Simply stated, if organ-threatening disease is present and steroids are not prescribed, the patient can lose function in that organ. If mild disease activity is present, other therapeutic alternatives with or without steroids are available, but many physicians have little experience in using these alternatives and tend to overuse steroids.

So how did things get this way? Let us begin our story in 1855, when Thomas Addison noticed that the adrenal gland above the kidney had physiologic functions. Even though it was soon shown that the hypothalamus and pituitary gland controlled some of these functions, the adrenal gland's ability to act independently on occasion excited interest in this area. Tissue from adrenal cortex extracts was broken down and analyzed. By 1942 the structures of 28 steroids from the adrenal cortex had been elucidated. Ultimately, five of them were shown to be biologically active: in other words, they did something. Enter Phillip Hench, one of two rheumatologists to win the Nobel Prize in Medicine. As early as 1929, he had observed that patients with rheumatoid arthritis went into remission during pregnancy, and he speculated that a metabolite was responsible. As soon as Hench became aware of the ongoing research on the adrenal cortex, he speculated that these steroids might be the "metabolite" he was looking for. In 1949 Dr. Hench and his colleagues at the Mayo Clinic gave cortisone to a patient with rheumatoid arthritis, and the patient had a dramatic response. Numerous steroid preparations became available during the 1950s, and rheumatologists eventually determined—largely as a result of trial and error—which preparations should be used and in what amounts for inflammation. Lupus patients first received cortisone in 1950, and they have been using its derivatives ever since.

### How Do Steroids Work?

Steroids are hormones that play an important role in the body, regulating *physiologic* functions. Doses above and beyond what the body makes have different actions, termed *pharmacologic* functions. The pharmacologic activities of steroids include stabilizing cells so that they are less likely to become involved in inflammatory processes. Steroids block numerous chemical pathways. They also decrease the number of circulating lymphocytes, the white blood cells responsible for immunologic memory.

Within the brain lies the hypothalamus, an organ that makes a chemical called *corticotropin-releasing hormone* (CRH). This hormone travels downstream a short distance to the pituitary gland and induces the pituitary to make *adrenocorticotropic hormone* (ACTH). The ACTH then stimulates the adrenal cortex to make steroids. This network, known as the *hypothalamic–pituitary–adrenal axis*, governs how much steroid our body makes. An average adrenal gland makes the equivalent of 7.5 milligrams of prednisone a day. Through a negative feedback loop, patients taking more than 7.5 milligrams of prednisone daily prevent the release of CRH and ACTH, which stops the adrenal gland from making steroids. This is why steroids cannot be discontinued suddenly; it takes months for the hypothalamic–pituitary–adrenal axis to return to normal after steroid doses drop below 7.5 milligrams of prednisone a day.

Adrenal insufficiency, also called Addison's disease (named after the discoverer of the adrenal cortex), is a potentially serious condition characterized by a critical shortage of steroids in the body. Dosages of prednisone in the 10- to 15-milligram range usually do not completely shut down the adrenal gland but make it sluggish; on this dosage, the adrenal cortex may make only 2 to 5 milligrams instead of 7.5 milligrams a day. Taking more than 15 milligrams of prednisone for a month usually shuts off the hypothalamic–pituitary–adrenal axis, and no steroid is made by the body. Figure 17.1 illustrates these concepts.

## Why Are There So Many Different Kinds of Steroids?

In addition to the numerous natural steroid derivatives, specially engineered synthetic steroids have become available. The most important preparations are listed in Table 27.1. Prednisone is the most commonly used oral preparation, followed by prednisolone and dexamethasone. Prednisolone is almost the same as prednisone, but some patients tolerate it better, and it can be the steroid of choice for children and patients with liver disease. These agents are usually given once a day, but in the presence of acute inflammation, they are metabolized (or used up) more quickly and must be given two to four times a day. Dexamethasone enters the central nervous system better than prednisone or prednisolone and is the steroid of choice and sometimes used neurosurgeons treating postoperative swelling. It has

**Table 27.1.** *Some Oral, Injectable, and Intravenous Steroid Preparations*

| Hormone Preparation | Equivalent in Milligrams | Comment |
|---|---|---|
| ACTH (Acthar) | | Injectable form that stimulates adrenal synthesis from steroids |
| Cortisone acetates (Cortone) | 25 | Very short-acting; must be given every 6 hours |
| Hydrocortisone (Hydrocortone; Solu-Cortef) | 20 | Short-acting; works within minutes |
| Prednisone | 5 | Takes 2 to 4 hours to work and lasts 18 hours; most popular preparation |
| Prednisolone | 4 | Almost the same as prednisone; preferred if liver disease is present |
| Methylprednisone (Medrol) | 4 | Similar to prednisone and prednisolone; used intravenously as Solumedrol |
| Triamcinolone (Aristocort; Kenalog) | 4 | Popular as an injection and as a dermatologic preparation for rashes |
| Dexamethasone (Decadron) | 0.75 | Lasts 24 to 36 hours; good penetration in the central nervous system |
| Betamethasone (Celestone) | 0.6 | Popular as an injection and for rashes; matures fetal lungs in pregnant patients with lupus at risk for delivering prematurely |
| Budesonide (Entocort) EC | 1.8 | Used for asthma and allergies as inhalers; oral preparation for inflammatory bowel disease |

a longer duration of action: dexamethasone is prescribed no more often than once a day and sometimes just several times a week.

Oral steroids can be taken daily or on an alternate-day schedule. Taking twice the dose every other day has the theoretical advantage of decreasing the risk of infection and should only be considered once a patient's clinical condition is stabilized.

*Local steroids* are used for skin involvement of lupus. They are of two types, fluorinated and nonfluorinated, and they are available in several forms: creams, gels, solutions, ointments, and occlusive dressings. Fluorinated steroids are very potent; if used too often, they cause skin thinning and atrophy. They should never be applied to the face continuously for more than 2 weeks at a time. Nonfluorinated steroids are very safe but much weaker, can be purchased without a prescription, and are used for facial rashes. The most effective topical salves are ointments. Though oily and gloppy, they are 80 percent absorbed. Creams are the best tolerated. They dry the skin but are only 20 percent absorbed and are therefore less effective than ointments. A dermatologist can also deliver steroids by intralesional injections or occlusive dressings. This highly effective technique means using thin needles to inject discoid lesions and areas of hair loss with steroid solutions.

*Pulse steroids* are administered in high doses intravenously. Examples include methylprednisolone (Solumedrol) and dexamethasone (Decadron). These are given in dosages equivalent to 1,000 milligrams of prednisone per day to achieve high anti-inflammatory levels in critically ill patients. The effect of pulse steroids often lasts for weeks. Patients who cannot tolerate oral steroids may occasionally be given monthly pulse steroids. Hospitalized patients who cannot take any medications by mouth (e.g., after surgery) are given intravenous steroids in lower doses that simulate a corresponding oral dosage.

Steroids can also be given *intra-articularly* or *intramuscularly*—in other words, into a joint or muscle. Steroids injected into joints consist of preparations that have more of a water or oil base. Water-based preparations do not stay in the joint and quickly enter the bloodstream. These include hydrocortisone, dexamethasone, and methylprednisolone (e.g., Depo-Medrol). Thicker preparations stay in joints for weeks (betamethasone or triamcinolone [Celestone, Kenalog, Aristocort]), and one triamcinolone preparation, Aristospan, never really enters the bloodstream and stays in a joint for months. The choice of steroid depends on the patient's clinical picture: If the problem is limited to one joint, Aristospan may be advised; but if a patient complains especially of knee pain but also hurts all over, Kenalog is used. Aristospan is not widely prescribed because of its expense and intermittent availability. I am frequently asked how often steroids can be injected into joints, tendons, or ligaments. Studies have suggested that injecting a joint with a steroid more often than every 3 months destroys cartilage and is not advisable. Too many injections into tendons or ligaments can weaken or rupture these structures.

## What Types of Steroid Regimens Are Used to Treat Lupus?

Active, organ-threatening lupus should always be treated with steroids. Involvement of lupus in the heart, lung, kidneys, liver, or blood (autoimmune hemolytic anemia or thrombocytopenia) is managed with *high-dose steroids*— 1 milligram per kilogram of body weight (1 kilogram = 2.2 pounds) per day of prednisone for at least several weeks. This usually averages out to 40 to 80 milligrams a day. Doses above 40 milligrams a day are considered high. Acute central nervous system vasculitis is treated with high-dose steroids for shorter periods of time, often with additional pulse therapy (see Why Are There So Many Different Kinds of Steroids?).

Severe flare-ups of non-organ-threatening disease warrant *moderate doses*, or 20 to 40 milligrams of prednisone a day. This circumstance arises when a patient complains of severe chest or heart pains that turn out to be pleurisy or pericarditis, manifests active skin disease, or has a severe flare of joint inflammation. These moderate doses are maintained for a few days to several weeks.

Chronic, mild, non-organ-threatening disease responds to daily doses of 2 to 20 milligrams of prednisone. This is considered *low-dose therapy*. Most patients with non-organ-threatening disease on low- or moderate-dose steroids have other agents added and ultimately are switched over to NSAIDs, antimalarials, or methotrexate, all of which are safer than using long-term steroids unless the doses are very low.

## What Are Surgical and Stress Doses of Steroids?

The adrenal gland helps compensate the body for stress by releasing extra adrenalin (epinephrine and norepinephrine) and steroid. Surgery, for example, stresses the body, and we all need extra adrenalin and steroids to handle it. When lupus patients undergo surgery or face any stressful procedure, doctors usually give two to three times the usual daily dose of steroids on the day of the event to ease stress; sometimes it takes a few days before the cortisone doses are back to their original levels.

## What Can Steroids Do That's Bad?

Steroids are a blessing and curse. Without them, many lupus patients would die, but with them, serious complications can arise. Certain reactions to steroids occur immediately, whereas other reactions occur in patients who have had higher doses of the drugs or have taken lower doses for longer periods of time. One immediate reaction to steroids is a sense of energy. However, steroids can also cause palpitations, agitation, and rapid heart rates, and they can make it hard to sleep. Many of my patients tell me that they clean house at 3 AM after starting moderate-dose steroids. Heartburn is an early side effect in patients beginning steroids.

As time passes, numerous additional side effects occur that can best be categorized by organ systems. The *skin* becomes thin and wrinkles easily. Bruises appear and hair loss in the male pattern of baldness from the scalp is noted (in the temples and the upper back of the head), whereas facial hair increases, along with facial acne. Wound healing is impaired, and sores take longer to disappear. Stretch marks are noted throughout the skin, especially on the abdomen. *Musculoskeletal* problems include muscle weakness and loss of calcium in bones (which can lead to osteoporosis). Clots of fat released by steroids can settle in the blood supply of bones, leading to a condition known as avascular necrosis or "dead bone." The skin and muscles become very sensitive to the touch and fibromyalgia may ensue.

Because steroids are hormones, the *endocrine/metabolic system* is affected. Among the complications caused by steroids are glucose intolerance, which eventually becomes diabetes; menstrual irregularity; and central obesity, wherein one's body weight is redistributed toward the belly and buttocks and away from the extremities. Steroids can stunt the growth of children taking them, and—as discussed earlier—they can suppress the hypothalamic–pituitary–adrenal axis. The production of fats, especially cholesterol and triglycerides, is increased. Cataracts form, and glaucoma develops in the *eyes.*

The *central nervous system* is stimulated, which produces agitation, confusion, and difficulty in concentrating, and it may even result in psychotic behavior. Patients may become moody and irritable. Some of the *cardiovascular–renal* effects lead to salt and water retention with bloating and puffiness, especially in the face and ankles. Potassium blood levels decrease, often necessitating oral replacement of this mineral. Salt retention causes blood pressure to rise. The *gastrointestinal system* is involved, as continued steroid use causes heartburn to lead to ulcers. Steroids thin intestinal walls and increase the risk of perforation, especially of diverticula (pouchings) in the colon. The pancreas can also become inflamed by corticosteroids. Finally, the risk of *infection* is much greater, because steroids prevent antibodies from killing bacteria, viruses, fungi, and parasites.

Not everybody develops all of these complications, and many individuals who are steroid-dependent develop none of them. It is impossible to predict which complication will occur in whom, except that those who have taken these drugs in higher doses are more likely to note some of these side effects.

### How Does One Get off Steroids?

Unless a person has been on steroids for less than a month, the drugs should be removed slowly. Acute lupus flare-ups can be treated with short courses of steroids, given as a methylprednisolone pack (Medrol Dosepak), by which higher doses are dropped to zero within a week. Or steroids can be injected into the buttocks with betamethasone, triamcinolone, or dexamethasone, whereby the drug is out of the system within several weeks. These short-term treatment courses are rarely if ever associated with serious problems.

The ideal way for a doctor to taper steroids if a patient has been on the drug for at least a month is to decrease the dose by 10 percent a week until adrenal replacement levels are reached (7.5 milligrams of prednisone daily). A *steroid withdrawal syndrome* simulating fibromyalgia frequently mimics disease flare-ups and must be differentiated from active lupus. This syndrome is self-limited and disappears within 2 to 3 weeks of keeping the steroid doses at the same level. When adrenal replacement levels are reached, the doctor may wish to taper more slowly (e.g., 10 percent reductions every few weeks or reduced doses of 5 percent every week or 10 days). On occasion, the doctor may order a *cortrosyn stimulation test*, which evaluates the sluggishness of the adrenal glands (*adrenal insufficiency*) and offers guidance as to how fast or slowly the medication can be tapered. Many of the side effects listed, especially those of weight gain and bloating, can persist for several months after the drugs have been discontinued.

### How Do Doctors Minimize the Side Effects of Steroids?

Because doctors know what can happen when they start patients on cortisone, is there anything they can do to minimize the reactions that have just been discussed? The answer is yes, to a certain degree. For example, I sometimes prescribe antacids, H2 blockers (e.g., ranitidine), or proton-pump inhibitors (e.g., omeprazole), along with steroids. Patients are urged to keep to a low-sodium, low-fat, and low-carbohydrate diet and to limit their calorie intake. Sometimes diuretics are prescribed to deal with bloating and fluid retention. Steroid-dependent patients should take in at least 1 gram of calcium daily and vitamin D to protect their bones. Mild sedatives allow patients to get some rest at night, and families are counseled to be supportive rather than upset at the appearance or behavior of their loved ones. I also urge my patients to keep active, which minimizes muscle atrophy and osteoporosis (see Chapter 29), and I counsel them to stay away from friends or colleagues who have colds or other infections. No environment is ideal for a patient taking steroids, but it can be tailored to some extent to make life more comfortable.

### TRADITIONAL IMMUNOSUPPRESSIVE THERAPIES

"Chemotherapy" can be a scary-sounding word. Some rheumatologists instead use the terms "immunosuppressive," "cytotoxic," or "steroid-sparing" therapy. Essentially, these therapies are used when serious organ-threatening disease is present and steroids alone are not sufficient to deal with the problem. They are also employed when a patient cannot tolerate high doses of steroids, because chemotherapies reduce steroid requirements. Chemotherapies are not as scary as they sound and are very useful agents in the treatment of SLE.

## Alkylating Agents

In 1947, a patient with severe discoid lupus had *nitrogen mustard* ointment applied to the skin, and the rashes healed. Shortly thereafter—and in the days before dialysis—this agent was given to patients with severe kidney disease and proved to be life-saving. However, nitrogen mustard is messy and inconvenient; the doctor has to wear a Darth Vader–like space suit to apply the ointment, and intravenous mustard must be given in the hospital, and patients become quite ill from it. Efforts were made to improve upon this useful compound, and this led to the introduction of *cyclophosphamide* (CYP; Cytoxan) in the early 1960s. CYP is chemically similar to nitrogen mustard but much better tolerated. Until the early 1980s, CYP was given as a daily pill. Even though it proved to be effective in managing severe lupus and it was steroid-sparing, several problems arose. First, patients had to drink gallons of water daily to prevent a condition known as hemorrhagic cystitis. This was manifested by bloody urine and sometimes evolved into bladder cancer. Also, many patients lost so much hair they had to wear wigs. Further, some young women stopped menstruating and became sterile. CYP also upset the stomach and lowered blood counts, which made patients more susceptible to infection. Finally, CYP use for several years was associated with a 5 to 10 percent risk of developing a malignancy in 10 to 20 years.

CYP and nitrogen mustard are alkylating agents; their effects simulate total-body irradiation. In the early 1980s, a kinder, gentler way of administering CYP was found. This involved a once-a-month high dose or every 2-week low dose (Eurolupus) regimen intravenous administration. When CYP was used in a cyclical fashion, the incidence of hemorrhagic cystitis dropped to less than 5 percent; patients did not lose their hair; newer medicines that minimized nausea are available (e.g., ondansetron, also known as Zofran); the malignancy risk decreased to less than 1 percent; and fewer patients became sterile from it. However, most female patients over the age of 30 who take at least nine monthly doses of cyclophosphamide in a 1-year period stop menstruating, unless leuprolide (Lupron) is given as a shot 2 weeks before the CYP is due.

Patients with organ-threatening disease who do not quickly respond to steroids benefit from the addition of intravenous, intermittent CYP. For severe kidney disease (Chapter 19), doctors usually give CYP once a month for 6 months (or every 2 weeks for six doses) and then every 2 to 3 months until 2 years have elapsed, unless mycophenolate or azathioprine is added. CYP does not always work; up to 30 percent of patients who take the drug benefit from the addition of a second agent or therapy such as azathioprine.

*Chlorambucil* is an oral alkylating agent commonly used in Europe and developing countries, but it is rarely prescribed in the United States and only for patients who are allergic to or cannot tolerate CYP. It is much better tolerated than oral CYP; however, it is less effective and more dangerous than intravenous CYP because its long-term use makes it a potent carcinogen.

## Immune Suppressives

In the early 1960s, an agent became available that prevented patients with kidney transplants from rejecting them. Not a chemotherapy, because it does not treat cancer, *azathioprine* (AZA; Imuran) has turned out to be a solid addition to the rheumatologist's therapeutic arsenal. A slight modification of *6-mercaptopurine*, which is used for inflammatory bowel disease, AZA blocks inflammation pathways and is FDA-approved for rheumatoid arthritis. Numerous studies examining the role of AZA in SLE have shown that it has modest effects on serious lupus but has the advantage of reducing steroid requirements.

Azathioprine ends up being used frequently as a compromise between potent chemotherapies and an ongoing requirement for high doses of oral steroids. Imuran is generally well tolerated; about 15 to 20 percent of patients have some stomach upset, which can be managed by dividing the doses or lowering them. AZA does not alter fertility, and although it is not without risk, and many kidney transplant patients have had normal children while taking the drug (Chapter 30). Abnormal liver function tests and low blood counts can be found with AZA and should be monitored every month at the beginning of treatment and ultimately every few months. A blood test, known popularly as "TPMT," is now available and can predict who will have difficulty tolerating the drug. Azathioprine, like all immunosuppressive therapies, increases one's susceptibility to infection. Although AZA can be carcinogenic after many years of use, administration of the drug for 2 to 4 years in patients with active SLE is not associated with increased cancer risk.

A popular rheumatoid arthritis drug, *methotrexate*, has been on the market since the 1940s. In high doses, it is a very effective agent in managing numerous types of cancer. The drug is popular because it works within weeks and is taken only once a week. Acting via its inhibition of inflammatory chemicals that are necessary for cell growth, low doses of methotrexate decrease joint inflammation and have been used in SLE. However, several problems have been encountered. Methotrexate appears to have little effect on organ-threatening disease. Additionally, the drug is handled by the kidneys. Therefore, if renal disease is present, the doses have to be drastically reduced to prevent a precipitous drop in blood counts. Anyone taking methotrexate must refrain from drinking alcohol and must have blood and liver function tests made at regular intervals. Nausea, mouth sores, and headaches are the most common side effects of methotrexate, some of which can be minimized by daily doses of folic acid and generally well tolerated. Methotrexate's is generally used in lupus patients who have active joint inflammation without significant skin or organ-threatening disease.

Mycophenolate mofetil (MMF; Cell Cept) is an immunosuppressive agent that is similar to azathioprine. It has been used since the early 1990s for organ transplant rejection. Taken orally in doses of 1,000 to 3,000 mg daily in divided doses, MMF has been shown to be as effective in some studies as CYP for renal disease. Some lupus practitioners use it in lieu of CYP or as an add-on after several months of CYP, at which point it is held or tapered off. MMF is usually well tolerated, but up to 20 percent of users complain of gastrointestinal upset, particularly in higher doses. A modified form of MMF known as mycophenolic acid (Myfortic) is gentler on the gastrointestinal tract, MMF is contraindicated in pregnancy, and it has not been well studied for lupus outside of the kidney.

*Leflunomide* (Arava) inhibits pyrimidine production, one of the building blocks of DNA. As effective as methotrexate in managing rheumatoid arthritis, it has been suggested that this agent helps lupus arthritis as well. Leflunomide is approved in China in high doses for lupus nephritis, but there is little experience with this drug outside of Asia. The major side effects of leflunomide are hair thinning and diarrhea.

### Calcineurin Inhibitors

Agents that block interleukin-2 and T cell activation are often used to prevent renal transplant rejection in SLE. *Cyclosporin* (Neoral, Genfraf) prevents organ transplant rejections in part by blocking the cytokine interleukin-2. Inflammatory rheumatoidlike arthritis responds this drug, which, however, is rarely used for this. Cyclosporin A was avoided for use in lupus for a long time because it raises blood pressure, causes unwanted hair growth, and elevates lipid and creatinine (kidney function) blood levels in tests. However, most lupus patients who take the drug after a kidney transplant have tolerated it surprisingly well, with few adverse reactions. Class V (membranous) lupus nephritis responds particularly well to this agent. Cyclosporin also helps patients with suppressed bone marrow activity who have difficulty making red blood cells or platelets and some lupus patients with urticaria, mouth sores, or welts. A similar agent known as *tacrolimus* (Prograf) may improve inflammatory arthritis or kidney disease. A topical preparation of tacrolimus (Protopic), as well as the closely related *pinecrolimus* (Elidel), has been used for cutaneous lupus. Tacrolimus is relatively safe in pregnancy. *Rapamycin (sirolimus, Rapamune)* and *everolimus* have not been well studied in lupus but may have promising effects on cell surface receptor pathways that block inflammation.

### SUMMING UP

Antimalarials are prescribed for non-organ-threatening disease and to relieve skin, joint, pleural, and fatigue symptoms. They take many months to work and probably decrease the risk of lupus spreading to critical organs. I give them to all newly diagnosed lupus patients without organ-threatening disease. Corticosteroids are used in high doses for critical organ disease; otherwise, function in that organ might be lost. They can be prescribed for mild to moderate disease, but antimalarials, NSAIDs, and methotrexate should be started at the same time, allowing steroids to be discontinued as soon as possible. Chemotherapies and immune suppressives are used for patients with serious, active disease. They work with corticosteroids in decreasing disease activity and also allow steroid doses to be tapered. Corticosteroids and immuno-suppressives are very toxic, and careful monitoring during their use is necessary.

## FURTHER READING

1. Wallace DJ, Gudsoorkar VS, Weisman MH, Venuturupalli SR. New insights into mechanisms of therpateutic effects of antimalarial agents in SLE. *Nat Rev Rheumatol.* 2012;8(9):522–533.
2. Marmor MF, Kellner U, Lai TY, Melles RB, Mieler WF; American Academy of Ophthalmology. Recommenations on screening for chloroquine and hydroxychloroquine retinopathy (2016 revision). *Ophthalmology.* 2016;123(6):1386–1394.
3. Canadian Hydroxychloroquine Study Group. A randomized study of of the effect of withdrawing hydroxychloroquine sulfate in systemic lupus erythematosus. *N Engl J Med.* 1991;324(3):150–154.
4. Thamer M, Hernán MA, Zhang Y, Cotter D, Petri M. Prleldnisone, lupus activity and permnanent organ damage. *J Rheumatol.* 2009;36(3):560–564.
5. Dooley MA, Jayne D, Ginzler EM, et al; ALMS Group. Mycophenolate versus azathioprine as maintenance therapy for lupus nephritis. *N Engl J Med.* 2011;365(20):1886–1895.
6. Croyle L, Morand EF. Optimizing the use of existing therapies in lupus. *Int J Rheum Dis.* 2015;18(2):129–137.

# 28

# *Other Treatment Options: Treatments Occasionally Used to Manage Lupus*

In addition to the disease-modifying drugs discussed in the last chapter, many other agents have a place in managing different aspects of lupus. These drugs or therapies fall into the cracks or have limited uses under special circumstances. Most of them have a "bridging" function: they are used for short periods of time until one of the disease-modifying agents discussed in the previous chapter becomes effective. This section offers a brief overview of these niche therapies.

## NONCONTRACEPTIVE HORMONES

The use of estrogen-containing hormones for contraceptive purposes has been the focus of many discussions of lupus. Far less attention has been given to other hormones that may be useful in systemic lupus erythematosus (SLE).

Because 90 percent of lupus patients are women, rheumatologists logically thought that male hormones might help them. *Testosterone* was given to female lupus patients without success as early as 1948, and numerous unsuccessful findings have been published since. This might stand to reason, because males with lupus often fare worse than females. Newer formulations of testosterone patches were not effective for lupus. However, evidence that estrogen decreases the immune response and male hormones increase it suggests that certain male hormone products might be useful. A male-type hormone made by the adrenal gland known as *dehydroepiandrosterone* (DHEA) has a role in the treatment of mild to moderate lupus; it may be particularly useful in patients with cognitive dysfunction and fatigue. It may also decrease the rate of bone loss. Doses at 50 to 200 milligrams a day are effective; higher doses are associated with facial hair growth or outbreaks of acne. It is available over the counter as a food supplement or at a compounding pharmacy.

Even though there has been only rare reports in the world's literature of a lupus flare from *estrogens* given to manage menopausal symptoms (e.g., Estrace, estrogen patches), many physicians are needlessly reluctant to prescribe these replacement hormones. This is partly because, unlike birth control pills (discussed in Chapter 30), replacement hormones are not associated with clinically relevant blood clotting abnormalities, probably because they have only 20 percent as much estrogen as birth control pills. These agents are generally tolerated very well by my patients and also have a place in treating osteoporosis. *Osteoporosis* is the loss of calcium in bones and is more common in lupus, due to chronic inflammation and corticosteroid therapy. Severe bone loss leads to painful bony fractures (Chapters 13 and 29).

Stimulating the adrenal gland to make more of one's own cortisone (steroids) has been used to manage lupus since the 1950s and is approved by the Food and Drug Administration for this indication. *ACTH (Acthar)* also contains amelano cortin peptide (which prednisone does not have) and it has been hypothesized that this compound might be additionally advantageous in managing lupus.

*Danazol* (Danocrine), marketed for endometriosis, is an antiestrogen that, for unclear reasons, can improve autoimmune hemolytic anemia and low platelet counts associated with SLE. I rarely use it for patients with low platelet counts who have no lupus disease activity elsewhere in the body. *Bromocriptine* (Parlodel) and cabergoline (Dostinex) inhibit the secretion of breast milk by blocking the actions of prolactin, the hormone that stimulates the production of breast milk. Considerable evidence has accumulated indicating that many lupus patients have elevated prolactin levels. This, in turn, is associated with an immune dysfunction. Unfortunately, patients of mine who have taken bromocriptine have had no improvement in their clinical lupus.

## RETINOIDS

*Retinoids* are vitamin A derivatives that block cell growth and act as anti-inflammatories. Retinoids were not used in the past in part because they, with the exception of beta carotene, tend to increase sun sensitivity. Reports indicate that retinoids are very effective in managing subacute cutaneous lupus and refractory discoid lesions if they are used with sun blocks, and this has changed doctors' thinking. Retinoids, including *13-cis-retinoic acid* (Accutane) and *acitretin* (Soriatane), are potent agents usually used to treat psoriasis or acne, and they also have anti-lupus effects. All these agents can raise lipid levels (especially triglycerides) and are very drying. None of these drugs should be prescribed for women who might become pregnant because they induce birth defects. Their effects last only as long as they are taken; they do not have the disease-modifying properties of the antimalarials. As with antileprosy drugs, retinoids are used concurrently with antimalarials until the rashes improve to the degree that the drugs can be discontinued.

*Beta carotene* is a nonprescription retinoid health supplement that acts as a mild sun block, but it has little if any effect upon lupus.

## ANTILEPROSY DRUGS

*Leprosy*—a bacterial infection primarily involving the skin, joints, and peripheral nervous system—provokes a mild autoimmune reaction. Cutaneous leprosy and discoid lupus can be difficult to tell apart.

Antileprosy drugs have actions similar to those of antimalarial agents and are useful for resistant skin and joint problems. However, they have no place in treating serious systemic activity. *Dapsone* is the most commonly used drug in this class. It has been helpful in managing hard-to-treat skin and joint lupus, especially if a particular rash called *bullous lupus* or *lupus panniculitis* is present. Bullous lupus resembles chickenpox except that its distribution is different and the blisters tend to be larger. If it is left untreated, serious systemic complications can develop, especially dehydration. Patients taking dapsone (who have an initial negative screening blood test for an abnormality known as G6PD) should have liver tests and blood counts monitored at regular intervals. A G6PD deficiency is a contraindication to the use of dapsone because it can cause hemolytic anemia.

A third limited-use alternative, *thalidomide*, was introduced in Europe as a mild sedative in the late 1950s. A worldwide scandal exploded in the early 1960s when the agent was implicated in causing birth defects and numerous children were born with limbs missing in whole or in part. Patients who might become pregnant must not even consider trying this agent. However, the drug has remained available for leprosy patients who had no other alternatives. And in the mid-1970s, dermatologists documented its benefits for antimalarial-resistant cutaneous lupus. Thalidomide has sedating effects and should be taken at night. Up to 10 percent of patients develop a peripheral neuropathy, which can be rather annoying, as it produces continuous numbness and tingling. Abnormal blood clotting can occur in higher doses. Further, even though thalidomide clears most lupus lesions, its benefits usually wear off as soon as the drug is stopped. Most rheumatologists use antileprosy drugs along with antimalarials and stop the former as soon as the patient improves to the point that antimalarials alone can control the problem. A similar drug used for myeloma, *lenalodomide*, is also being tested in lupus.

## SPECIALIZED TREATMENTS FOR KIDNEY DISEASE

*Dialysis* involves using a machine to remove wastes from the blood that are normally cleared by the kidney. Patients with lupus and kidney failure make up about 5 percent of the SLE population and need dialysis to stay alive. This can be performed with *hemodialysis*, by which the patient's blood is cleansed three times a week for several hours, or *peritoneal dialysis*, which is often performed continuously at home, with a catheter connected in the abdominal area. Although moderately unpleasant and time consuming, both procedures are usually well tolerated, but hemodialysis may be better at helping decrease lupus disease activity and allowing patients to discontinue steroids.

The ideal management for end-stage renal disease is a *kidney transplant*. One third of lupus patients on dialysis are able to undergo a transplant successfully. The best results are seen when the kidney donor is a sibling under the age of 60 who has normal blood pressure and matches the patient's blood type. Cadaver transplants are a second choice. Lupus only rarely returns to the transplanted kidney, and more than 85 percent of all transplants prove to be successful after 5 years of follow-up.

Several preparations help kidney disease by decreasing urine protein leakage, improving blood flow to the kidney, and lowering blood pressure. These agents include *angiotensin converting enzyme (ACE) inhibitors* and *angiotensin receptor blockers* (ARBs) such as captopril, lisinopril, or losartan.

## GAMMA GLOBULIN

Gamma globulin is a protein that circulates in the blood, boosts immunity, and helps fight and prevent infection. It has been used for years as an intramuscular injection with modest results. Once the technical problems were overcome in the late 1970s, much larger amounts of the immune globulin could be administered intravenously (IV). Intravenous gamma globulin has several mechanisms of action, among the most important of which is its ability to prevent the spleen from destroying platelets.

Though expensive, IV gamma globulin or administered subcutaneously in lupus is helpful only for short-term use in autoimmune thrombocytopenia (low platelets) until other agents can become effective and for use in inflammatory nerve conditions. It may be used monthly for the occasional lupus patient who has recurrent infections and low gamma globulin levels or immunoglobin G subclass deficiencies (most lupus patients have elevated gamma globulin levels). The majority of studies published to date suggest that IV gamma globulin has no place in the management of fibromyalgia or chronic fatigue.

## APHERESIS, THERAPEUTIC BLOOD, OR LYMPH GLAND FILTERING

Lymphocytes are white blood cells that help control the immune response. Because steroids and chemotherapy work partly by destroying lymphocytes, it seemed logical that removing lymphocytes from the body with a filtering machine might be effective and reduce inflammation with fewer side effects. In the late 1960s, investigators found that draining lymphocytes from the thoracic duct (a lymph gland collection site near the left collarbone) was feasible. *Thoracic duct drainage*, as it was called, drained billions of lymphocytes from patients and decreased disease activity for about 4 months. This led researchers to attempt the removal of lymphocytes directly from the blood, a process called *lymphapheresis*. Performed on a blood filtering device, *apheresis* (meaning "to remove by force" in Greek) was difficult to perform in SLE patients. This is because they had antilymphocyte antibodies that, along with steroids and chemotherapy, decreased lymphocyte counts to such a low level that the machine could not remove enough cells to make a difference. Investigators at Harvard University and Stanford University then attempted to irradiate lymphocytes in the lymph glands. Known as *total lymphoid irradiation* (TLI), it resulted in improvements that lasted for several years. However, 80 percent of the patients developed shingles; they also lost an average of 20 pounds and 10 teeth. Furthermore, the use of TLI prevented further useful chemotherapy from being employed when the disease ultimately flared. (Prior radiation mixed with alkylating agents such as cyclophosphamide or chlorambucil greatly increases a patient's risk for developing cancer.)

Attention was then shifted to depleting plasma on a cell-separator device that resembles a dairy creamer. Removing plasma from whole blood and returning red blood cells, white blood cells, and platelets to the patient is called *plasmapheresis*. Because many proteins and antibodies promote inflammation, plasmapheresis was tried in a variety of critical lupus complications. This expensive procedure is beneficial and lifesaving for some lupus patients with thrombotic thrombocytopenic purpura (TTP), hyperviscosity syndrome, alveolar hemorrhage, inflammatory polyneuropathy, and cryoglobulinemia. However, attempts to use plasmapheresis for serious organ-threatening complications of lupus such as nephritis or central nervous system disease have generally been disappointing, although occasional results have been dramatically successful. Researchers are currently manipulating concurrent medications, replacement products, and plasmapheresis schedules to improve its efficacy.

Despite all the scary-sounding procedures mentioned in this section, the technical aspects of plasma or lymphocyte removal are generally well tolerated, with only a 3 percent rate of serious complications, which is very good considering that doctors are dealing with seriously ill patients. Apheresis produces some temporary light-headedness, dizziness, and cramping; moreover, vascular access—the ability to find a vein for intravenous infusions—can be a problem.

## SUMMING UP

Even though NSAIDs, antimalarials, corticosteroids, and chemotherapy account for the overwhelming majority of all lupus therapies, other treatments are occasionally useful. Antileprosy drugs help resistant skin lesions and joint inflammation; retinoids are also useful for refractory skin rashes. These preparations are only helpful temporarily and act as an adjunct to antimalarials. The only hormones that have a role in SLE are danazol for low platelet counts and certain anemias and postmenopausal estrogen replacement therapy. Immune stimulants are disappointing. Gamma globulin helps fight immune deficiencies that promote infection, and it can raise low platelet counts. Machines can act as artificial kidneys or be used to remove antibodies, cells, or proteins from the body. The role of maintenance dialysis is firmly established, but many uses of apheresis are still controversial.

## FURTHER READING

1. Wallace DJ. Apheresis for lupus erythematosus: state of the art. *Lupus.* 2001;10(3): 193–196.
2. Petri M, Kim MY, Kalunian KC, et al; OC-SELENA Trial. Combined oral contraceptives in women with systemic lupus erythematosus. *N Engl J Med.* 2005;353(24):2550–2558.
3. Watad A, Amital H, Shoenfeld Y. Intravenous immunoglobulin: a biological corticosteroid-sparing agent in some autoimmune conditions. *Lupus.* 2017;26(10):1015–1022.
4. Sabucedo AJ, Contreras G. ESKD, transplantation and dialysis in lupus nephritis. *Semin Nephrol.* 2015;35(5):500–508.

## 29

# Fighting Infections, Allergies, and Osteoporosis

After most recent surveys, infection has now been rated the second most common cause of death among lupus patients, after cardiovascular complications. Why are lupus patients so susceptible to infection, and what can be done about it? Should at-risk patients receive vaccinations, or would that make the disease worse? And what about allergies and allergy shots? Moreover, one of the major problems facing women after they go through menopause is osteoporosis, and women with lupus are especially vulnerable to this disease. This chapter outlines a practical approach for dealing with infections and vaccines while promoting awareness of the issues involved in infection, allergy, and lupus. Finally, the management of osteoporosis is reviewed as it applies to lupus.

## WHAT IS AN INFECTION?

Patients with systemic lupus have altered abilities to fight common infections and are susceptible to attack by uncommon organisms that rarely affect healthy people. Infections of this kind are called *opportunistic*. Opportunistic infections are usually seen only in cancer patients receiving chemotherapy, individuals suffering from HIV infection, and those who have altered immune systems. Autoimmune diseases fall into the last category, particularly when immunosuppressives or steroids are being used.

Microbes can attack cells and, in turn, kill cells and damage tissue. The body produces antibodies to these microbial antigens, killing foreign organisms as part of an anti-inflammatory and occasionally an allergic response. Many different kinds of organisms can infect the body. Depending on size, structure, life cycle, and ability to produce certain chemicals, they are called bacteria, viruses, parasites, fungi, or protozoans. Common infections, from streptococcal or staphylococcal bacteria, affect healthy people all the time.

## ARE LUPUS PATIENTS MORE VULNERABLE TO INFECTION?

Because 80 percent of patients with systemic lupus erythematosus (SLE) take corticosteroids during the course of their disease and 10 to 30 percent undergo chemotherapy, it stands to reason that lupus patients are vulnerable to infectious processes. NSAIDs and antimalarials do not increase susceptibility to infection. Even if you are not receiving steroids or chemotherapy, you are still susceptible to unusual infections. Lupus patients attacked by common microbes frequently require treatment for longer periods of time and often project a more severe clinical picture. Their susceptibility is changed in several ways. First, the microbial killing function of neutrophils, a type of white blood cell, is altered, and second, certain complement components critical in the killing process are inhibited. Third, there is evidence to indicate that many lupus patients have circulating blood factors that inhibit a component of complement (C5) from being attracted to an inflamed cell. Finally, cytokine dysfunction in SLE (Chapter 5) decreases the body's ability to kill foreign organisms.

Additionally, corticosteroids block cells from destroying other cells and thus from diminishing inflammation. Chemotherapies prevent the reproduction of cells with immunologic memories, which can signal the body to kill microbes and decrease the numbers of cells themselves.

## WHAT KIND OF INFECTIONS MIGHT A LUPUS PATIENT GET?

The principal bacterial infections seen in lupus affect the respiratory tract (*Streptococcus, Staphylococcus*) and urinary tract (*Escherichia coli*). As a lupus patient, you could also be at special risk for developing infections in your joints (septic arthritis), tuberculosis, or salmonellosis. In addition to cold viruses, you might be especially susceptible to herpes zoster (shingles). Epstein–Barr virus, hepatitis viruses, and cytomegalovirus may be slightly more prevalent in SLE. The most common fungal process in lupus patients is *Candida*, or yeast. This cheesy-white infiltrate is seen in the throat and esophagus (causing sore throat and difficulty swallowing) and in the vagina. Rarely, unusual fungal infections such as those caused by *Cryptococcus, Coccidioides immitis*, and *Nocardia* are observed. In the United States, the principal parasitic pathogen seen in lupus patients is called *Strongyloides*, and the protozoan to be aware of is *Pneumocystis carinii*, which is frequently found in HIV infection patients.

## HOW ARE INFECTIONS DIAGNOSED?

Active lupus mimics infection and infectious processes not only mimic lupus but can also flare it. Infections can be difficult to diagnose. The principal manifestations of infections include fever, sweats, and shaking chills. If you have a high fever for more than a few days, you should be thoroughly evaluated, especially if you are also taking NSAIDs or steroids, which lower the body temperature. I try to take a thorough medical history of a patient with a possible infection, noting symptoms and inquiring about recent travel (especially abroad), exposure to illness, purchase of a new pet, and occupation-related illnesses. I often order a throat, urine, blood, or stool culture in addition to a complete blood count or chest X-ray. Other causes of fevers such as active lupus, cancer, allergy, or a drug reaction must be considered. Some physicians find a C-reactive protein (CRP) blood test helpful in differentiating active lupus from infection, but this is controversial. Anybody with a suspected life-threatening infection from an unknown source may have to be observed and have cultures taken in a hospital where, if necessary, specialized scanning, bone marrow biopsy, lymph node biopsy, or obtaining lung tissue can be performed to make a critical diagnosis as safely and quickly as possible and where intravenous antibiotics are readily available.

## HOW ARE INFECTIONS TREATED?

Many rheumatologists have noted that patients with SLE need higher doses of antibiotics for longer periods of time than healthy people need. Most infections can be treated on an outpatient basis, but serious bacterial processes and many opportunistic infections necessitate a period of in-hospital intravenous antimicrobial therapy. Antimicrobial agents fight numerous types of organisms. Antibiotics attack bacteria and prevent them from reproducing. Antiviral, antiparasitic, antiprotozoan, and antifungal drugs are also available. Although steroids may delay the response to antibiotics, the two can be taken together, because lupus frequently flares up when the patient becomes infected.

## CAN INFECTIONS BE PREVENTED?

Some prevention is possible and just requires common sense. For example, a lupus patient's exposure to people with colds or other infections should be minimized. Antibiotics are sometimes given to such patients as a preventive measure before, during, or after certain surgical and dental procedures. A patient's dentist should know that he or she has lupus. Dental procedures in those with heart murmurs or phospholipid antibodies or endocarditis are managed with at least 2 to 4 grams of ampicillin or amoxicillin equivalent 2 hours before, and, if necessary, the dose can be divided so that some is given 4 to 6 hours afterward. If a patient is allergic to penicillin, there are substitutes available.

I occasionally encounter lupus patients who develop repeated colds or infections. Some of them have low gamma globulin (immunoglobin G [IgG] subclass, low IgG) levels and need replacement with intravenous immune globulin (IVIg). *Chronic variable immune deficiency (CVID)* is found in 1 to 5 percent of SLE patients and may warrant IVIg. Exposure to a person with influenza usually warrants a 48-hour course of oseltamivir (Tamiflu) 75 milligrams twice a day for 2 days to prevent the development of symptoms. The key to prevention is to be aware of the conditions in your environment and make sure your doctors and dentist know you have lupus so they can take necessary steps to protect you.

## WHAT ABOUT VACCINES?

Occasional reports have appeared of healthy persons developing lupus after receiving a routine vaccination. The concept of vaccinating patients with small amounts of a provoking substance, with the goal of having them make antibodies to an infectious agent, dates back to Edward Jenner's experiments with smallpox in the 1700s. Nearly all individuals with SLE have been vaccinated against a variety of diseases with little difficulty. Some vaccines use live organisms (e.g., virus), and others do not. Vaccines against measles, whooping cough (pertussis), mumps, and polio, among others, use live viruses. Even though there is a theoretical risk in exposing a lupus patient to a live virus or to a family member who has received a live-virus vaccine, there has never been a case report of the patient contracting the disease. Passive immunization with nonspecific antibodies such as gamma globulin poses no problems in patients with SLE. Relatedly, I have frequently been asked whether patients can develop lupus from a vaccine. Though this is theoretically possible, it is a very rare occurrence and probably happens in no more than one out of several thousand genetically predisposed persons.

Most lupus patients should consider having a shingles vaccine (Shinglex). As with most vaccines, this is best administered before starting an immune suppressive. Even though it's a live virus, it appears to be well tolerated. Some practitioners advise their patients not to take immune suppressive or targeted therapies one month before and one month after receiving Shingrix. Difficulties have been encountered with some types of immunization in a small number of lupus patients. Some investigators have observed that certain patients who received tetanus or flu vaccines, for example, also made antibodies to DNA or other lupus autoantigens. It seems that flu vaccines do not work as well if the patient has active SLE; antibodies achieve most of the desired levels. Additionally, up to 10 percent of those with SLE may feel sick or achy for a few days, which is double the incidence in the general population. These patients should consult their physicians before they receive any vaccine. Most rheumatologists give their lupus patients flu shots; others choose to prevent influenza with antiviral antibiotics when their patients are exposed. Patients on immune suppressive medication such as belimumab, rituximab, or tocilizumab tolerate vaccinations well but they may be less effective. In potentially serious circumstances, however, rheumatologists rarely hesitate to give necessary vaccinations. As a general practice, I give routine flu, hepatitis, meningitis, tetanus, and pneumonia shots to patients with stable, relatively inactive lupus.

## ARE LUPUS PATIENTS MORE LIKELY TO HAVE ALLERGIES?

Generalized allergies or increased sensitivities to environmental chemicals or drugs are observed in 10 percent of the general population and in 20 to 25 percent of those with SLE. Patients with lupus are more liable to have drug, insect, and skin allergies as well as asthma. What does this mean for the patient? On the one hand, allergic lupus patients have no difficulty using the antihistamines, inhalers, nasal sprays, pseudoephedrine-containing decongestants, or steroids that many otherwise healthy allergy-prone patients take from time to time. On the other hand, sulfa antibiotics can make them more sun sensitive and cause more allergic reactions; they should be used cautiously. (These antibiotics are arylamine sulfas; most lupus patients do fine with nonarylamine sulfa-based medicines.) Also, a minority of lupus patients who receive *allergy shots* (immunotherapy) make more autoantibodies and experience disease flare-ups. However, 90 percent of my patients do fine with this treatment.

## WHAT IS OSTEOPOROSIS?

With the passage of time, all of us are likely to have some thinning of our bones. Manifested by a loss of calcium in bone mineral, osteoporosis can lead to fractures, bone pain, and shorter stature. The consequence can be an inability to live independently. Lupus patients are especially susceptible to this demineralization process.

We have two types of bone: cortical (as in the hips) and trabecular (as in the vertebrae of the spine). With age, men and women become osteoporotic, or lose calcium in their cortical bones. Additionally, the onset of menopause selectively demineralizes trabecular bone. Therefore, women are more susceptible to osteoporosis in general. Persons who are Caucasian, have thin builds, or abuse tobacco or alcohol—as well as those with a genetic predisposition—are also at increased risk. Inflammation from lupus and the use of corticosteroids accelerate this process, which is why osteoporosis is so common in SLE. Further complicating this picture is the general hesitancy of doctors to prescribe hormones to lupus patients and evidence that certain chemotherapies can bring on premature menopause.

### How Is Osteoporosis Managed in Systemic Lupus?

Despite all the gloomy risk factors previously detailed, an intelligent woman with lupus who works with her healthcare team can frequently prevent the serious complications induced by osteoporosis (e.g., fractures from thin bones). I usually order a *bone densitometry study* (DEXA) in women at risk to help me decide what management is optimal. They are inexpensive, painless, take 15 minutes to perform, and provide a lot of information. I usually order them at 1- to 2-year intervals in high-risk patients, in patients who will be on steroids for at least several months, and at the onset of menopause. One has osteopenia if her base mineralization is 1 to 2.5 standard deviations below the mean, and osteoporosis if greater than 2.5.

Women with early SLE should initiate preventive measures such as taking 1 to 1.5 grams of calcium by mouth daily in divided doses. Along with a well-balanced diet, preparations such as Citrical, Tums EX, Os-Cal, and Posture are easily obtainable without a prescription. A regular exercise program, as reviewed in Chapter 24, also decreases demineralization rates. The role of postmenopausal replacement estrogen therapy is reviewed in Chapter 28. These agents are well tolerated in lupus. The American College of Rheumatology has issued guidelines suggesting that patients on 5 milligrams of prednisone a day be considered for bisphosphonate therapy. The oral administration of alendronate (Fosamax), risedronate (Actonel), ibandronate (Boniva), or yearly, intravenous infusions of zoledronic acid (Zometa Reclast) is appropriate for lupus patients on corticosteroids, those with osteoporosis, or those with active disease and osteopenia. There is a small risk for avascular necrosis of the jaw, and patients should consult their rheumatologist if they require significant dental work. Denosumab (Prolia) is efficacious for patients who cannot tolerate bisphosphonates. It is given as a subcutaneous injection every 6 months. Patients with severe osteoporosis or recurrent fractures should consider parathyroid hormone injections (teriparatide [Forteo], abaloparatide [Tymlos]) for 2 years without a bisphosphonate. Raloxifene (Evista) and nasal calcitonin are weak agents that may increase trabecular mineralization and are occasionally useful. Table 29.1 summarizes available approaches. The most important thing

**Table 29.1.** *The Management of Osteoporosis in Systemic Lupus Erythematosus*

1. Try to eat foods with high calcium contents (the average US diet contains 600 mg a day)

| | |
|---|---|
| Milk, 8 oz., 300 mg | Hard cheese, 1 oz., 200 mg |
| Ice cream, 1 cup, 176 mg | Oysters, ½ cup, raw, 113 mg |
| Broccoli, 1 cup, 136 mg | Sardines, canned, 3 oz., 372 mg |
| One large orange, 78 mg | Spinach, ½ cup raw, 111 mg |
| Yogurt, 8 oz., 400 mg | |

2. Take oral calcium supplements. They should never be taken in over 600 mg doses at a time. The body does not absorb more. Reserve some calcium for bedtime.
   Calcium carbonate (OsCal, Tums, Titrilac, Maalox)
   Calcium citrate (Citrical, Caltrate)
   Calcium lactate (store brands)
   Calcium gluconate (store brands)
3. Vitamin D improves the absorption of calcium by the gastrointestinal tract. The easiest way to derive enough vitamin D is by taking two multivitamin tablets a day.
4. If appropriate, Calcitonin, estrogen replacement therapy, or Evista can be prescribed and have modest effects on bone mineralization.
5. Bisphosphonates are the agents of choice for lupus-associated demineralization.
6. Parathyroid injections without bisphosphonates are used to manage severe osteoporosis.

one can do regarding osteoporosis is to be aware of the risk of this condition and try to prevent it.

## SUMMING UP

Lupus is complicated by an increased susceptibility to infection, and this is associated with a greater risk of disease-related complications. A rheumatologist or family physician should be consulted (at least by telephone or electronically) before a patient with SLE takes an antibiotic or receives a vaccine. Prudent preventive measures help prevent problems later. When there is a question of serious, life-threatening infection, careful evaluation (and perhaps hospitalization) is essential. Patients with lupus have stronger reactions to allergies, drugs, insects, and chemicals. Extreme caution should be exercised before taking allergy shots or sulfa antibiotics. Patients who have risk factors for osteoporosis should arrange to have themselves tested and, if necessary, treated, because this condition occurs more frequently with lupus.

## FURTHER READING

1. Bragazzi NL, Watad A, Sharif K, et al. Advances in our understanding of immunization and vaccines for patients weieth systemic lupus erythematotus, *Expert Rev Clin Immunol.* 2017;13(10):939–949.
2. Bultink IE, Lems WF. Lupus and fractures. *Curr Opin Rheumatol.* 2016;28(4):426–432.
3. Aceves-Avila FJ, Benites-Godínez V. Drug allergies may be more frequent in systemic lupus erythematosus than in rheumatoid arthritis. *J Clin Rheumatol.* 2008;14(5):261–263.

# 30

## *Can a Woman with Lupus Have a Baby?*

Ninety percent of patients with lupus are female, and 90 percent develop the disease during their reproductive years. And most women with SLE want to have children. Unfortunately, many of my colleagues advise lupus patients not to become pregnant on the basis of incorrect or outdated information. In addition, doctors are notorious for lacking a special sensitivity that is often needed when pregnancy is ill advised. The good news is that the overwhelming majority of lupus patients can have normal babies. However, there are circumstances in which pregnancy presents increased risks. This chapter attempts to confront and clarify misconceptions and notions often held by both patients and doctors about pregnancy and lupus.

### DOES LUPUS ALTER THE ABILITY TO CONCEIVE?

The ability to procreate, or fertility, is usually normal in systemic lupus erythematosus (SLE). Discoid lupus and drug-induced lupus per se are not associated with fertility problems. But several specific circumstances relevant to SLE may affect fertility. These include disease activity, renal failure, and drugs.

Patients with very active disease frequently have irregular periods or none at all. This is the body's reaction to stress; menstrual regularity is restored when the disease is under adequate control. Thirty percent of patients with SLE have significant kidney disease, and 10 to 20 percent of them evolve end-stage renal disease, necessitating dialysis over a 10-year observation period. Dialysis is associated with scanty or no menstrual cycles. A successful kidney transplant obviates the need for dialysis and may restore regular periods. Finally, certain chemotherapy drugs interfere with ovulation (Chapter 27). Cyclophosphamide causes premature menopause in 25 to 50 percent of the women in their 20s who receive it for at least a year, and in 80 percent of the women who take it in their later 30s. Azathioprine, cyclosporin, tacrolimus, rituximab, methotrexate, and mycophenolate mofetil are not associated with loss of periods in women with SLE. Some women need to take cyclophosphamide to be made hormonally "prepubertal" with leuprolide (Lupron), the equivalent of having their eggs removed and stored for later use.

What about male fertility? Sperm counts (but not libido) decrease in men who take chemotherapies. Although sterility is uncommon, I urge males with SLE who require chemotherapy to bank (store) their sperm before starting treatment.

## THE MOTHER: WHAT WILL HAPPEN INSIDE OF HER?

### The Overall View

Our group conducted a survey and chart review of 307 women with SLE who had 634 pregnancies and were seen in our office. Eighty patients (26 percent) never conceived; this is three times the national average. Of the 634 pregnancies, 439 (69 percent) resulted in live births, 106 (17 percent) in therapeutic abortions, and 95 (15 percent) in spontaneous abortions. These patients fell into low-risk, high-risk, and moderate-risk categories.

### Low-Risk Mothers

Those who fall into the low-risk group have nothing to worry about, because their risk of a problem pregnancy is the same as that in the general population (one in six pregnancies in healthy women fail). These women include those with discoid lupus, those with drug-induced lupus, and those with SLE who have mild disease and are in remission, off all medication, and lack the Ro (SSA) antibody and anticardiolipin antibody.

### High-Risk Mothers

A small group of women face an extremely high risk of fetal demise and maternal organ failure if they become pregnant. Overall, up to 3 percent of high-risk pregnant women with SLE die. This group includes patients with active lupus myocarditis, antiphospholipid syndrome, pulmonary hypertension, active lupus nephritis with an elevated serum creatinine, severe and uncontrollable high blood pressure, and those who need to receive chemotherapy during their pregnancy. Myocarditis is usually aggravated during pregnancy and leads to heart failure. Many lupus patients with active nephritis and an elevated serum creatinine will require dialysis, and that hikes the risk of fetal demise to over 80 percent. Pre-existing hypertension is aggravated during most pregnancies and, if not well controlled, can lead to stroke.

Despite these odds, I continuously come across brave women who wish to exercise their biological prerogative to procreate and don't care that the odds are greatly stacked against them. About 20 percent of the mothers make it through, have a normal baby, and come out unscathed. Most mothers with these risk factors miscarry; the remaining 20 percent develop serious complications. Lupus patients with serious, organ-threatening disease who wish to have children should be encouraged to consider adoption or a surrogacy.

## MOMS WHO SHOULD PROCEED WITH CAUTION

Individuals who are not at especially high risk but for whom a pregnancy might well present problems fall into the most common category for young female patients. This section provides a clear road map for them to follow.

### What Will Happen to the Lupus?

Patients whose lupus is mild or moderately active at the time of conception have a 60 percent chance of having no change in their disease, a 20 percent chance of flaring, and a 20 percent chance of improving. The fetus makes cortisone, and by the second trimester, mild disease may improve as the mother receives this extra dose of steroids. However, various chemicals released in pregnancy can also promote inflammation. Most flares are mild and easy to manage. Serious flares rarely occur in this group, but mild cutaneous or musculoskeletal postpartum flares are common, especially between the second and eighth weeks after delivery. The withdrawal of fetal steroids from the body, delivery of the placenta, and less adrenal stimulation to the new mother may have something to do with this. Sometimes steroids are given for a few days to weeks during this period.

### What Lupus Medications Can Patients Take during a Pregnancy?

*Regular-dose aspirin or daily nonsteroidal anti-inflammatory drugs (NSAIDs)* are not advisable during a pregnancy because they may induce bleeding, which leads to miscarriage, prolongs labor, and causes early closure of the opening between the pulmonary artery and descending aorta near the fetal heart. However, these dangers are not applicable to patients taking low-dose aspirin who have antiphospholipid antibodies. A patient who is pregnant and has intermittent NSAIDs or NSAIDs on a short-term basis is at no increased risk.

Numerous surveys published since 2000 have demonstrated the safety of *hydroxychloroquine (Plaquenil)* in pregnancy and breast feeding, and some even advocate its use. Historically, *antimalarials* were not advisable in pregnancy, and the manufacturers list pregnancy as a contraindication. The administration of chloroquine is associated with a very small risk of causing blindness or deafness in the fetus. Several reports of congenital malformations with quinacrine have appeared. Moderate- or low-dose *corticosteroids* (less than 40 milligrams of prednisone a day) appear to be relatively innocuous and free of significant problems in pregnancy. This is probably because they are natural hormones made by both mother and fetus. A steroid preparation called betamethasone (sometimes injected into joints as Celestone) crosses the placenta particularly well and is used by obstetricians to improve the maturity of fetal lungs in mothers who show signs of delivering prematurely.

The following agents are safe in pregnancy: prednisone, hydroxychloroquine, intermittent NSAIDs, apheresis and intravenous immune globulin.

The following agents have an acceptable safety profile but need to be closely monitored: cyclosporine, tacrolimus, azathioprine, belimumab, tocilizumab, abatacept.

Rituximab may be used carefully in pregnancies with serious complications.

The following agents should never be used with pregnancy: methotrexate, leflunomide, cyclophosphamide, and mycophenolate mofetil, unless the benefits outweigh the risks.

### How Can Complications Related to the Antiphospholipid Syndrome Be Prevented?

The antiphospholipid syndrome (Chapter 21) is associated with an increased risk of fetal death and miscarriage. One-third of those with SLE have antiphospholipid antibodies (especially anticardiolipin), and in these patients the risk of spontaneous abortion ranges from 20 to 50 percent. *Antiphospholipid antibodies* cross the placenta and promote clots in it, which results in fetal death. I usually screen all newly pregnant patients for antiphospholipid antibodies if they have not been tested previously. Occasionally, doctors come across a patient who is antiphospholipid-negative but becomes positive only during the pregnancy.

There is no agreed-upon way to manage pregnant women with antiphospholipid antibodies. If the antibody is present in a patient with no prior miscarriages, I prescribe one baby aspirin a day (81 milligrams) during the pregnancy until the 28th week, when it is stopped to allow the baby's heart channel to close. There is a much greater risk that immunoglobin G antibodies above 25 to cardiolipin will induce abortion than that immunoglobin M or A antibodies (dangerous if levels are above 100) will do so. If the mother miscarries despite baby aspirin therapy, the next time she conceives I initiate therapy with daily subcutaneous injections of enoxaparin (Lovenox), which also has anti-inflammatory properties. Oral heparins can be used as well. Oral warfarin (Coumadin), which is usually used when patients with these antibodies have systemic blood clots while taking baby aspirin, is not advised in pregnancy.

### What Should Patients Who Carry the Ro (SSA) Antibody Do?

Between 20 percent and 30 percent of those with SLE carry the Ro (SSA) antibody. Many of these patients also carry the La (SSB) antibody; the presence of this antibody by itself is very rare. Anti-Ro and anti-La can cross the placenta and induce two syndromes: neonatal lupus and congenital heart dysfunction or block. (Both are discussed in detail in Chapter 23.) These antibodies present no risk to the mother. The chance of developing either of these syndromes is very small, and cutaneous neonatal lupus is a mild, self-limited process. Even though congenital heart block in the infant is found in less than 5 percent of pregnancies of Ro-positive mothers, pregnant women should be screened for it with a fetal echocardiogram (ultrasound of the heart) at weeks 18 through 24. The administration of betamethasone (a steroid that crosses the placenta), dexamethasone, or intravenous gamma globulin may be useful.

### What about Patients with Active Kidney Disease?

Renal disease present at the beginning of pregnancy is associated with a 50 percent flare rate, a 25 percent incidence of pregnancy-related hypertension including pre-eclampsia, and a 25 percent risk of kidney failure requiring dialysis during the pregnancy. Patients who have normal renal function (creatinines of less than 1.5 milligrams per deciliter) should be closely monitored, with doctor visits approximately every 2 weeks. Rigid blood pressure control (with the caveat that angiotensin converting enzyme [ACE] inhibitors and angiotensin receptor blockers [ARB] agents are contraindicated), salt restriction, and increased doses of steroids if renal function worsens or serum complements fall are desirable. Patients with elevated serum creatinines are at an even greater risk and must follow these precautions.

### How Should Pregnant Patients Feel and What Should They Do?

Pregnant patients with lupus behave and feel like most healthy pregnant women. There is no reason why they cannot work or exercise if they wish to and are able. No special dietary considerations apply. There is a chance that if they have mild to moderate disease, their lupus symptoms could worsen during the first trimester. The fetus's adrenal gland and the placenta start making cortisone during the second trimester, and the mother will probably start feeling better at that time. The child's father should be included on the healthcare team so that he can help and support the mother when she needs rest or doesn't feel up to doing things. Flare-ups can be treated with acetaminophen (Tylenol), if fever or musculoskeletal aching is involved, and with steroids if the flare-ups are more serious.

### What Laboratory Tests Should Be Obtained during a Lupus Pregnancy?

When a patient tells me she is pregnant, I ask her (and the father) to come into my office so I can explain the situation and answer many of the questions raised in this chapter. In addition to examining the patient, I also perform baseline laboratory studies. These include a complete blood count, platelet count, blood chemistry panel, urinalysis, anticardiolipin antibody, lupus anticoagulant, complement studies, C-reactive protein (CRP), anti-DNA, and anti-Ro (SSA) and anti-La (SSB) antibodies. The Westergren sedimentation rate is falsely elevated in all normal pregnancies and is not reliable. I try to see my pregnant lupus patients once each trimester and more often if necessary. Blood pressures and weight are monitored at each visit. Pregnancy is associated with a physiologic anemia that occurs as red blood cells are diluted out with the increased volume of body fluids. Therefore, the development of anemia must be significant to be a concern. At follow-up visits, I check a complete blood count, dipstick the urine (which screens for protein and sugar), and obtain C3 and C4 complement levels. A fall in complement values is an excellent indicator of disease flares in pregnancy. Additional testing is done only if the patient's complaints or medical history warrant it. The patient's doctor should make every effort to communicate regularly with her obstetrician so that they can work together as a team.

### What Can the Patient Who Is Breastfeeding Take?

Up to 20 percent of the NSAIDs taken by a mother who breast feeds reaches the infant and may cause a bleeding tendency or acidosis; therefore, these agents are not advised. Even though only 1 percent of antimalarial drugs are excreted in breast milk, studies suggest that hydroxychloroquine (HCQ) is compatible with breastfeeding. It would also be dangerous to expose any infant to chemotherapy unnecessarily. The only anti-lupus drug that is safe to use with breastfeeding is prednisone. Studies have shown that doses of up to 30 milligrams daily taken by the mother have no untoward effects on the baby. The advantage of breast feeding an infant applies only for the first 3 months of life. Breastfeeding after that time can limit the physician's ability to intervene in managing lupus activity.

### THE FETUS

### What Are the Chances That the Baby Will Have Lupus?

The risk that any child born to a mother with SLE will develop the disease is small. The "lupus gene" or sets of genes predisposing to lupus has what doctors call "a low penetrance." In other words, fewer than 10 percent of patients who carry a lupus gene will ever develop the disease.

If anti-Ro (SSA) and anti-La (SSB) are absent, the risk of being born with lupus is negligible. These rare occurrences are associated with the anti-RNP antibody (see Chapters 6 and 11 for a review). Cutaneous neonatal lupus is seen in less than 5 percent of patients with anti-Ro or anti-La and is a self-limited, benign process that disappears within weeks to months. Congenital heart dysfunction or block is discussed in Chapter 22.

The chance that an offspring of a lupus patient will develop the disease in childhood and adult life is 10 percent for females and 2 percent for males. However, up to 50 percent will carry autoantibodies in their blood (especially antinuclear antibodies [ANA]), and up to 25 percent will develop an autoimmune disease (including lupus) in their lifetime. The most common non-lupus autoimmune process is thyroiditis, which is usually mild and benign, followed by rheumatoid arthritis.

### What Are the Chances of a Successful Pregnancy?

Among nonterminated pregnancies of mothers with SLE in the United States, the frequency of miscarriage is 17.5 percent; stillbirth, 6.9 percent; prematurity, 29 percent; and neonatal death, 8 percent. The last category includes babies who die within 30 days of birth. All told, two thirds, or 67 percent, of all lupus pregnancies produce a successful birth. This is considerably less than the national rate of 85 percent. Most of the miscarriages can be traced to the antiphospholipid antibodies, which, if identified, can lead to successful treatment during the next pregnancy. High blood pressure, systemic lupus activity, and gestational diabetes from steroid therapy also contribute to prenatal deaths. Prematurity, defined as birth before the 37th week of gestation, is quite common in SLE cases and is usually associated with an active maternal disease. There are, however, other factors for premature births, as evidenced by many of my healthy mothers who deliver early.

### Is Termination Safe, and When Should It Be Considered?

Therapeutic termination poses no special risks for lupus patients. However, the decision to terminate a pregnancy should not be taken lightly, and moral, religious, ethical, financial, and social considerations must be discussed with the patient and her family. Speaking personally, the only times I advise termination is when the life or critical well-being of the mother is at stake. This usually occurs when the only way to reverse serious organ-threatening disease, reduce hypertension, or prevent the mother from going on dialysis is to terminate the pregnancy.

### Family Planning and Birth Control

I've noted that, barring unusual circumstances, lupus patients are normally fertile. Women with SLE should ideally plan their pregnancies during a period of disease remission or relative inactivity that has been sustained for several months. Barrier methods of contraception such as diaphragms or condoms are generally effective. Though less efficacious, spermicidal creams, sponges, or jellies are also safe. Intrauterine devices (IUDs) should be used with caution, because they are associated with an increased risk of pelvic infection, and with the difficulty lupus patients have with fighting infection, this could be problematic.

## Can Lupus Patients Take Birth Control Pills?

When estrogen-containing birth control pills first became available in the early 1960s, there were numerous reports of young women either developing lupus or having their pre-existing lupus flare while taking these agents. By the early 1970s, these reports completely disappeared. Nevertheless, many physicians trained during this period who have not kept up with the rheumatology literature advise their lupus patients against taking oral contraceptives. What was responsible for the initial reports? First, birth control preparations in the 1960s contained much more estrogen than they do today. Also, estrogen-containing contraceptives during that era had tartrazine preservatives, which are no longer used. As discussed in Chapter 8, aromatic amines such as tartrazines are known to induce lupus.

Even though hundreds of my lupus patients have taken birth control preparations without difficulty, there are certain individuals who should not take them. *Estrogen-containing contraceptives are not recommended for patients with SLE who have antiphospholipid antibodies, high blood pressure, migraine headaches, a history of abnormal blood clotting, or very high lipid (cholesterol or triglyceride) levels.* These clinical subsets are associated with an increased risk of developing blood clots or having strokes. Beyond these groups, there is no evidence that contemporary oral contraceptives induce lupus in a genetically susceptible patient. A large clinical trial concluded that the overwhelming majority of women with SLE can take birth control pills if they do not have any of these contraindications. Also, several surveys have shown that ANAs do not develop as a result of taking birth control pills. Some published papers have suggested that estrogen-containing contraceptives induce disease flares in a minority of patients, but other studies have failed to show any relationship. It appears that mild, reversible flares can occur in a small number of lupus patients taking birth control pills. Progesterone-only methods of birth control appear to present no specific risks in SLE patients.

## The Delivery and Postpartum Period

Mothers and their obstetricians should aim for a vaginal delivery. The incidence of Cesarean sections in lupus patients is the same as in the general population except for unusually high-risk medical situations (e.g., uncontrollable blood pressure). Once the placenta is delivered, steroid levels drop. Two to eight weeks after childbirth, the body goes into a steroid withdrawal. If that extra fetal steroid boost was suppressing the lupus, this is the time when lupus flares. To prevent this, as previously noted, I frequently see my lupus patients 10 to 14 days after delivery and give them 60 milligrams of triamcinolone (Kenalog) intramuscularly. This modestly dosed time-release steroid prevents steroid withdrawal symptoms from occurring and decreases the risks of a postpartum flare.

## SUMMING UP

Lupus patients are normally fertile unless they have very active systemic disease or have received chemotherapy. Lupus pregnancies are successful 67 percent of the time; 13 percent fail due to antiphospholipid antibodies; and up to 30 percent of all deliveries are premature. If frequent competent clinical evaluations, blood testing, and good obstetric care are available, most lupus patients with mild to moderately active disease do quite well. Oral contraceptives should not necessarily be ruled out in family planning. Steroids can be safely used for exacerbations of lupus during pregnancy or for postpartum flares in those who choose to breastfeed.

## FURTHER READING

1. Fischer-Betz R, Specker C. Pregnancy in systemic lupus erythematosus and antiphospholipid syndrome. *Best Pract Res Clin Rheumatol.* 2017;31(3):397–414.
2. Lightstone L, Hladunewich MA. Lupus nephritis and pregnancy: concerns and management. *Semin Nephrol.* 2017;37(4):347–353.
3. Andreoli L, Bertsias GK, Agmon-Levin N, et al. EULAR recommendations for women's health and the management of famiy planning, assisted reproduction, pregnancy and menopause in patients with systemic lupus erythematosus and/or antiphospholipid syndrome. *Ann Rheum Dis.* 2017;76(3):476–485.
4. Götestam Skorpen C, Hoeltzenbein M, Tincani A, et al. The EULAR points to consider for use of antirheumatic drugs before pregnancy and during pregnancy and lactation. *Ann Rheum Dis.* 2016;75(5):795–810.
5. Noviani M, Wasserman S, Clowse ME. Breastfeeding in mothers in systemic lupus erythematosus. *Lupus.* 2016;25(9):973–979.

# 31

## *Economic Impact of Lupus in the United States and Disability Issues*

Lupus costs the American public approximately $20 billion a year in lost wages, disability, hospitalizations, medical visits, and medication. Direct costs account of one third and indirect costs, two thirds of this amount. The average lupus patient has an average of $10,000 to $20,000 in healthcare-related expenses annually.

### CAN LUPUS PATIENTS WORK?

A citizen's ability to work has a significant impact on our nation's economy and productivity. Fortunately, most lupus patients who wish to work are employed. Perhaps this sweeping generalization should be approached the opposite way. Why can't some lupus patients work? The answers include fatigue, inflammation, and swollen joints that prevent the ability to perform required tasks; medications that alter the ability to function or think clearly; cognitive dysfunction from lupus; heart or lung impairment affecting stamina or endurance; a lupus-related seizure disorder resulting in a restricted driver's license; or difficulty coping with the disease. It's hard to get a good handle on numbers because most lupus patients are women, and some are quite young. Therefore, many are classified as students, and still others as homemakers. Also, some lupus patients are in the retirement age group.

Patients with cutaneous lupus can almost always work, drug-induced lupus is transient, and systemic lupus erythematosus (SLE) is divided into organ- and non-organ-threatening disease. Several surveys have shown that fewer than 20 percent of lupus patients without heart, lung, kidney, liver, or central nervous system disease; autoimmune hemolytic anemia; or thrombocytopenia are listed as being disabled. Social Security guidelines make it relatively easy for lupus patients with organ-threatening disease to obtain disability and Medicare benefits. However, fewer than half the patients in this category take advantage of what's available and most work full time. This calculation is also not accurate because many lupus patients work part time or have had to change jobs or job descriptions have their needs accommodated.

In a 2012 study, 33 percent of individuals with SLE stopped working within 4 years of being diagnosed. This was largely due to musculoskeletal, neuropsychiatric issues, or blood clots.

## What's the Best Way to Be Able to Work?

In interviewing for a prospective position, be up front with your employer. Be positive and tell your employer all the things you can do and do well. Most lupus patients work best in an environment in which their hours are flexible and rest periods are available when needed. Professionals such as physicians, attorneys, or accountants can often set their own hours, which takes their needs into account. Others can seek out occupations in which they don't have to "clock in and clock out," or in which they can work from home when they feel up to it. These include being a real estate agent, travel agent, home-based computer consultant, or telephone salesperson.

Companies with more than 15 employees must comply with the Americans with Disabilities Act, which mandates making a reasonable accommodation for individuals with special needs. Some of these accommodations might include minimizing sun exposure, a warmer environment for those with Raynaud's, restricting heavy lifting or repetitive motions in individuals with swollen joints, providing enough rest periods during the day or more time to perform a task, and allowing employees to make time for doctor appointments.

Many lupus patients also have a household to maintain in addition to working outside the home. It's hard to maintain these two jobs. Nevertheless, working improves self-esteem, acts as a healthy form of distraction, and gives one a sense of accomplishment, and depression and social isolation is less common among those who are employed.

## When You Cannot Work

Some lupus patients are no longer able to work or simply cannot be employed. Disability can be temporary and total, temporary and partial, permanent and partial, or permanent and total. Temporary disability allows one to receive benefits while undergoing a medical or surgical treatment. If disability is permanent and partial, revising one's job description or responsibilities should be considered. Total, permanent disability usually qualifies one for Social Security disability allowances and Medicare health benefits after 2 years of not working. Private plans and state disability plans usually provide benefits until that time.

To qualify for benefits, the Social Security Administration will review your medical file and often have one of their consulting physicians examine you. Individuals with organ-threatening disease infrequently have a problem being awarded benefits. If you are turned down, you have a right to appeal. Ask your doctor to write a note on your behalf. (I have rarely encountered a "consulting physician" for disability who is a rheumatologist. Most consultants welcome a rheumatologist's input.) At this point, consider hiring an attorney. Disability attorneys don't get paid by you; if successful, their bill is fixed as a percentage of your benefits for a limited period of time. Vocational rehabilitation is offered by most private disability carriers and includes job retraining, tuition payments for career-oriented college classes, and work-function assessments to see what skills you can offer in the work force. Infrequently, lupus patients are covered by insurance and disability provided by worker's compensation, automobile, or homeowner's insurance carriers, which is beyond the scope of this discussion.

## FURTHER READING

1. Li T, Carls GS, Panopalis P, Wang S, Gibson TB, Goetzel RZ. Long-term medical costs and resource utiliziation in systemic lupus erythematosus and lupus nephritis: a five year analysis of a large medicated population. *Arthritis Rheum.* 2009;61(6):755–763.
2. Yelin E, Tonner C, Trupin L, et al. Longitudinal study of the impact of incident organ manifestations and increased disease activity on work loss among persons with systemic lupus erythematosus. *Arthritis Care Res* (Hoboken). 2012;64(2):169–175.
3. Agarwal N, Kumar V. Burden of lupus on work: issues in the employment of individuals with lupus. *Work.* 2016;55(2):429–439.

# 32
# What's the Prognosis?

When I first diagnose a patient with systemic lupus, she frequently enquires about the bottom line. She wants to know outcomes. Will I live? Can I have children? Is this crippling or deforming? Many lupus patients have excellent outcomes, live normal lives, and generally feel well. Others have serious impairments. I have to tell my patients that the prognosis varies from individual to individual, and it is dependent on many factors.

## WE'VE COME A LONG WAY!

I still come across newly diagnosed patients who are convinced that lupus is a fatal disease and that they only have 6 months to live. This nonsense is based on perceptions by some older physicians, who have had limited recent exposure to lupus patients. It also stems from the many outdated encyclopedias and reference books that line our family bookshelves. The first lupus survival study was published in 1949; it stated that half these patients were dead within 2 years. This 50 percent survival figure has constantly been revised. In 1955 half the patients were dead within 4 years, and by 1969, within 10 years. *In fact, at the present time, more than 90 percent of all lupus patients live more than 10 years after diagnosis*, although—if organ-threatening disease is present—only 60 percent survive 15 to 20 years. (This is a worldwide overall average.)

How can we account for these improvements? First, the discovery of the lupus erythematosus prep in 1948 and antinuclear antibodies in 1957 allowed milder cases to be diagnosed, which increased the number of people with the disease. This increased the pool of SLE patients, and those with mild cases naturally have longer life spans. Also, the widespread availability of steroids by 1950, chemotherapy by 1955, and dialysis by 1970 extended life spans. Though less dramatic, additional factors have also greatly improved survival: doctors have newer antibiotics to treat a variety of infections, better agents to attack high blood pressure, and broader experience in managing disease complications.

## OUTCOME AND TYPE OF LUPUS

As you might expect, certain types of lupus have better outcomes than others. Cutaneous (discoid) lupus and drug-induced lupus are associated with a normal life expectancy. Patients with non-organ-threatening SLE can expect the same outcome as that of a person without lupus; more than 95 percent survive at least 10 years after diagnosis.

The "prognostic variables," as lupus specialists like to call them, depend on several major considerations. *Methods of healthcare delivery* have an impact on determining outcome. For example, a Veterans Administration lupus study would include a disproportionate number of males. Several Kaiser-Permanente HMO lupus surveys limit themselves to analyzing trends among middle-class, insurable, working families. Hospital-based surveys focus on a sicker population of lupus patients. Publicly funded patients (e.g., Medicaid, county hospital patients) clearly have worse outcomes. Bluntly stated, if patients can read or write, afford food and medications, have transportation to clinics and access to rheumatologists who know their cases, and have been educated about the disease, their prognosis improves. *Epidemiologic factors* include race, geography, environmental exposure, and age. For example, more Asians (especially Chinese) develop SLE, but African Americans have a more severe process. Native Americans are also particularly prone to develop lupus. Lupus is rare on the African continent but observed in 1 of 300 African American women. Childhood SLE is more organ threatening and severe; lupus is much milder in patients over the age of 60. Environmental considerations reveal the influence of climate, occupation, smoking, diet, and exercise; none of these has been adequately surveyed in lupus.

*Genetic factors* influence outcome. Males make up only 10 percent of all lupus patients but may have more severe disease. Also, a family history of autoimmune disease increases awareness of lupus, which can lead to earlier diagnosis and intervention.

*Clinical and laboratory variables* (findings from blood and other testing) suggest that organ-threatening disease has a worse outcome. High blood pressure, low platelet counts, anemia, elevated cholesterols, and renal involvement—especially with nephrotic syndrome—require more attentive and aggressive care. The presence of certain autoantibodies such as anti-Ro (SSA), anticardiolipin antibody, and anti-RNP can be seen as distinguishing different types of lupus with distinct treatments and outcomes.

Finally, *treatment variables* influence the course of the disease. Some rheumatologists rarely prescribe chemotherapies for kidney disease and restrict their patients to corticosteroids. When these investigators publish survival studies, they must be interpreted differently from those of centers that intervene liberally with azathioprine, mycophenolate, or cyclophosphamide. There is no right or wrong treatment, only different outlooks and viewpoints. More subtle "adjunctive" measures—such as whether or not doctors prescribe birth control pills, immunizations, antimalarials, special diets, and so forth—can also affect quality of life and survival.

## PROACTIVE AND PREVENTIVE STRATEGIES FOR MANAGING LUPUS WITHOUT USING LUPUS MEDICINE

The last two decades have been characterized by the development of lupus consortia and cohorts. Organizations such as the Systemic Lupus International Collaborative Clinics (SLICC) have spearheaded "outcomes" research, wherein patients with SLE are followed prospectively for years and a variety of factors are analyzed to ascertain which groups do better. This research has shown that the prognosis of lupus can be improved by implementing measures that don't involve using medicine. These are enumerated in the following discussion.

*Educating the patient* about lupus makes a difference. If you know the side effects of a medication, what symptoms and signs to look for if lupus is flaring, what to do if you develop a fever, how to pace yourself, and how to keep physically and emotionally fit, the risk of complications is less and your quality of life improves.

Believe it or not, a prescription is actually filled and taken only 70 percent of the time a doctor prescribes a lupus medication. Even fewer patients take the medicine as prescribed. Increasingly, lupus doctors have become aware that lack of patient *adherence* is a major impediment to optimal care. Perhaps we don't explain what we are doing to the patient as well as we should. It is possible that you get scared by what we have to say and want to think about it. Studies have shown that lupus clinics have a high no-show rate and that adolescents with lupus take their medicine as prescribed only 50 percent of the time. Individuals who are not compliant have a worse prognosis than those who are.

*Access to lupus specialists* is critical. Not all lupus specialists are rheumatologists, and for reasons of personal interest and research, 80 percent of lupus is managed by 20 percent of the rheumatologists in the United States. Just as with heart surgery, outcomes improve with larger numbers of lupus patients a rheumatologist treats and has experience with. Ask your primary care doctor, local lupus society, or Arthritis Foundation chapter who is taking new lupus patients and providing good care for them. Unfortunately, the problem more often is that in a managed care setting, access to a lupus specialist is restricted to a single or occasional visit or simply not available. Don't take no for an answer. Be aggressive and pushy and take the lead to make sure that your lupus care is handled by a competent, caring, knowledgeable physician who can see you whenever necessary.

*Exercise programs* can improve outcomes by diminishing muscle atrophy, complications from injuries, and bone demineralization. The use of antiresorptive therapies in patients with active lupus or in those on corticosteroids can prevent and treat *osteoporosis*. Fewer fractures lead to greater mobility, independence, and self-esteem.

There is increasing evidence that lupus patients with cognitive impairment function better after a program of *biofeedback, mindfulness* and *cognitive behavioral therapy*. These modalities allow lupus patients to better cope with anxiety and stress, function better in society, and improve productivity, which, in turn, improves outcomes.

All lupus patients should be screened for *antiphospholipid antibodies* as well as the lupus anticoagulant. Because 12 percent of lupus patients sustain a thromboembolic event (e.g., stroke, pulmonary embolus) in their lifetime, individuals at risk can usually be identified and treated with low-dose aspirin, antimalarials, or other platelet inhibitors as needed.

Half of all lupus patients take alternative medicines on a regular basis, but many never tell their doctor about it. Some of these medicines contain potentially harmful materials such as phenylbutazone, corticosteroids, echinacea, sulfa derivatives, alfalfa sprouts, or ephedra components, as well as impurities that can flare the disease. When your doctor asks what medicines you are taking, please be sure to list nonprescription ones as well.

Finally, a lot of attention has focused on preventing heart disease, especially in patients taking corticosteroids. (Lupus patients not on corticosteroids are at a slightly increased risk for atherosclerotic and thromboembolic complications due to chronic inflammation.) Measures that make a difference include blood pressure screening and treatment, cessation of smoking, weight reduction, and regularly following blood sugar and lipid tests. Individuals who have cardiovascular risk factors should have an electrocardiogram, baseline 2-D echocardiogram to screen for pulmonary hypertension, imaging studies to look for atherosclerosis (heart scanning, duplex scanning of the carotids), and periodic stress testing (e.g., treadmill).

Implementing the strategies in this section has the potential of decreasing the mortality rate of lupus by at least 50 percent, and it can do so without the use of lupus medicine. (See Table 32.1.)

### DOES LUPUS EVER GO AWAY ON ITS OWN?

Every few months, I come across a newly diagnosed lupus patient who listens patiently to my 30-minute speech on the disease, followed by specific therapeutic recommendations, and says, "Doctor, I appreciate everything you are telling me, but I am going to take vitamins and herbs, eat a well-balanced diet, exercise, and see what happens." What happens to these patients? Can their disease go away on its own? Spontaneous remissions in lupus were reported as early as 1954. Non-organ-threatening disease has a 2 to 10 percent disappearance rate without medication. These are long-shot odds, and I do not recommend taking the chance, because non-organ-threatening disease also has a 20 percent chance of becoming organ-threatening within 5 years. I believe that antimalarial therapies decrease

**Table 32.1.** *Preventive Strategies That Improve Prognosis without Using Lupus Medicines*

1. Patient education
2. Improved adherence to medication programs
3. Exercise programs
4. Osteoporosis preventive and treatment measures
5. Cognitive therapy, mindfulness and biofeedback: optimizing coping mechanisms
6. Antiphospholipid antibody screening with preventive measures
7. Smart use of alternative medications
8. Screening for hypertension, hyperlipidemia, hyperglycemia
9. Smoking cessation
10. Weight control and dietary measures
11. Cardiac screening measures (e.g., electrocardiogram, heart scanning, stress test, 2-D echocardiogram, carotid duplex)
12. Coordination of care between primary care physician and lupus specialist

this risk. The spontaneous disappearance of lupus in the heart, lung, kidney, liver, or hematologic systems is so rare that when one well-documented patient with severe lupus prayed to Father Junipero Serra (founder of the Spanish missions in California in the 1700s) and had her organ-threatening disease disappear, this evidence was submitted to the Vatican, where Serra was ultimately sanctified.

In non-organ-threatening disease, lupus tends to burn itself out with time. Also, the onset of menopause is associated with milder disease. I occasionally allow reluctant patients with long-standing mild lupus to avoid medicine unless they are at risk for major complications.

## WHAT DO LUPUS PATIENTS DIE FROM?

The natural course of SLE has been extensively studied, and researchers have come to some interesting conclusions. The concept of a "bimodal survival curve" was first proposed in the 1970s and subsequently validated. This means that some lupus patients who die from the disease do so within the first 2 to 3 years of developing it. These individuals have active, aggressive lupus that responds poorly to therapy. After the third year, however, there's a lengthy hiatus of 10 to 15 years with few lupus-related deaths. But at 15 to 20 years, the effects of years of disease and medication seem to catch up with some patients, and a second mortality "hump" is observed. For example, young women who have active disease and are given moderate to high doses of steroids when they are 20 do well for a while, but eventually they may experience complications from ongoing steroid therapy. This leads to diabetes, high blood pressure, elevated cholesterols, and obesity—which may result in heart attacks by the time they are 40, as in Bonnie's case (Chapter 14).

More than 90 percent of lupus patients with SLE die from one of five causes: complications of kidney disease, infections, central nervous system lupus, blood clots, or cardiovascular complications. For unknown reasons, fatal cancer is rare among lupus patients. Several trends have become evident since survival curves were first published in the 1950s. Improved methods of dialysis and the introduction of transplantation have substantially decreased kidney-related deaths. Superior methods of detecting and managing central nervous system lupus have also greatly decreased mortality from this complication. Unfortunately, infections are still a major cause of death, especially among patients receiving steroids or immune suppressives. The discovery of antiphospholipid antibodies in the 1980s and the use of blood thinning to prevent serious clots and strokes in patients is making a difference. Some types of lupus are still very difficult to treat, and insufficient progress has been made to improve survival. These subsets include those patients with pulmonary hypertension, pulmonary hypertension, mesenteric vasculitis, and thrombotic thrombocytopenic purpura (TTP). Bimodal survival curves are still relevant, but far fewer lupus patients are dying in the first 2 years after diagnosis.

## SUMMING UP

The outcome of SLE depends on who is treating the disease; which ethnic, racial, or geographically defined populations have the disease; their socioeconomic status and consequent access to subspecialty care; and the treatment philosophy of the healthcare provider. More than 90 percent of all lupus patients in the United States live more than 10 years after being diagnosed. The survival of patients with organ-threatening disease is still an unsatisfactory 60 percent at 15 years. Patients with high blood pressure, low platelet counts, kidney disease, and severe anemia have a poorer outcome and should be managed aggressively. Even mild lupus is associated with alterations in quality of life and occasionally disappears spontaneously; serious lupus may ease up but does not go away without treatment. Deaths from lupus generally occur early on from active disease or later from continuously active inflammation or complications of therapy. Finally, despite all that has been said, I have found that patients who have a positive attitude and good coping mechanisms and who employ proactive strategies with their physicians have a better prognosis.

## FURTHER READING

1. Bernatsky S, Boivin JF, Joseph L, et al. Mortality in systemic lupus erythematosus. *Arthritis Rheum.* 2006;54(8):2550–2557.
2. Wallace DJ. Improving the prognosis of SLE without prescribing lupus drugs and the primary care paradox. *Lupus.* 2008;17(2):91–92.

# 33
## *Clinical Trials, New Therapies for Lupus, and Future Directions*

What advances will take place in the next 15 years? Will we be able to cure lupus or prevent it? Is there anything to look forward to? Let's take a look at what the future holds—and it is indeed promising!

If developments proceed at the expected rate, my crystal ball suggests that by 2030, an integrated healthcare system will be in place, allowing all lupus patients to receive optimal treatment regardless of socioeconomic status or medical insurability. A national data network should reveal exactly how many lupus patients there are as well as their gender and their racial, ethnic, and occupational background. The gene or combination of genes that predispose one to systemic lupus erythematosus (SLE) and the environmental factors (viruses, chemicals, drugs, etc.) that turn these genes on will be known. We will learn more about the microbiome, and a specific lupus diet will be available. It should be possible to identify individuals at risk for developing the disease and perhaps to vaccinate them so as to prevent autoimmune reactions. By 2030, we will know why 90 percent of patients with lupus are women, and we'll be able to manipulate hormones to decrease the disease's severity.

Existing therapies for lupus will be fine-tuned and improved upon. An ideal nonsteroidal anti-inflammatory drug (NSAID) that treats mild inflammation without any adverse reactions will be marketed. New-generation antimalarials and steroids that eliminate most of the side effects and could be more effective will become available.

Our current immune suppressive approaches are very general: they suppress all types of white blood cells and do not substantially focus on any single "bad guy" subset. Increased use of combinations of targeted or biologic therapies and immune suppressives that act at different levels of the inflammatory and immune process will be commonplace. The major advances in lupus therapy will emphasize tolerization as well cellular and antibody manipulation.

## HOW ARE DRUGS STUDIED FOR LUPUS?

Until belimumab (Benlysta) was approved in 2011, no new drug had been sanctioned by the Food and Drug Administration (FDA) for lupus since the 1950s. The only drugs approved for lupus are hydroxychloroquine (Plaquenil), prednisolone (Medrol, a relative of prednisone), and aspirin. In 2005, the FDA sponsored hearings that led to development of a guidance document (revised in 2010) that jump-started interest in testing new drugs for the disease. Though highly flawed, the document recognized the importance of a variety of disease activity and outcome measures, and advanced the conversation about how to best do a lupus trial.

### Classification of Lupus

Any patient participating in a clinical SLE trial will have to fulfill one of the criteria for lupus. All are 90 percent sensitive and specific for diagnosing the disease (see Chapter 2).

### Clinical Activity Indices

Since the mid-1980s, several centers have developed indices that assess disease activity. By giving points for specific symptoms, signs, and laboratory abnormalities, these indices allow investigators to follow improvement or worsening of the disease through a composite score. They include the British Isles Lupus Assessment Group (BILAG), Systemic Lupus Erythematosus Disease Activity Index (SLEDAI; see Table 33.1), Systemic Lupus Activity Measure (SLAM), and European Consensus Lupus Activity Measurement (ECLAM). However, these measures were derived before modern clinical trials were started in the 1990s and are not as comprehensive or as accurate as they should be. Currently, pharmaceutical companies are using a composite index that contains elements of both the BILAG and SLEDAI (the BILAG Based Combined Lupus Assessment [BICLA] and the Systemic Lupus Erythematosus Response Index [SRI]) with physician assessments of activity. An example of such an instrument is the Systemic Lupus Responder Index (SRI) endorsed by the FDA for belimumab. It included a reduction of disease activity, no new organ involvement, and improvement in blinded physician assessments. There is an ongoing initiative to use pooled data from completed clinical trials whose goal is to develop a newer, more accurate lupus activity and index.

### Quality of Life

Several instruments that have been validated for other diseases have been shown to be helpful in lupus as well. These include measuring health-related quality of life using the SF-36, which evaluates physical functioning, physical role,

**Table 33.1.** *One Version of the SLEDAI (Systemic Lupus Erythematosus Disease Activity Index)*

| Weight | Descriptor | Definition |
|---|---|---|
| 8 | Seizure | Recent onset (last 10 days). Exclude metabolic, infectious drug cause, or seizure due to past irreversible central nervous system damage. |
| 8 | Psychosis | Altered ability to function in normal activity due to severe disturbance in the perception of reality. Include hallucinations, incoherence, marked loose associations, impoverished thought content, marked illogical thinking, bizarre, disorganized, or catatonic behavior. Exclude uremia and drug causes. |
| 8 | Organic brain syndrome | Altered mental function with impaired orientation, memory, or other intellectual function |
| 8 | Visual disturbance | Retinal and eye changes of systemic lupus erythematosus. Include cytoid bodies, retinal hemorrhages, serious exudate of hemorrhage in the choroid, optic neuritis, scleritis, or episcleritis. Exclude hypertension, infection, or drug causes. |
| 8 | Cranial nerve disorder | New-onset sensory or motor neuropathy involving cranial nerves. Include vertigo due to lupus. |
| 8 | Lupus headache | Severe persistent headache: may be migrainous but must be nonresponsive to narcotic analgesia. |
| 8 | Cerebrovascular accident | New onset of cerebrovascular accident(s). Exclude arteriosclerosis or hypertensive causes. |
| 8 | Vasculitis | Ulceration, gangrene, tender finger nodules, periungual infarction, splinter hemorrhages, or biopsy or angiogram proof of vasculitis. |
| 4 | Arthritis | More than two joints with pain and signs of inflammation (i.e., tenderness, swelling, or effusion). |
| 4 | Myositis | Proximal muscle aching/weakness associated with elevated creatine phosphokinase/aldolase or electromyogram changes or a biopsy showing myositis. |
| 4 | Urinary casts | Heme-granular or red blood cell casts. |
| 4 | Hematuria | >5 red blood cells/high power field. Exclude kidney stone, infection, or other causes. |
| 4 | Proteinuria | New-onset or recent increase of >0.5 g/24 hours. |
| 4 | Pyuria | >5 white blood cells/high power field. Exclude infection. |
| 2 | Rash | New or ongoing inflammatory lupus rash. |
| 2 | Alopecia | New or ongoing abnormal, patchy, or diffuse loss of hair due to active lupus. |
| 2 | Mucosal ulcers | New or ongoing oral or nasal ulcerations due to active lupus. |
| 2 | Pleurisy | Classic and severe pleuritic chest pain or pleural rub or effusion, or new pleural thickening due to lupus. |
| 2 | Pericarditis | Classic and severe pericardial pain or rub or effusion, or electrocardiogram confirmation. |
| 2 | Low complement | Decrease in CH50, C3, or C4 below the lower limit of normal for testing laboratory. |
| 2 | Increased DNA binding | >25% binding by Farr assay or above normal range for testing laboratory. |
| 1 | Fever | >38°C. Exclude infectious cause. |
| 1 | Thrombocytopenia | <100,000 platelets/mm$^3$. |
| 1 | Leukopenia | <3,000 white blood cells/mm$^3$. Exclude drug causes. |
| | **TOTAL SCORE** | (Sum of weights next to descriptors marked present.) |

Score if descriptor is present at time of visit or in the preceding 10 days.

bodily pain, general health, vitality, social functioning, emotional roles, and mental health; Health Assessment Questionnaire (HAQ) score; patient and physician assessments of the disease and disability; and the Functional Assessment in Chronic Illness–Fatigue Scale (FACIT). However, these metrics are lupus nonspecific and the measures and can reflect hypertension, depression, steroid use, and fibromyalgia activity. Most studies are using a Lupus quality of life (QOL) measure or Lupus Impact Tracker (LIT) for now. The National Institutes of Health PROMIS (Patient Reported Outcomes Measurement System) initiative, for example has a goal of developing such an inventory.

### Drug Safety and Pharmacoeconomic Impact

A new agent must not only be effective, it must also be safe. How do new drugs influence hospitalizations? Adverse events from a drug's administration must be outweighed by its potential benefits. Further does it reduce death rates and is it cost effective? When can the drug be stopped?

### Damage Indices

The American College of Rheumatology (ACR) and Systemic Lupus International Collaborating Clinics (SLICC) have endorsed and validated a damage index. Prior inflammation can scar the kidneys, heart, lung, kidney, or liver, producing irreversible changes. If a drug can prevent new damage by slowing the rate of increase of a damage index, it is potentially useful.

### Biomarker or Surrogate Markers

In the past, clinicians used sedimentation rates, C3 complement, and anti-DNA levels to assess disease activity and adjusted medication based on these values. It turns out that some of these markers, or a combination of these markers, correlates with long-term outcome. If a new drug can improve these markers, it may decrease the time necessary to test it, because it often takes 10 years of observation to know whether a treatment protocol for the kidneys, for example, prevents one from needing dialysis. The use of traditional and newly developed markers are being evaluated in lupus drug testing evaluations. Some of the furthest along include looking at the innate immune system by testing for the interferon signature and urinary biomarkers.

### The Bottom Line

For a new drug to be approved for lupus, it should ideally decrease clinical disease activity by clinical indices or biomarkers, prevent damage, be safe, and improve one's quality of life.

## WHAT ABOUT TARGETED AND BIOLOGIC THERAPIES?

Most drugs traditionally used for serious lupus are immunosuppressives. In other words, they lower blood counts and kill cells. However, these agents kill good cells as well as bad cells. Targeted therapies (biologics) kill bad cells without killing good ones. See Table 33.2.

### Targeted Therapies Used in SLE Currently Approved by the FDA

*Belimumab* (Benlysta) is approved for patients with SLE who are autoantibody-positive. Given as an intravenous monthly or as a weekly injection, 70 percent of patients improve after 3 to 6 months. It is steroid and immune suppressive sparing and improves quality of life. Belimumab has an excellent safety profile and is very well tolerated. It is generally used for patients with active disease despite having steroids, antimalarials, and immune suppressives or for those intolerant of these agents.

Agents that block *anti-TNF* (e.g., remicade [Infliximab], etanercept [Enbrel], adalimumab [Humira]) have been available since 1998 and are widely prescribed for rheumatoid arthritis, inflammatory bowel disease, psoriasis, psoriatic arthritis, uveitis, and juvenile inflammatory arthritis. Many lupus patients have used these drugs. A summary of experience suggests that patients with prominent inflammatory arthritis (swollen joints) may do well with anti-TNFs, especially if there is a lupus/rheumatoid overlap. However, some individuals experience increases in anti-DNA, antinuclear antibodies, and anticardiolipin antibodies as well as more infections.

*Rituximab* (Rituxan) is a B-cell depletion drug that is given intravenously every 6 months or as needed. It is generally well tolerated, but one must monitor counts and be vigilant in looking out for infections. There is a wealth of experience demonstrating that lupus patients with severe arthritis, central nervous system

**Table 33.2.** *Targets for New Therapies in Systemic Lupus Erythematosus*

| | |
|---|---|
| T cells | CTLA4-Ig; modified CD40L monoclonal antibody, ICOS inhibition |
| B cells, anti-double-stranded DNA antibodies | Monoclonal antibodies to CD19,CD20, CD22; anti-BLyS TACI-Ig; BAFF-RFc; blockade of plasma cells |
| Complement | Anti-C5a |
| Cytokines | Monoclonal antibodies to IL-6R, IL-6, IL-10, IL-17 |
| Promote regulatory cells | Expand CD4+CD25+ cells, CD8+CD28– cells |
| Inhibition of interferon, toll receptors | Anti-IFN-alpha; TLR7 and TLR9 antagonists |
| T cell regulation of autoantibody production, tolerogens | Peptides derived from nucleosomes; SmAg Igs; 16/6 idiotype |
| Cell surface receptor activation inhibition | Syk-kinase inhibition; JAK inhibition, BTK inhibition and kinome directed therapies, rapamycin |

vasculitis, low platelet counts, inflammatory polyneuropathies, and hemolytic anemia do well with this agent.

*Tociluzumab* (Actemra) is an antibody to interleukin-6 (IL-6) and a favorable trial conducted at the National Institutes of Health was published. Approved for rheumatoid arthritis, this agent helps lupus arthritis and other anti-IL-6 compounds have been studied with promising results.

*Abatacept* (Orencia) inhibits the T cell co-stimulatory pathway and is approved for rheumatoid arthritis. It can be given as an intravenous once a month or as a weekly injection. Abatacept is very well tolerated, and it may play a role in patients with serious SLE who would benefit from steroid and immune suppressive sparing approaches.

*Stem cell transplantation* is expensive and risky. Patients are prone to infections; need medicines that stimulate red cell, white cell, or platelet production; evolve graft-versus-host reactions; and can have disease recurrence. *Mesenchymal cell therapy* may also be promising and is safer. It is too early to tell how these patients will do over the next few years.

## TARGETED THERAPIES CURRENTLY IN DEVELOPMENT

There are numerous biologic therapies that are currently being studied in SLE and are listed in Table 33.3. I am hopeful that some of these agents will be approved by the FDA in the next few years.

### Looking beyond the Next Few Years

Lupus is characterized by "dyslexic T cells," which lead to alterations in immune trafficking. In addition to the biologics being studied, several other investigational

**Table 33.3.** *Innovative Approaches under Study*

1. T-cell vaccination
2. Agents that target cytokines (IL-12,13,15,16,17,18, 21,23), growth factors or chemokines
3. Peptide tolerogens to proteins such as HLA molecules, Sm, Immunoglobulin
4. Promotion of T regulatory cells
5. Gene therapies
6. Up-regulation of TGF-beta
7. Targeting Fc receptors
8. Developing a lupus derived from manipulation of the microbiome
9. Targeting cell surface receptors (human kinome) such as TYK, BTK, JAKs, SYK, MAP kinases
10. Mesenchymal stem cell transplantation
11. Agents that influence mTOR regulation
12. Inhibition of adhesion molecules
13. Inhibitors of co-stimulation
14. Blocking activation of inflammatory mechanisms in the tubulointerstitium
15. Combination B cell therapies (e.g., rituximab with belimumab)
16. Targeting complement activation

lines are under scrutiny (Table 33.3). These include antibodies or blockers of an array of cytokines, agents that block adhesion molecules (the cellular glue that attracts inflammatory factors to cells from blood). A class of medicines that "tolerize" the body and prevent patients from making antibodies to themselves is being studied. Small oral molecules targeting genes in the human kinome interacting with cell surface receptors are available for rheumatoid arthritis and are under intense study in lupus. Additional approaches include small molecules (peptides), antibodies against antigen-binding sites (anti-idiotypic antibodies), and T cell receptors. Special vaccines with specifically designed payloads can not only alter immunity as we know it but also create new immune environments.

Albert Einstein said that God does not play dice with the universe. Some astounding developments now support this philosophical remark. The concept of apoptosis, or programmed cell death, has taken center stage in the last few years. A variety of apoptosis genes sometimes seem to work at cross purposes, but the bottom line is that cells that are damaged and should die fail to do so in lupus. The persistence of cellular debris or altered cells promotes the production of autoantibodies, perpetuating autoimmunity. Is lupus related to some grand design?

Down the line, we will be able to fashion new immune environments that may eliminate lupus. Not only will people who carry lupus genes be vaccinated to prevent the disease's activation, but gene therapies (placing messages into cells to produce or not produce proteins) will become important. Improved new ways of performing stem cell transplantation are theoretically capable of giving us an entirely new immune system programmed not to allow lupus to exist or become active. These are indeed exciting times for a lupologist!

Our concepts of cell immunology change every year. Some ethicists and philosophers in our discipline postulate that a higher authority created an immunotheology that can be manipulated only with rigid discipline if it is to be of any help to patients. We may hope that, by 2030, some lupus can be prevented, no one will die from it, and treatment will be both effective and safe.

## FURTHER READING

1. Wallace DJ. Improved strategies for designing lupus trials with targeted therapies: learning from 65 years of experience. *Lupus.* 2016;25(10):1141–1149.
2. Touma Z, Gladman DD. Current and future therapies for SLE: obstacles and reommendations for the development of novel treatments. *Lupus Sci Med.* 2017;4(1):e000239.

# Glossary

**ACR/American College of Rheumatology**  A professional association of 7,000 American rheumatologists. Criteria, or definitions for many **rheumatic diseases**, are called the ACR criteria.

**Acute**  Of short duration and coming on suddenly.

**Adaptive immunity**  An evolved system of immune responses.

**Adenopathy**  A swelling of lymph nodes.

**Adrenal glands**  Small organs, located above the kidney, that produce many **hormones**, including **corticosteroids** and epinephrine.

**Albumin**  A **protein** that circulates in the blood and carries materials to cells.

**Albuminuria**  A **protein** in urine.

**Alopecia**  Hair loss.

**Analgesic**  A drug that alleviates pain.

**Anemia**  A condition resulting from low red blood cell counts.

**Antibodies**  Special **protein** substances made by the body's white cells for defense against bacteria and other foreign substances.

**Anticardiolipin antibody**  An **antiphospholipid antibody**.

**Anticentromere antibody**  **Antibodies** to a part of the cell's **nucleus**; associated with a form of **scleroderma** called **CREST syndrome**.

**Anti-double-stranded DNA (anti-DNA)**  **Antibodies** to **DNA**; seen in half of those with **systemic** lupus and implies serious disease.

**Anti-ENA**  Old term for extractable nuclear **antibodies**, which largely consist of **anti-Sm** and **anti-RNP** antibodies.

**Antigen**  A substance that stimulates antibody formation; in lupus, this can be a foreign substance or a product of the patient's own body.

**Anti-inflammatory**  An agent that counteracts or suppresses **inflammation**.

**Antimalarials**  Drugs originally used to treat malaria that are helpful for lupus.

**Antinuclear antibodies (ANA)**  **Proteins** in the blood that react with the nuclei of cells; seen in 96 percent of those with **systemic** lupus erythematosus (SLE), in 5 percent of healthy individuals, and in most patients with autoimmune diseases.

**Antiphospholipid antibodies    Antibodies** to a constituent of cell membranes seen in one third of those with SLE. In the presence of a cofactor, these **antibodies** can alter clotting and lead to strokes, blood clots, miscarriages, and low **platelet** counts. Also detected as the **lupus anticoagulant**.

**Anti-RNP**    Antibody to ribonucleoprotein; seen in SLE and **mixed connective tissue disease**.

**Anti-Sm**    Anti-Smith antibody; found only in lupus.

**Anti-SSA**    Also known as the **Ro antibody**; associated with **Sjögren's syndrome**, sun sensitivity, neonatal lupus, and **congenital heart block**.

**Anti-SSB**    Also known as the **La antibody**; almost always seen with **anti-SSA**.

**Apheresis**    See **plasmapheresis**.

**Apoptosis**    Programmed cell death.

**Artery**    A blood vessel that transports blood from the heart to the tissues.

**Arthralgia**    Pain in a joint.

**Arthritis    Inflammation** of a joint.

**Ascites**    An abnormal collection of abdominal fluid.

**Aspirin**    An **anti-inflammatory** drug with pain-killing properties.

**Atrophy**    A thinning of the surface; a form of wasting.

**Autoantibody**    An antibody to one's own tissues or cells.

**Autoimmune hemolytic anemia**    See **hemolytic anemia**.

**Autoimmunity**    Allergy to one's own tissues.

**B lymphocyte or B cell**    A white blood cell that makes **antibodies**.

**Biologic**    A substance made from a living organism or its products used in the prevention, diagnosis or treatment of disease

**Biopsy**    Removal of a bit of tissue for examination under the microscope.

**Bursa**    A sac of **synovial fluid** between **tendons**, muscles, and bones that promotes easier movement.

**Butterfly rash**    Reddish facial eruption over the bridge of the nose and cheeks, resembling a butterfly in flight.

**Capillaries**    Small blood vessels connecting the arteries and veins.

**Candida**    A yeast.

**Cartilage**    Tissue material covering bone. The nose, outer ears, and trachea consist primarily of cartilage.

**Chronic**    Persisting over a long period of time.

**CNS**    Central nervous system.

**Collagen**    Structural **protein** found in bone, **cartilage**, and skin.

**Collagen vascular disease; connective tissue disease**    Antibody-mediated inflammatory process of the connective tissues, especially the joints, skin, and muscle.

**Complement**    A group of **proteins** that, when activated, promote and are consumed during **inflammation**.

**Complete blood count (CBC)**    A blood test that measures the amount of red blood cells (**RBCs**), white blood cells (**WBCs**), and **platelets** in the body.

**Congenital heart block**　Dysfunction of the rate/rhythm conduction system in the fetal or infant heart.

**Connective tissue**　The "glue" that holds muscles, skin, and joints together.

**Corticosteroid**　Any natural **anti-inflammatory** hormone made by the adrenal cortex; also can be made synthetically.

**Cortisone**　A synthetic **corticosteroid**.

**Creatinine**　A blood test that measures kidney function.

**Creatinine clearance**　A 24-hour urine collection that measures kidney function.

**CREST syndrome**　A form of limited **scleroderma** characterized by C (calcium deposits under the skin), R (**Raynaud's phenomenon**), E (esophageal dysfunction), S (sclerodactyly or tight skin), and T (a rash called telangiectasia).

**Crossover syndrome**　An autoimmune process that has features of more than one **rheumatic disease** (e.g., lupus and **scleroderma**).

**Cryoglobulins**　**Protein** complexes circulating in the blood that are precipitated by cold.

**Cutaneous**　Relating to the skin.

**Cytokines**　A group of chemicals that signal cells to perform certain actions.

**Dermatologist**　A physician specializing in skin diseases.

**Dermatomyositis**　An autoimmune process directed against muscles associated with skin rashes.

**Discoid lupus**　A thick, plaquelike rash seen in 20 percent of those with SLE. If the patient has the rash but not SLE, he or she is said to have **cutaneous** (discoid) lupus erythematosus.

**Diuretics**　Medications that increase the body's ability to rid itself of fluids.

**DNA (deoxyribonucleic acid)**　The body's building blocks; a molecule responsible for the production of all the body's **proteins**.

**Dysphagia**　Difficulty in swallowing.

**Ecchymosis**　Purplish patch caused by oozing of blood into the skin.

**Edema**　Swelling caused by retention of fluid.

**ELISA (enzyme-linked immunosorbent assay)**　A very sensitive blood test for detecting the presence of **autoantibodies**.

**Enzyme**　A **protein** that accelerates chemical reactions.

**Epigenetics**　Influence of the environment upon **genes**.

**Erythema**　A reddish hue.

**Erythematous**　Having a reddish hue.

**Estrogen**　Female hormone produced by the ovaries.

**Exacerbations**　**Symptoms** reappear; a **flare**.

**False-positive serologic test (STS)**　A blood test revealing an antibody that may be found in patients with syphilis and that gives false-positive results in 15 percent of patients with SLE; associated with the **lupus anticoagulant** and **antiphospholipid antibodies**.

**FANA**　Another term for **ANA**.

**Fibrositis; fibromyalgia**  A pain amplification syndrome characterized by fatigue, a sleep disorder, and tender points in the soft tissues; can be caused by **steroids** and mistaken for lupus, although 20 percent of those with lupus have fibrositis.

**Flare**  **Symptoms** reappear; another word for **exacerbation**.

**Genes**  Consisting of **DNA**, they are the basic unit of inherited information in our cells.

**Glomerulonephritis**  **Inflammation** of the glomerulus of the kidney; seen in one-third of patients with lupus.

**Hematocrit**  A measurement of red blood cell levels. Low levels produce **anemia**.

**Hemoglobin**  Oxygen-carrying **protein** of red blood cells. Low levels produce anemia.

**Hemolytic anemia**  **Anemia** caused by premature destruction of red blood cells due to **antibodies** to the red blood cell surface. Also called **autoimmune hemolytic anemia**.

**Hepatitis**  **Inflammation** of the liver.

**HLA (human leukocyte antigen)**  Molecules inside the **macrophage** that binds to an antigenic peptide. Controlled by **genes** on the sixth chromosome. They can amplify or perpetuate certain immune and inflammatory responses.

**Hormones**  Chemical messengers—including thyroid, **steroids**, insulin, **estrogen**, progesterone, and testosterone—made by the body.

**Immune complex**  An **antibody** and **antigen** together.

**Immunity**  The body's defense against foreign substances.

**Immunofluorescence**  A means of detecting immune processes with a fluorescent stain and a special microscope.

**Immunoglobulins**  **Protein** fraction of **serum** responsible for antibody activity.

**Immunosuppressive**  A medication such as cyclophosphamide or azathioprine, which treats lupus by suppressing the immune system.

**Inflammation**  Swelling, heat, and redness resulting from the infiltration of white blood cells into tissues.

**Innate immunity**  Primitive responses to bacteria and viruses.

**Interferon**  A **protein** made to protect the body from infection that is overactive in lupus.

**Kinome**  **Protein** kinases recorded in our **genes** that regulate cell signaling

**Kidney biopsy**  Removal of a bit of kidney tissue for microscopic analysis.

**La antibody**  Also called **anti-SSB**, a **Sjögren's** antibody.

**LE cell**  Specific cell found in blood specimens of most lupus patients.

**Ligament**  A tether attaching bone to bone, giving them stability.

**Lupus anticoagulant**  A means of detecting **antiphospholipid antibodies** from prolonged clotting times.

**Lupus vulgaris**  Tuberculosis of the skin; not related to **systemic** or **discoid lupus**.

**Lymph**  Fluid collected from tissues that flows through lymph nodes.

**Lymphocyte**  Type of white blood cell that fights infection and mediates the immune response.

**Macrophage**  A cell that kills foreign material and presents information to lymphocytes.

**MHC (major histocompatibility complex)**  In humans, it is the same as **HLA**.

**Microbiome**  Bacterial and microbial makeup of our gut (intestines)

**Mixed connective tissue disease (MCTD)**  Exists when a patient who carries the **anti-RNP** antibody has features of more than one autoimmune disease.

**Natural killer cell**  A white blood cell that kills other cells.

**Nephritis**  **Inflammation** of the kidney.

**NETs (neutrophil extracellular traps)**  Networks of extracellular fibers composed of DNA from neutrophiils, which bind pathogens

**Neutrophil**  A granulated white blood cell involved in bacterial killing and **acute inflammation**.

**NSAID (nonsteroidal anti-inflammatory drug)**  Drug or agent that fights **inflammation** by blocking the actions of prostaglandin. Examples include **aspirin**, ibuprofen, and naproxen.

**Nucleus**  The center of a cell that contains **DNA**.

**Orthopedic surgeon**  A doctor who operates on musculoskeletal structures.

**Pathogenic**  Causing disease or abnormal reactions.

**Pathology**  Abnormal cellular or anatomic features.

**Pericardial effusion**  Fluid around the sac of the heart.

**Pericarditis**  **Inflammation** of the **pericardium**.

**Pericardium**  A sac lining the heart.

**Petechiae**  Small red spots under the skin.

**Photosensitivity**  Sensitivity to ultraviolet light.

**Plasma**  The fluid portion of blood.

**Plasmapheresis**  Filtration of blood **plasma** through a machine to remove **proteins** that may aggravate lupus.

**Platelet**  A component of blood responsible for clotting.

**Pleura**  A sac lining the lung.

**Pleural effusion**  Fluid in the sac lining the lung.

**Pleuritis**  Irritation or **inflammation** of the lining of the lung.

**Polyarteritis**  A disease closely related to lupus, featuring **inflammation** of medium- and small-sized blood vessels.

**Polymyalgia rheumatica**  An autoimmune disease of the joints and muscles seen in older patients with high sedimentation rates who have severe aching in their shoulders, upper arms, hips, and upper legs.

**Polymyositis**  An autoimmune disease that targets muscles.

**Prednisone; prednisolone**  Synthetic steroids.

**Protein**  A collection of amino acids. **Antibodies** are proteins.

**Proteinuria**  Excess **protein** levels in the urine (also called **albuminuria**).

**Pulse steroids** Very high doses of **corticosteroids** given intravenously over 1 to 3 days to critically ill patients.

**Purpura** Hemorrhage into the skin.

**Raynaud's disease** Isolated **Raynaud's phenomenon**; not part of any other disease.

**Raynaud's phenomenon** Discoloration of the hands or feet (they turn blue, white, or red), especially with cold temperatures; a feature of an autoimmune disease.

**RBC** Red blood cell count.

**Remission** Quiet period free from **symptoms** but not necessarily representing a cure.

**Rheumatic disease** Any of 150 disorders affecting the immune or musculoskeletal systems; about 30 of these are also autoimmune.

**Rheumatoid arthritis** **Chronic** disease of the joints marked by inflammatory changes in the joint-lining membranes, which may give positive results on tests of rheumatoid factor and **ANA**.

**Rheumatoid factor** **Autoantibodies** that react with Immunoglobin G; seen in most patients with **rheumatoid arthritis** and 25 percent of those with SLE.

**Rheumatologist** An internal medicine specialist who has completed at least a 2-year fellowship studying **rheumatic disease**.

**Ro antibody** See **anti-SSA**.

**Salicylates** Aspirinlike drugs.

**Scleroderma** An autoimmune disease featuring rheumatoid-type **inflammation**, tight skin, and vascular problems (e.g., **Raynaud's**).

**Sedimentation rate** Test that measures the precipitation of red cells in a column of blood; high rates usually indicate increased disease activity.

**Serum** Clear liquid portion of the blood after removal of clotting factors.

**Sjögren's syndrome** Dry eyes, dry mouth, and **arthritis** observed with most autoimmune disorders or by itself (termed primary Sjögren's).

**Steroids** Usually a shortened term for **corticosteroids**, which are **anti-inflammatory hormones** produced by the adrenal cortex or synthetically.

**Symptoms** Changes patients feel.

**Synovial fluid** Joint fluid.

**Synovitis** **Inflammation** of the tissues lining a joint.

**Synovium** Tissue that lines the joint.

**Systemic** Pertaining to or affecting the body as a whole.

**T cell** A lymphocyte responsible for immunologic memory.

**Targeted therapy** Molecularly designed treatment for disease

**Temporal arteritis** **Inflammation** of the temporal **artery** (located in the scalp) associated with high sedimentation rates, **systemic symptoms**, and sometimes loss of vision.

**Tendon** Structure that attaches muscle to bone.

**Thrombocytopenia** Low **platelet** counts.

**Thymus**   A gland in the neck area responsible for immunologic maturity.

**Titer**   Amount of a substance, such as **ANA**.

**Tolerance**   The failure to make **antibodies** to an **antigen**.

**Toleragen**   Agent that promotes **tolerance**—where non self is not rejected

**Toll receptor**   A pattern-recognition feature of the innate immune system.

**UCTD (undifferentiated connective tissue disease)**   Features of **autoimmu-nity** in a patient who does meet established criteria for lupus**, rheumatoid arthritis**, **scleroderma**, or inflammatory myositis.

**Uremia**   Marked kidney insufficiency, frequently necessitating dialysis.

**Urinalysis**   Analysis of urine.

**Urine, 24-hour collection**   The collection of all urine passed in a 24-hour period; it is examined for **protein** and **creatinine** to determine how well the kidneys are functioning.

**Urticaria**   Hives.

**UV light**   Ultraviolet light. Its spectrum includes UVA (320–400 nanometers), UVB (290–320 nm), and UVC (200–290 nm) wavelengths.

**Vasculitis**   **Inflammation** of the blood vessels.

**WBC**   White blood cell.

# Appendix: Lupus Resource Materials

**How can I find more information about what I just read in *The Lupus Book* when there are no references?**

1. Consult any of the rheumatology textbooks listed in this appendix. Two books in the list that are authored by this writer are exhaustively referenced.
2. Consult websites of the lupus support organizations listed herein.
3. On your computer, access the website for the National Library of Medicine, http://www.ncbi.nlm.nih.gov/pubmed. Type in the keywords of the topic you wish to obtain references for. This is a free service.

**What organizations provide patient support in the United States? (Many such organizations exist; only those with a research budget of over $1 million are listed.)**

**Arthritis Foundation**, 1335 Peachtree St NE #600, Atlanta, GA 30309, 1-800-283-7800. There are 56 US chapters hat provide research monies, publish literature, and offer patient support for arthritis and related conditions such as lupus. Website: http://www.arthritis.org

**Lupus Foundation of America, Inc. (LFA)**, 2121 K St NW #200, Washington, DC 20039, 1-202-349-1155 or 1-800-558-0121 (Spanish line, 1-800-558-0123). With 50 chapters and 220 support groups in 32 states, the LFA is the nation's leading nonprofit voluntary health organization dedicated to finding the cause and cure for lupus. Website: http://www.lupus.org

**In addition to the previously listed organizations, where else can reliable information about lupus be obtained?**

**American College of Rheumatology (ACR) and Association of Rheumatology Health Professionals (ARHP)**, 2200 Lake Blvd NE, Atlanta, GA 30329, 1-404-633-3777. This is the professional organization to which nearly all US and many international rheumatologists belong. Website: http://www.rheumatology.org

**National Institute of Arthritis and Musculoskeletal and Skin Diseases (NIAMS)**, 1 AMS Circle Bethesda, MD 20892, 1-301-495-4484. Toll free: 877-22NIAMS. Part of the National Institutes of Health, NIAMS had a budget of $542 million in 2017 and funds nearly $100 million in lupus relevant research each year at the Bethesda campus and elsewhere in the country. Website: http://www.niams.nih.gov

**In addition to the previously listed organizations, what other organizations fund lupus research? (Many such organizations exist; this list is restricted to those that give more than $1 million a year to lupus-related research at more than one institution.)**

**Rheumatology Research Foundation of the American College of Rheumatology**, 2200 Lake Boulevard NE, Atlanta, GA 30319, 1-800-346-4753, 404 365 1373. The research funding arm of the ACR provides money for rheumatology training and research programs that are vital to the care of patients suffering from rheumatic diseases. Website: http://www.rheumatology.org/ref

**Lupus Research Alliance**, 275 Madison Ave, 10th Floor, New York, NY 10016. This alliance has 11 affiliate organizations and spends $10 million a year on lupus research related initiatives. Email: info@lupusresearch.org

**How can I find out about lupus support outside the United States?**

**Lupus Europe**. All efforts in Europe are coordinated through a central office. Affiliate groups are located in Belgium, Finland, France, Germany, Great Britain, Iceland, Ireland, Israel, Italy, Netherlands, Norway, Portugal, Spain, Sweden, and Switzerland. Email: Tony Bonello. Website: http://www.lupus-europe.org

**Lupus Canada** (the national organization), 3555 14th Avenue, Unit #3, Markham, Ontario L3R 0H5, Canada 1-905-513-0004 or toll free in Canada, 1-800-661-1468. Website: http://www.lupuscanada.org (in French and English)

**Panamerican League of Associations for Rheumatology**. Comprises the scientific societies of rheumatology health professionals and rheumatic patient association in all the Americas.

**Which organizations serve patients with lupus-related disorders?**

**Fibromyalgia Network**, P.O. Box 31750, Tucson, AZ 85751-1750, 1-520-290-5508 or 1-800-853-2929. This organization supports research through the American Fibromyalgia Syndrome Association. Website: http://www.fmnetnews.com

**Scleroderma Foundation**, 300 Rosewood Drive, #105, Danvers, MA 01923, 1-978-463-5843 or 1-800-722-4673. Website: http://www.scleroderma.org.

**Sjögren's Syndrome Foundation**, 6707 Democracy Blvd, #325, Bethesda, MD 20817. Toll free: 800-475-6473 Website: http://www.sjogrens.org

**What about rheumatology or lupus textbooks?**

Tsokos G, *Systemic Lupus Erythematosus* Amsterdam: Academic Press; 2016.

Wallace DJ. *Lupus*: The Essential Clinician's Guide. New York: Oxford University Press; 2014.

Wallace DJ, Hahn BH. *Dubois' Lupus Erythematosus*. 9th ed. Philadelphia: Elsevier; 2018. The definitive text on the topic.

The best general rheumatology textbooks are as follows:

GS Firestein, R Budd, *Kelley* and Firestein's *Textbook of Rheumatology*. 2 vols. Philadelphia: Elsevier; 2016.

Hochberg MC, Gravellese EM *Rheumatology*. 6th ed. 2 vols. Philadelphia: Elsevier; 2018.

**How can I find another good book for lupus patients?** Over 100 books have been published aimed at lupus patients. They vary widely in their quality, focus, and expertise. A few simple rules will help in navigating Amazon, Barnes and Noble, and other listings.

1. Avoid all books that have "cure" in the title.
2. Individual testimonials can be compelling but are only occasionally applicable to the reader; no two lupus cases or circumstances are the same.
3. Books endorsed by the Arthritis Foundation, Lupus Foundation of America, or the SLE Foundation have been peer reviewed by experts and generally are of superior quality.
4. Try to find books written by an MD who is involved in lupus research or patient care, especially if they are the first author. Some efforts have an introduction or foreword by a lupus specialist, and the reader can be misled from the book jacket that the specialist actually wrote the book.
5. Avoid books more than 10 years old; the advice may be outdated or no longer valid.
6. New books are appearing all the time; consult the websites of lupus support organizations listed in this appendix for updated listings.
7. There is no proven lupus diet or alternative therapy regimen. This is a serious disorder; consult your lupus specialist before embarking on any of these regimens.

This writer highly recommends: D Thomas, The Lupus Encyclopedia, Johns Hopkins U Press, 2014.

# Index